PRINCIPLES AND PRACTICE OF CARDIOTHORACIC SURGERY

Edited by **Michael S. Firstenberg**

Principles and Practice of Cardiothoracic Surgery
http://dx.doi.org/10.5772/56726
Edited by Michael S. Firstenberg

Contributors

Wickii Thambiah Vigneswaran, Ronaldo Velasquez Purugganan, January Tsai, Teresa Moon, Shital Vachhani, Peter H. Norman, Javier Lasala, Hidir Esme, Mustafa Calik, Krishnan Subramaniam, Neville Solomon, Nikolaos Barbetakis, Christos Asteriou, Athanassios Kleontas, Sumit Yadav, Anand Iyer, Francesco Formica, Calvin Sze Hang Ng, Kelvin Lau, Vladimir Shipulin, Ihsan Alloubi, Haralabos Parissis, Alan Soo, Bassel Al-Alao, P. Michael McFadden, Dawn Hui, Arman Kilic, Ahmet Kilic, Tomoaki Suzuki, Tohru Asai, Daniel Eiferman, R. Nathan Cotterman, Michael S Firstenberg, Karen Nelson, Kevin Kissling, Stanislaw P. A. Stawicki, David Lindsey, Jennifer Schwartz, Hooman Khabiri

Published by InTech

Janeza Trdine 9, 51000 Rijeka, Croatia

Publishing Process Manager Ana Pantar
Technical Editor InTech DTP team
Cover InTech Design team

Additional hard copies can be obtained from orders@intechopen.com

Principles and Practice of Cardiothoracic Surgery, Edited by Michael S. Firstenberg
p. cm.
ISBN 978-953-51-1156-6

For EU product safety concerns:
IN TECH d.o.o., Prolaz Marije Krucifikse Kozulić 3, 51000 Rijeka, Croatia,
info@intechopen.com or visit our website at intechopen.com.

Meet the editor

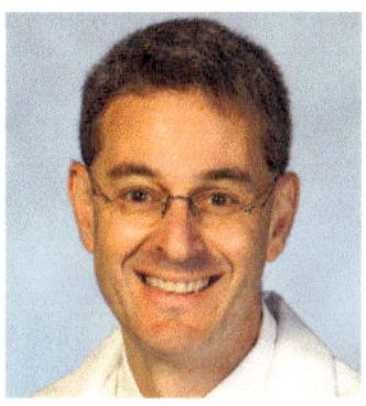

Michael S. Firstenberg, MD is currently an Assistant Professor of Surgery and Integrative Medicine at the Northeast Ohio Medical University and a full-time Cardiothoracic surgeon at Akron City Hospital. He was previously on the faculty at The Ohio State University where, in addition to being an active cardiac surgeon, he was active on numerous University, College, and Health system committees. He received his Thoracic surgery training at Ohio State with additional training at The Cleveland Clinic. Michael is currently active within numerous other professional organizations and has co-authored >100 manuscripts, lectured worldwide on extra-corporeal support, and he serves on the editorial board of several Journals. He was recently nominated for the prestigious Thoracic Surgery Resident Association Socrates Teaching Award.

Contents

Preface

The field of thoracic and cardiovascular surgery continues to evolve at a pace in which almost by definition any idea that is published is instantly out-of-date. Ideas are in constant evolution and new, exciting, and innovative technologies are often featured not only in mainstream Journals, but the lay-press media as well. While such progress is exciting–particularly for those at the forefront of such developments–unfortunately, it often takes years for some of these technologies to mature to the point in which they are safely and readily available to our patients. Many of these developments sometimes become restricted to specialized centers and occasionally only available to those patients with access to referrals and resources. Furthermore, it is also unclear the extent in which such advances may actually benefit patients as some of the most significant, exciting, and expensive therapies are indicated for potentially only a small number of patients. Nevertheless, there are still numerous problems–beyond some of the basics - in which the management continues to challenge all of those who are involved in the care of the cardiothoracic patient. As more and more of these problems require the management of multi-disciplinary Teams, the ability to speak a common language and understand complex problems becomes even more important. Furthermore, as patients–for many reasons–present in various stages of their diseases, some very early and some very late–combined with the challenges of dealing with more complex co-morbidities, unusual problems are becoming more common and common problems are presenting in more unusual ways.

The goal of Principles and Practice of Cardiothoracic Surgery is not to be an all encompassing text of an endless field, but rather to highlight some of the challenges that might be facing the Team that is often faced with dealing with the wide-spectrum of problems that can, and often are, encountered at centers throughout the world on a daily basis. Obviously topics like percutaneous valves, long-term ventricular assist devices, and thoracic organ transplantation continue to fascinate those who follow our field–but unfortunately, for many reasons, these topics, not only are constantly changing, but are rarely available outside of major medical centers and have limited availability to patients. Entire textbooks have been dedicated to these individual topics. As such, they can be of limited practical interest to the practicing surgeon who is not already at a center that performs these procedures or, conversely, who is still in training or trying to figure out how to get involved with a field that might be moving too quickly–and potentially in too many different directions.

This text is divided into 3 sections – Thoracic Surgery, Cardiac Surgery, and Great-vessel Surgery – with not only state of the art discussions of the current literature on some of the topics, but as importantly and emphasis on the basic"tried and true"approaches to the management of some unusual and difficult to manage problems such as the mesothelioma and post-myocardial infarction ventricular septal defects. In addition, chapters on such topics ranging from extra-corporeal membrane oxygenation and surgery for massive acute pulmonary embolism are also presented as potentially valuable references for those clinicians who rarely encounter such problems, but when they do, immediate access to a standard reference with a recipe for success is critical in the setting of an acutely life-threatening problem.

In addition, chapters that focus specifically on the peri-operative management of these patients and their complex problems are also included. The field of anesthesia for thoracic surgery is constantly changing as clinicians continue to strive to make the task of single lung ventilation and even general anesthesia for pulmonary resections safer. The insights from this chapter are of value to surgeon and anesthesiologist alike as there are few areas in medicine in which it is so critical that physicians from different specialties be able to communicate in a common language. Similarly, the chapters that discuss the management of complications after thoracic procedures and potentially catastrophic gastrointestinal problems after cardiac surgery are also included to serve as a reference point for dealing with these issues when their arise.

Of course, no text on cardiothoracic surgery would be complete without a foundation in the complex anatomy and the embryologic development of the heart to assist in putting any procedure into a proper context. A fundamental understanding of anatomy and embryology is critical to our field and one can never be too educated on this topic–in fact, I am sure most practicing physicians could always benefit from further education in this area.

The international and diverse nature of the authors allows the reader to also avoid some of the inherent regional bias that comes from texts in which the opinions and experiences of a single center are discussed. While such experiences are of considerable value and are considered sometimes"state of the art", there are concerns about whether some of the techniques and outcomes can be translated into common and daily practice–and in the spectrum of environments that might be represented by the anticipated audience.

The open-access model of this text also addresses some of the practice concerns to providing knowledge to those who need it most but who are typically the least likely to have access to it (typically due to financial constraints of scientific publishing). While physical copies of this text are available, the real benefit stems for the ability to access and download individual chapters on an as-needed basis from anywhere in the world and without charge. The benefits of this model of distribution of medical knowledge will only continue to grow in the future as more and more medial, in general, is distributed electronically and availability is provided anywhere, anytime, for anyone–and without cost.

Principles and Practice of Cardiothoracic Surgery will only be one of countless texts on the topic. The information, like all texts, will reflect a"snap-shot"of the understanding of the topics presented at a point in time. While it would be foolish of any author or editor to claim their work is the definitive, complete, and final word on any topic–the true goal of this work is to provide a foundation of knowledge of common, unusual, and intriguing problems that will hopefully spark further curiosity on the various topics, serve as a new baseline for further growth in the field, and most importantly–help clinicians to help patients, sometimes at their time of greatest need and uncertainty. Basically, the hope is that this text will be a starting point for a life-long journey.

Michael S. Firstenberg, MD FACC
Department of Surgery (Cardiothoracic)
Summa Health Care System – Akron City Hospital
Assistant Professor of Surgery and Integrative Medicine
Northeast Ohio Medical University, USA

Section 1

Thoracic Surgery

Chapter 1

Anesthesia for Thoracic Surgical Procedures

January Tsai, Teresa Moon, Shital Vachhani,
Javier Lasala, Peter H Norman and
Ronaldo Purugganan

Additional information is available at the end of the chapter

http://dx.doi.org/10.5772/56104

1. Introduction

As thoracic surgery evolved, anesthesia evolved in parallel, allowing even the most complicated surgical procedures to be performed relatively safely. This co-evolution mirrors the close association of the thoracic surgeon and anesthesiologist when caring for their patients. This unique association is predicated on the nature of thoracic procedures, where the surgeon and anesthesiologist share a "thoracic workspace" - the surgeon operating on vital thoracic structures and the anesthesiologist managing ventilation, oxygenation, and hemodynamics. Because of this close partnering, it is valuable for thoracic surgeons to be familiar with anesthetic considerations exclusive to their patients.

2. Considerations for One-Lung Ventilation (OLV)

Thoracic Surgery poses unique challenges to the anesthesiologist, including surgery in the lateral decubitus position, an open thorax, manipulation of thoracic organs, potential for major bleeding, and, unique among all potential surgery scenarios, the need for lung isolation.

2.1. Physiologic effects of lung isolation

Successful lung isolation (one-lung ventilation, OLV) requires the management of oxygenation, ventilation, and pulmonary blood flow. Remarkably, OLV decreases total minute ventilation minimally. In fact, it has been shown that the non-isolated lung receives close to the same minute ventilation as ventilation to two lungs. The rate of CO_2 elimination undergoes minimal changes because CO_2 is readily diffusible and has no plateau in its dissociation curve.

When a patient is placed on OLV, inevitably a shunt is developed. The non-dependent lung is no longer being ventilated but is still perfused, resulting in a right to left shunt. When this occurs, the pulmonary system has physiological adaptations to decrease this shunt. Given that the patient is in the lateral decubitus position, one of the responses is a decrease in blood flow to the non-dependent lung due to gravitational forces. These effects are significant because the pulmonary system has a much lower blood pressure than the systemic circulation. Another adaptation is hypoxic pulmonary vasoconstriction of the vascular supply in the non-dependent lung. Hypoxic pulmonary vasoconstriction is a physiological phenomenon in which pulmonary arteries constrict in the presence of hypoxia (unlike the systemic circulation), redirecting blood flow to the dependent lung. Surgical compression of the non-dependent lung can also serve as a way of decreasing shunt as the pulmonary vasculature is compressed. One last factor contributing to a decrease in shunt fraction is apneic oxygenation—residual oxygen in the non-dependent isolated lung diffusing into the pulmonary circulation. All these factors combined allow for better oxygenation during OLV.

2.2. Preoperative anesthetic evaluation of the thoracic surgery patient

Patients undergoing OLV should undergo a perioperative assessment of their respiratory function that includes testing of lung mechanical function, pulmonary parenchymal function, and cardiopulmonary reserve. The best assessment of respiratory function comes from a history of the patient's quality of life [1]. It is useful to think of respiratory function in three related but independent areas: respiratory mechanics, gas exchange, and cardio-respiratory interaction [2].

The most valid test for perioperative assessment of respiratory mechanics is the predicted post-operative forced expiratory volume in one second (ppoFEV1). This test is the best at predicting post thoracotomy respiratory complications [3].

Percentage of predicted postoperative (ppo) FEV1 after lobectomy is given by

$$ppoFEV1 = preoperative\ FEV1\ x\ \frac{No.\,of\ segments\ remaining}{total\ No.\,of\ segments}$$

Nakahara et al found that patients with a ppoFEV1 of more than 40% had no or only minor post resection respiratory complications [4]. Major respiratory complications were only seen in the sub group with ppoFEV1 < 40%; post-operative mechanical ventilator support was seen in those < 30%.

For the assessment of lung parenchymal function, the most useful test of the gas exchange capacity is the diffusing capacity for carbon monoxide (DLCO). This test correlates with the total functioning surface of the alveolar-capillary interface. The DLCO is used to calculate a post resection value using the same calculation as FEV1. A ppoDLCO less than 40% of predicted correlates with increased cardiac and respiratory complications and is relatively independent of the FEV1 [5].

Stair climbing is the most traditional test of respiratory function in the assessment of cardio-pulmonary interaction. Ability to climb three flights or more is closely associated with a decrease in morbidity and mortality. The ability to climb fewer than two flights is associated with a very high risk [6]. The "gold standard" for assessment is formal laboratory exercise testing with maximal oxygen consumption. Climbing five flights of stairs approximates a VO_2 max value of >20 ml/kg/min and less than one flight is associated with values <10 ml/kg/min (S9). Ventilation-perfusion (V/Q) scintigraphy can also be used as a preoperative assessment when pulmonary resection is to be undertaken. This modality is particularly helpful for patients undergoing pneumonectomy or any patient with a ppoFEV1 less than 40% [2].

Slinger et al. proposed a "3-legged" stool of pre-thoracotomy respiratory assessment, which encompasses the prior mentioned pre-operative tests [7]. This model summarizes the results of those tests and reveals that patients have lower expected post-operative morbidity if they have a ppoFEV1 > 40%, cardio-pulmonary reserve with a VO_2 max >15 ml/kg/min, and lung parenchymal function with a ppoDLCO >40%. These three tests are the most valid for pre-operative assessment. Other tests that can be used are maximal volume ventilation (MVV), residual volume/total lung capacity (RV/TLC), and forced vital capacity (FVC), but these are less valid for respiratory mechanics. Stair climbing (two flights), a 6-minute walk, and measurement in the change in SpO_2 (<4%) during exercise are other tests that can be used to measure cardio-pulmonary reserve. Measurement of arterial blood gas values can also serve as a respiratory assessment; indicators of good prognosis are PaO_2 > 60 and a $PaCO_2$ < 45.

In regards to post-thoracotomy anesthetic management, Slinger et al. devised an algorithm derived from pre-operative assessment using ppoFEV1 [7]. If the patient's ppoFEV1 is > 40% and the patient is awake, alert, warm, and comfortable, immediate postoperative extubation is recommended. If the ppoFEV1 is between 30-40%, extubation should be considered based on exercise tolerance, DLCO, V/Q scan, and associated diseases. If the ppoFEV1 < 30%, staged weaning from mechanical ventilation is recommended. However, when the patient has a functioning thoracic epidural catheter providing adequate analgesia, extubation may be attempted even at ppoFEV1 values as low as 20% [7].

2.3. Tracheo-bronchial anatomy for lung isolation

Knowledge of tracheo-bronchial anatomy is important for achieving and maintaining proper lung isolation. Other chapters in this text describe lung and bronchial anatomy in detail. Features of the anatomy that are relevant to anesthetic considerations are presented here.

A critical landmark when placing lung isolation devices is the primary carina, where the trachea splits into two main bronchi. The diversion angle differs between these main bronchi, with the right bronchi angled at 25 degrees and the left bronchus at 45 degrees. Because of the steeper angle of diversion of the right main bronchus, foreign bodies (including lung isolation devices) are more likely to travel into this bronchus. Left and right side double lumen tubes (DLTs) are designed with curvatures to accommodate left or right main bronchi diversion angles to make intubation into the specified main bronchi easier (Figure 1).

Because of the steeper angle of the right mainstem bronchus, it is not uncommon to inadvertently intubate the right mainstem when intending to intubate the left mainstem with a DLT (using blind or non fiberoptic guided placement techniques). Operators unfamiliar with distal bronchial anatomy sometimes confuse secondary carinas with the primary carina. For example, the right main bronchus divides at the secondary carina into the upper lobar

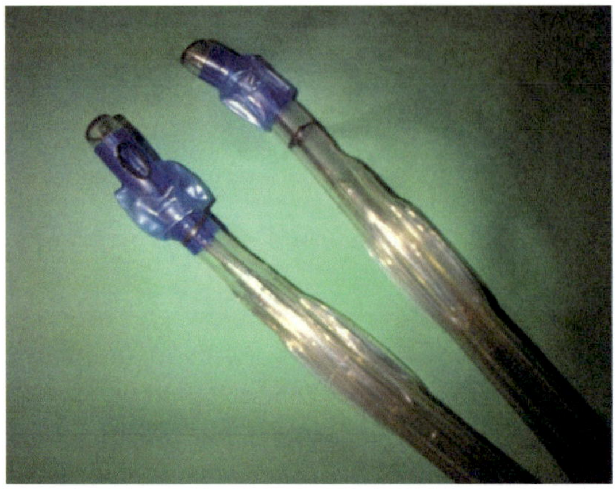

Figure 1. Left (top) and right (bottom) conformations of double lumen tubes. Note the right upper lobe ventilation lumen on the right conformation tube.

bronchus and bronchus intermedius; this secondary carina may be mistaken for the primary carina when viewed under bronchoscopy. Therefore, knowledge of distal bronchial anatomy is fundamental in confirming correct placement as well as in correcting misplacement.

Knowledge of distal bronchial anatomy is essential for additional reasons. First, the operator must recognize that a right DLT has an additional slot to allow for ventilation of the right upper lobe and must place it at the correct depth and rotational alignment to assure adequate ventilation of all three lobes. Secondly, anatomy is abnormal in a small percentage of patients. For example, in up to 2% of patients, the right bronchus originates directly from the supra carinal trachea (a so-called bronchus suis) [8]. Abnormal anatomy is also seen in patients who have had previous lung surgeries. The operator must be able to recognize and respond to abnormal anatomy by selecting the appropriate device to provide effect lung isolation in any scenario.

2.4. Indications for lung isolation

Patient pathology and/or operative requirements determine the indication for OLV. Patients with lung pathology may need lung protection. For example, OLV may be used to protect the unaffected lung from contamination with pus or blood from the affected lung. Alternatively, OLV may be used to provide differential lung ventilation to minimize volutrauma and barotrauma to the affected lung while optimizing ventilation to the non-affected lung. Certain operative scenarios require OLV. Because it optimizes visualization of the operative site, OLV is absolutely indicated in closed procedures (for example, thoracoscopic surgery) but is also useful in open procedures to maximize exposure.

2.5. Lung isolation devices

Three standard methods for lung isolation include DLT, bronchial blockers, and mainstem intubation.

2.5.1. DLT

The standard device for providing lung isolation is the DLT. It provides reliable lung isolation, offers the ability to suction both lungs, allows for bilateral differential lung ventilation with minimal device manipulation, and allows for simple procedures such as bronchoalveolar lavage. DLTs range in size from 28 to 41 Fr. Posteroanterior (PA) chest x-ray is the standard method for sizing comparison between DLT, trachea, and bronchial diameter [9]. However, patient sex, age, and height are commonly used to choose DLT size. As discussed above, DLTs are made in right-side and left-side conformations to accommodate the differences in the anatomy of the right and left main bronchi (i.e., the right upper lobe branch).

2.5.2. SLT with bronchial blocker

Bronchial blockers used with conventional single lumen tubes have advantages in difficult airways, in patients with indwelling endotracheal or tracheostomy tubes, in patients who are nasally intubated with SLTs, and in cases where sub-segmental blockade may be required [10]. Bronchial blockers have several disadvantages, however. They are easier to displace and provide limited suction and drainage to the isolated lung, which may lead to an accumulation of pus, blood or secretions [11]. They are deployed in the operative lung, which may interfere with the surgical procedure, and the device must be repositioned for contralateral lung isolation.

Despite their specific enhancements, bronchial blockers are essentially modeled after vascular embolization catheters (albeit with high compliance low pressure cuffs and a deflation port). They are manufactured as separate units or units integrated with an endotracheal tube. Separate units include the Cohen Flexi-tip BB (Cook Critical Care), Fuji Uni-blocker (Fuji Systems, Tokyo) (Figure 2A) and the Arndt wire-guided BB (Cook Critical Care, Bloomington, IN) (Figure 2B). An example of an integrated unit is the Univent tube (Fuji Systems, Tokyo).

2.5.3. Mainstem intubation

Mainstem bronchial intubation with an SLT may be used for lung isolation in emergent scenarios or in pediatric cases. However, with this method, exhalation of the operative lung is limited, airway protection at the vocal cords is compromised, and the endotracheal tube tip is advanced into the operative lung; lastly, repositioning is required if contralateral isolation is needed. Furthermore, standard endotracheal tubes may be too short to effectively mainstem intubate either main bronchi; specialized longer tubes, such as Micro Laryngoscopy Tubes (MLTs), may be required.

2.6. Difficult airway and lung isolation

Campos describes two categories of patients at risk for difficult intubation during OLV: those with complications related to the upper airway and those related to the lower airway [12]. The former include a short neck and increased neck circumference, prominent upper incisors with a receding mandible, limited cervical mobility, limited jaw opening due to previous surgery, radiation therapy of the neck, previous hemiglossectomy or hemimandibulectomy, and

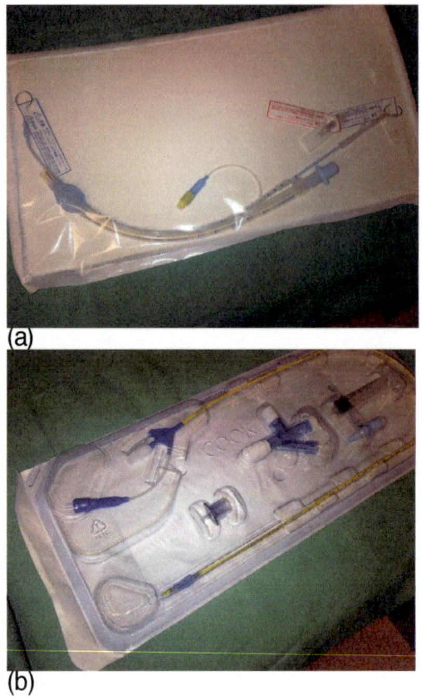

Figure 2. Examples of bronchial blockers. (A) Fuji Uni-blocker (Fuji Systems, Tokyo); (B) Arndt wire-guided BB (Cook Critical Care, Bloomington, IN).

tumors of the upper airway. Lower airway risk factors include an existing tracheotomy, a distorted tracheobronchial anatomy, and compression at the entrance of the left mainstem bronchus. Patients with any of the above conditions might pose a difficulty for lung isolation with a conventional DLT and might be candidates for SLT placement with subsequent lung isolation with a bronchial blocker. However, if a DLT is indicated, fiberoptic intubation may be used to facilitate placement [13]. However, because of the long length of the DLT, it is difficult to maintain distal control of the fiberscope, especially with patients having longer oral to vocal cord distance. Additionally, the small diameter bronchoscope required (to assure fit for the DLT) results in an inferior view and restricts suction capabilities. Therefore, new generation indirect laryngoscopes may be preferable. Indirect laryngoscopes (e.g., CMAC [Storz, Tuttlingen, Germany], GlideScope [Verathon,Bothell, WA], Airtraq (Prodol Meditec S.A., Vizcaya, Spain)) improve airway grade and have been shown to improve the ease of intubation with DLTs in patients with difficult airways [14].

2.7. Confirming proper lung isolation

Regardless of the device used for lung isolation, the anesthesiologist must confirm correct placement of the device. Chest auscultation has traditionally been used to confirm correct DLT placement. The process is straightforward in patients with normal pulmonary anatomy. First, inflate both tracheal and bronchial balloons and auscultate to confirm bilateral breath sounds (if bilateral breath sounds are absent, suspect malposition – the DLT may be too deep). Next, sequentially clamp the tracheal and bronchial inflow limbs of the DLT and auscultate the chest. Absent breath sounds corresponding to the tracheal or bronchial lumen clamped, should be confirmed. Different malposition scenarios may be deduced depending on type of DLT (L v. R), intended mainstem to be intubated, DLT lumen occluded and the absence or presence of breath sounds. Although auscultation is an important tool in situations where fiberoptic bronchoscopy is unavailable, studies have shown a large margin of positioning error when it is not used [15-18]. Fiberoptic confirmation is required for proper positioning of bronchial blockers because they lack basic ergonomic design features that enable blind placement (like curvature or specialized ventilation port configurations of DLTs). Furthermore, because malpositioned lung isolation devices may be potentially be fatal, and auscultation is usually not an option intraoperatively, fiberoptic bronchoscopy has become the standard for proper placement and maintenance of lung isolation devices.

3. Intraoperative care for the thoracic surgical patient

3.1. Ventilator strategies for one-lung ventilation

For thoracic surgery, the incidence of pulmonary complications now out-numbers that of cardiovascular complications [19], and pulmonary complications are the most common cause of postoperative death in esophageal cancer patients [20]. Injury from one-lung ventilation (OLV) can manifest as re-expansion pulmonary edema (REPE), acute lung injury (ALI), or acute respiratory distress syndrome (ARDS). While late causes of ALI (3-10 days after surgery) are secondary to bronchopneumonia or aspiration, early ALI is predicted by high intraoperative ventilation pressures, increased surgery duration, excessive intravenous volume replacement, pneumonectomy, and preoperative alcohol abuse [21]. Most likely, a combination of a patient's health status, intraoperative fluid management, the use of epidural analgesia, inflammatory responses due to surgical manipulation, alveolar recruitment, and reexpansion/ reperfusion lung injury [22, 23] underlie the development of ALI following OLV [24]. While chronic patient risk factors are difficult to modify, protective ventilatory strategies and judicious fluid use may decrease the incidence of ALI [21].

Prior ventilatory schemes focused on the detrimental effects of atelectasis, primarily increased pulmonary shunt via local alveolar hypoxia and hyperoxia. Tidal volumes of 10-12mL/kg were advocated, as it was previously held that tidal volumes <8mL/kg resulted in decreased functional residual capacity (FRC) and worsening atelectasis in the dependent lung. The lowest positive end-expiratory pressure (PEEP) for acceptable oxygenation and normal arterial CO_2 levels (35 to 38 mmHg) were suggested [24]. OLV was achieved with parameters similar to two-lung ventilation, with consequent stimulation of stretch-activated cation channels, oxygen-derived free radicals, activated neutrophils, and cytokine upregulation contributing to increased microvascular-alveolar permeability [25].

The current strategy to minimize OLV-associated lung injury utilizes so-called lung protective ventilation. Overdistension (volutrauma), excessive transpulmonary pressure resulting in barotrauma, repeated opening and closing of alveoli resulting in ateletotrauma, and biotrauma caused by inflammatory mediators are considered contributing factors to ventilator-induced lung injury (VILI). These factors combined may induce inflammatory changes in pulmonary alveolar and vascular endothelium, predisposing them to pathological apoptosis and necrosis. In this way, VILI can both exacerbate existing lung injury and sensitize the lung to further injury via a two-hit model [26]. Reduction of tidal volumes during OLV to 5ml/kg was shown to reduce alveolar concentration of TNF-α and sICAM-1 [27] (will it be obvious to the reader what implications this has?). Moreover, with fixed tidal volumes of 9mL/kg, the addition of 5cm H_2O PEEP was associated with better oxygenation and earlier extubation [28]. PEEP improves the (ventilation:perfusion) V:Q relationship via increased FRC at end expiration. However, excessive PEEP may redistribute blood flow away from the dependent ventilated lung. Thus, protective ventilation consists of:

- maintaining the fraction of inspired O_2 ($Fi0_2$) as low as possible to avoid absorption atelectasis and worsening shunt [29]
- PEEP above the lower inflection point on the static pressure-volume curve
- a tidal volume of 5-6 mL/kg, plateau pressures of less than 20 cm H_2O above the PEEP value
- peak inspiratory pressures less than 35 cm H_2O
- respiratory rate (RR) 10-18
- inspiratory:expiratory (I:E) ratio 1:2 to 1:3
- permissive hypercapnia
- preferential use of pressure-limited ventilatory modes [24].

Hypoxemia may require continuous positive airway pressure (CPAP) to the nondependent lung, allowing apneic oxygenation and increasing overall partial pressure of O_2 ($pa0_2$). Permissive hypercapnia is generally tolerated with protective ventilator strategies during OLV. Not only does hypocapnia worsen parenchymal and ischemia-reperfusion injury [30], but hypercapnia itself may have beneficial effects on serum cytokine levels, apoptosis, and free radical injury [31]. The optimal level of $paCO_2$ has not been determined.

Pressure controlled ventilation achieves lower airway pressure, and the homogeneous distribution of inspired gas allows recruitment of collapsed lung and improved oxygenation [32]. This method is thought to minimize end-inspiratory distension and collapse of lung units and has demonstrated a decreased inflammatory response, improved lung function, and earlier extubation [28]. As compared with conventional ventilation, this protective strategy was associated with improved survival at 28 days, a higher rate of weaning from mechanical ventilation, and a lower rate of barotrauma in patients with ARDS. However, protective ventilation was not associated with a higher rate of survival to hospital discharge [25]. Even with protective lung ventilatory strategies, it is possible that certain patchy segments of alveoli are intermittently and inconsistently recruited, resulting in impaired surfactant effectiveness and barotrauma.

Lung protective ventilation primarily refers to the dependent lung, which shows a more pronounced inflammatory response than the nonventilated lung [33, 34]. However, it is likely that the overall postoperative clinical picture amounts to the combination of differing insults to the operative and nonoperative lung. Hypoxia-induced lung inflammation [30] and stress-induced mechanical injury affects the operative lung as well, as the atelectatic, nonventilated lung is periodically inflated to assess air leaks. Additionally, the operative lung is subject to pulmonary contusion due to surgical manipulation and mechanical trauma. After 30 minutes of OLV, the collapsed lung releases inflammatory mediators into the epithelial lining fluid, indicating tissue insult and possibly resulting in systemic physiological changes [35]. Finally, barotrauma may occur at the end of OLV as previously atelectatic alveolar units are recruited.

The contribution of the type of anesthetic to the inflammatory response and clinical outcomes is currently unknown. Studies comparing propofol to volatile anesthetics such as sevoflurane and desflurane have yielded conflicting results [36]. Overall, differences in surgical time, duration of OLV, and laboratory techniques in existing studies have complicated interpretation of the data[24]. Volatile agents are thought to have immune-modulating effects. While previous work showed anti-inflammatory effects of propofol, recent studies have demonstrated decreased inflammatory markers in both the operative and nonoperative lung with volatile anesthesia[36-38]. Sugasawa and colleagues found that sevoflurane use was significantly associated with a suppressed inflammatory response compared to propofol [38]. Thus, the choice of anesthetic agent and other drugs such as ropivacaine, ketamine, thiopental, and dexmedetomidine may have anti-inflammatory effects that may be protective during lung surgery with OLV. Further study is needed to elucidate the role of these agents [39].

In conclusion, lung protective ventilator strategies which minimize $Fi0_2$, barotrauma, and volutrauma are currently being used during OLV. Optimal lung protection, however, is multifactorial and may also depend on fluid administration techniques and perioperative drug administration. Alternative lung protective strategies for experimental or rescue use, such as extracorporeal membrane oxygenation and high-frequency oscillatory ventilation are discussed elsewhere.

3.2. Fluid therapy — Goal directed therapy for thoracic surgery

Intravenous fluids are administered perioperatively in order to optimize systemic oxygen delivery to meet metabolic demands. Cardiac preload, afterload, and contractility are frequently used as surrogate indicators of global tissue perfusion. Inadequate intravascular volume can predispose to ischemia and end-organ dysfunction. Excessive fluid administration, on the other hand, can lead to tissue edema and compromised perfusion. In the operative setting, surgical insults may theoretically cause an inflammatory response characterized by alterations in microvascular integrity, allowing abnormal transmicrovascular fluid flux. Due to this increase in microvascular permeability, interstitial edema may develop, which decreases O_2 diffusion, resulting in hypoxic cell injury. This injury propagates a vicious cycle involving further cell death and the subsequent release of inflammatory cytokines.

In esophagectomy patients, the goal of intraoperative fluid administration is to balance perfusion pressure and oxygen delivery to vital organs including the gut mucosa, while preventing excessive fluid accumulation that may delay recovery of gastrointestinal function, impair wound and anastomotic healing, coagulation, and cardiac and respiratory function. Restrictive fluid regimens were thought to result in better gastrointestinal recovery time, reduced overall morbidity[40], improved respiratory parameters, decreased incidence of postoperative pulmonary complications, and shorter recovery periods [41]. Conversely, fluid overload had a direct negative relationship to function and structure of the intestinal anastomoses [42].

The thoracic surgery population is particularly prone to pulmonary complications, which have significant implications for patient outcomes. In the setting of pulmonary resection, for example, postoperative pulmonary edema confers a high mortality risk. Three significant risk factors include right pneumonectomy, increased perioperative intravenous fluids, and increased postoperative urine output [43]. Patel (1992) found that fluid replacement of greater than 3L in the 24 hours surrounding surgery was correlated with increased mortality [44]. While pulmonary edema is associated with fluid overload, there is no clear causal relationship [45]. With histology compatible with ARDS, postpneumonectomy pulmonary edema occurs despite a normal PAOP, and the high protein content of edema fluid points toward low-pressure endothelial damage[46]. Nevertheless, appropriate fluid administration may mitigate the deleterious effects of pulmonary pathology.

Traditional static cardiac preload measures such as CVP may fail to provide reliable estimations of actual preload and cardiac responses to fluid therapy. Studies on supine patients have demonstrated improved intraoperative hemodynamic stability, reduced ICU admissions, lower incidence of complications, and reduced mortality after major surgery with the use of dynamic preload indicators and goal-directed fluid therapy (GDT) [47, 48]. Commonly used monitors include esophageal Doppler monitoring and measures of arterial pulse pressure variation with respiration, such as the Lithium Dilution Cardiac Output (LiDCOplus) system and FloTrac/Vigileo. Using an esophageal Doppler probe, Gan (2002) found that GDT in patients undergoing major elective general, urologic, or gynecologic surgery with an anticipated blood loss of greater than 500mL resulted in an earlier return of bowel function, lower incidence of postoperative nausea and vomiting, and decreased length of postoperative hospital stay [49].

GDT does not consistently result in either increased or decreased amounts of fluid administered. One study[50] showed that the GDT group received more volume. However, in a cohort of septic patients, GDT patients received significantly more fluid during the first six hours than those assigned to standard therapy; but in the overall period from baseline to 72 hours after the start of treatment there was no significant difference between the two groups in the total amount of fluid administered. Early GDT provided significant outcome benefits: of the patients who survived to hospital discharge, those assigned to standard therapy had significantly longer hospital stays than those with early GDT[51].

Slinger describes one rational approach to fluid administration [45]. The thorax is not assumed to be a third space. Total positive fluid balance in the first 24 hours postoperatively should not exceed 20ml/kg or approximately 3L of crystalloid. Unless the patient is at high risk of developing renal insufficiency, urine output of greater than 0.5mL/kg/hr is probably unnecessary. In the case of reduced tissue perfusion, as in the case of epidural-induced sympathectomy, it is preferable to invasively monitor and use GDT. The use of inotropes may be preferable to aggressive fluid overload.

One limitation of GDT, however, involves the extrapolation of studies correlating cardiac output measurements via PACs with those obtained via dynamic indices during abdominal surgery to thoracotomy patients who are positioned laterally and subjected to varying intrathoracic conditions, such as exposure to atmospheric pressure and OLV. The value of dynamic preload indicators in the thoracic population has not been systematically examined. Possible problems with extending the use of this device to thoracic surgery patients include lung compliance and intrathoracic pressure variations during positioning changes or insufflation for RATS, laparoscopy and changing intraabdominal pressure, the open chest, pressure changes with VATS, and differing ventilatory settings (TV, PEEP, OLV, DLV). One study has shown that GDT is at least not deleterious or does not result in pulmonary fluid overload when used for thoracic surgery requiring lateral thoracotomy and OLV[52]. While changing from the supine to the reverse Trendelenburg or prone positions significantly alters SV and thus SVV, 30° left or right recumbent and supine positions do not appear to affect SV or SVV measurements [53]. Kobayashi concludes that SVV, as displayed on the Vigileo monitor, is considered an accurate predictor of intravascular hypovolemia and is a useful indicator for assessing the appropriateness and timing of applying fluid for improving circulatory stability, but only during the perioperative period after esophagectomy [54]. De Waal (2002) demonstrated that while PiCCO-derived dynamic preload indicators were able to predict fluid responsiveness under closed-chest conditions, both static and dynamic preload indicators failed to predict fluid responsiveness in open-chest conditions [55]. Stroke volume variation (SVV) and pulse pressure variation (PPV) seem to be critically dependent on the undisturbed transmission of these pressure changes to cardiovascular structures within the closed thorax [56]. For example, sternotomy alone decreases SVV [57]. Additionally, one study [58] found that SVV could predict fluid responsiveness in patients undergoing OLV with acceptable levels of sensitivity and specificity only when tidal volumes were at least 8mL/kg. They state that dynamic indices of preload are based on the concept that positive pressure ventilation induces variations in SV. By definition, this concept requires that the preload is significantly affected by cyclic changes in intrathoracic and transpulmonary pressures, and these changes may be too small when patients undergoing OLV are ventilated with low tidal volumes (i.e. 6mL/kg). In short, the ability of SVV to predict volume responsiveness in thoracotomy patients is currently unknown.

Finally, the optimal type of fluid is debatable. Some animal models have demonstrated greater interstitial edema with crystalloid administration and better preserved effective capillary cross-sectional area in the colloid group[59]. Other studies conclude that when given in similar volumes, colloids are more beneficial for anastomotic healing than crystalloid [24, 42]. Improved microcirculatory blood flow and tissue oxygen tension were observed after abdominal surgery in one animal model [60, 61]. However, no difference in anastomotic healing was found in another animal model of colloid use [62]. To date, no consensus has been reached as to the superiority of crystalloids versus colloids. Pulmonary edema due to excessive crystalloid may clear faster than that caused by colloids.

In summary, intelligent fluid administration is vital to maintaining tissue perfusion and minimizing edema in the perioperative period. New methods of GDT based on SVV may offer useful tools to guide clinicians during thoracic surgery cases. However, the applicability of this technology to the thoracic population has not been fully investigated. Most likely, avoiding fluid overload by tailoring GDT in an educated manner to the patient's specific deficit and type of fluid loss yields optimal results.

3.3. Special intraoperative monitoring

Since thoracic surgery involves hemodynamic shifts with a goal of tight, goal-directed fluid therapy, knowledge of cardiac output (CO) and fluid responsiveness is important in the perioperative period. The historical gold standard for evaluation of left ventricular end-diastolic pressure (LVEDP), thermodilution (TD) uses a pulmonary artery catheter (PAC) to generate a measured time/temperature curve, from which CO can be calculated. These measurements are averaged over 2-9 minutes, so monitoring is not continuous. Recent studies show that fluid management based on TD may not improve patient outcomes and may, in fact, increase morbidity and mortality. PAC use itself may be complicated by arrhythmia, infection, pulmonary artery rupture, and damage to right heart structures [63]. PAC use may be unreliable due to the low pressure environment of the pulmonary vascular tree and the interference by hydrostatic pressure. With pre-existent pulmonary hypertension PAC use may become more reliable but conversely have more chance of a complication. The standard deviation (SD) for TD is about 1 L/minute or about 20% of the average CO [64]. Clearly, reliable and less-invasive methods of measuring CO are needed. Current options include lithium dilution, esophageal Doppler monitoring (EDM), pulse contour cardiac output systems, partial CO_2 rebreathing, and thoracic electrical bioimpedance.

Two methods of generating continuous CO measurements require a central venous catheter (CVC), which is arguably invasive, though less so than pulmonary artery catheterization. PiCCO (PULSION Medical Systems AG, Munich, Germany) generates CO via thermodilution from a CVC to a femoral or axillary arterial line. Using the Stewart-Hamilton principle, cold-saline thermodilution is used to provide calibration of the continuous CO analysis. Similarly, PulseCO (LiDCO Ltd, London, England) uses the Stewart-Hamilton equations as applied to lithium chloride (0.15 - 0.3 mmol for an average adult) dilution from a CVC or peripheral vein to an arterial line. The arterial lithium concentration-time curve can be subject to error in the presence of certain muscle relaxants. Recalibration is recommended after changes in patient position, therapy or condition. Clinical studies have demonstrated that over a wide range of cardiac outputs the LiDCO method is at least as accurate as thermodilution [65, 66].

Esophageal doppler monitoring uses a continuous wave sensor on the end of a probe which measures the velocity of blood flow within the descending thoracic aorta. Nomogram estimated aortic cross-sectional area based on the patient's weight, height, and age enables calculation of left ventricular (LV) stroke volume (SV) from the area of the velocity-time waveform. The total time that blood is traveling in a forward direction within the area is the systolic flow time, which is corrected for heart rate to give the corrected flow time, which is a good index of systemic vascular resistance and is sensitive to changes in LV preload. There is positive correlation between measures of cardiac output made simultaneously with the esophageal doppler and a thermodilution PAC [67]. Limitations of this monitor include assumptions of the diameter of the aorta based on the weight and height of the patient, a learning curve requiring about 12 probe placements [68], the need for patient sedation, and inability to be used during esophagectomies. This method has good validation; however, it only measures aortic blood flow and not true CO, and this may be potentially influenced by disproportionate changes in blood flow between the upper and lower body, although this is only important at the extremes of CO.

Pulse pressure (PP) methods measure the pressure in an artery over time to derive a waveform and use this information to calculate cardiac performance. However, any measure from an artery includes the changes in pressure associated with changes in vascular characteristics such as compliance and impedance. Physiologic or therapeutic changes in vessel diameter seen in the arterial waveform are assumed to reflect changes in CO. The ambiguity of the combined results of CO and vascular tone limits the application of PP methods. The values obtained by the LiDCOplus can be calibrated daily based on CO values generated by the LiDCO using the CVC waveform. It can also be used independently, as with the FloTrac/Vigileo (Edwards Lifesciences LLC, U.S.A.), which is an uncalibrated pulse contour analysis-based hemodynamic monitor that estimates CO utilizing a standard arterial catheter. The device consists of a pressure transducer which derives left-sided CO from a sample of arterial pulsations using an algorithm which calculates the product of the standard deviation of the arterial pressure wave (AP) (over 20 seconds) and a vascular tone factor (Khi) to generate stroke volume. Khi is derived from computer analysis of the morphologic change of the arterial pressure waveforms on a bit by bit basis based on the principle that changes in compliance or resistance affect the shape of the arterial pressure waveform. The equation in simplified form is as follows: SV=std(AP) * Khi or BP x k(constant). CO is then derived utilizing the equation CO=HR*SV. Only perfused beats that generate an arterial waveform should be counted for HR. While these monitors do not require intracardiac catheterization with a pulmonary artery catheter, they do require an arterial line. The benefits of this technology include the short time required for set up and data acquisition.

Disadvantages include its inability to provide right-sided heart pressures or mixed venous oxygen saturation. In addition, arterial monitoring systems are unable to predict changes in vascular tone and can therefore only estimate changes in vascular compliance. Some consider the measurement of pressure in the artery to calculate flow in the heart physiologically oversimplified and of questionable accuracy and benefit [64, 69]. The sensor is only indicated for adult use and has not been validated in patients with ventricular assist devices or intra-aortic balloon pumps. Absolute values during aortic regurgitation may be affected although trending may be appropriate. This monitor is dependent upon a high fidelity pressure tracing, which is compromised by spontaneous ventilation, atrial fibrillation or ectopy, severe peripheral constriction with vasopressor use, hypothermia, or dynamic autonomic states such as sepsis. In those instances, femoral artery cannulation or insertion of a PAC may be considered. Finally, in a study comparing these devices, although the PAC, FloTrac, LiDCO and PiCCO display similar mean CO values, they trended differently in response to therapy and showed different interdevice agreement. In the clinically relevant low CO range (< 5 L/min), agreement improved slightly. Thus, utility and validation studies using only one CO device may potentially not be extrapolated to equivalency of using another similar device [70].

The Fick principle allows multiple substitutions for O_2 consumption, including CO_2 clearance. Based on the ratio of the change in end-tidal CO_2 ($etCO_2$) and CO_2 elimination, the Noninvasive Cardiac Output (NICO) device (Novametrix Medical Systems, Inc., Wallingford, CT, USA) calculates CO using a disposable rebreathing loop which allows intermittent partial rebreathing in 3 minute cycles. This system contains a CO_2 sensor which uses infrared light absorption, a disposable airflow sensor or differential pressure pneumotachometer, a specific disposable rebreathing loop, and a pulse oximeter. The production of CO_2 (VCO_2, mL/min) is calculated from minute ventilation and its instantaneous CO_2 content, where the $CaCO_2$ (mL/100 mL of blood) is estimated from $etCO_2$ (mmHg). The rebreathing cycle induces an increase in $etCO_2$ and mimics a drop in CO_2 production. CO_2 production is calculated as the product of CO_2 concentration and air flow during a breathing cycle, and the arterial content of CO_2 ($CaCO_2$) is derived from the $etCO_2$ and the CO_2 dissociation curve. The obtained differences of these values are then used to calculate CO, such that $CO = \Delta VCO_2 / (S \times \Delta etCO_2)$, where S is the slope of the CO2 dissociation curve. The NICO system provides rapid, reliable CO values for mechanically ventilated patients with minor lung abnormalities and stable ventilatory settings [71].

The NICO system is also limited. For example, intrapulmonary shunt can affect the estimation of CO. Also, in patients undergoing thoracic surgery with OLV, the device underestimated CO compared with thermodilution CO at all measurement times [72]. With worsening pulmonary injury or hemodynamic compromise contributing to increasing shunt and dead space, assumptions made for calculating CO are less likely to approximate actual values. This technique reliably measures CO in patients affected by diseases causing low levels of pulmonary shunt, but underestimates it in patients with shunt higher than 35% [73]. In summary, compared to TD methods, the partial CO_2 rebreathing technique is non-invasive, can easily be automated, and can provide real-time and continuous cardiac output monitoring. Large outcome studies demonstrating use of this device are still lacking.

Impedance cardiography (ICG) or thoracic electrical bioimpedance (TEB) uses changes in thoracic impedance over the cardiac cycle to generate CO. A constant magnitude, high frequency, low amplitude current is applied longitudinally across a segment of thorax. Using Ohm's Law, the voltage difference within the current field is proportional to the electrical impedance (Z). Contraction of the heart produces a cyclical change in transthoracic impedance of about 0.5%. Upon ventricular ejection, a time-dependent cardiac-synchronous pulsatile impedance change is observed, $\Delta Z(t)$, which constitutes the time-variable total transthoracic impedance Z(t), when electrically parallel to baseline impedance (Z_0). Lower impedance indicates greater intrathoracic fluid volume and blood flow. TEB has waveform characteristics representing points in the cardiac cycle. The first derivative (dz/dt) of the waveform is used to identify the maximum upslope point, which is used to calculate the Velocity Index (VI). The VI is indicative of aortic blood velocity, such that impaired contractility is reflected by a decreased VI. By synchronizing fluid volume changes with the cardiac cycle, the change in impedance can be used to calculate SV, CO, and systemic vascular resistance [74]. TEB equipment consists of both noninvasive and invasive devices, of which the former has gained more acceptance. Examples include the Bio-Z Dx (Sonosite Inc®, Bothell, WA) and the niccomo® (medis GmbH, Ilmenau, Germany). Some studies comparing TEB-derived CO to TD have found significant correlation between the methods, but inaccuracies were observed with severe tachycardia, low CO, or frequent arrhythmias [75]. Questions with respect to the reliability and validity of this technique have led some to advocate its use only in research settings [76]. The clinical use of TEB has yet to be established.

Transesophageal echocardiography (TEE) is a method of ultrasound-based cardiac imaging which allows real-time visualization of anatomic structure and function. In the specific setting of thoracic surgery, TEE can be used to monitor ventricular function, valvular function, and wall motion changes reflective of ischemia during positioning changes, volume shifts, OLV, or surgical resection. Intrathoracic tumors may be visible in some exams, and compression or infiltration of structures such as the pulmonary artery or innominate vein may be visualized. Tumor invasion of the heart may be appreciated, as can other anatomic abnormalities resulting from the underlying disease process or iatrogenic causes. Intraoperative hemodynamic instability of unknown cause and the need for evaluation of affected cardiac and pulmonary structures will likely satisfy the Appropriate Use Criteria for Echocardiography [77]. Common contraindications to TEE use include some features present in the thoracic surgery population such as known esophageal strictures, perforation, lacerations or large diverticula. Relative contraindications also obviate TEE use in esophagectomies: dysphagia or odynophagia, recent upper GI bleeding, extensive radiation to the chest and mediastinum, and esophageal varices.

In terms of global cardiac function, the transgastric short-axis view provides a snapshot of left and right ventricular ejection fraction. Calculation of CO is also possible with two-dimensional (2D) Doppler measurements, such that CO = Aortic valve area (AVA) x heart rate (HR) x velocity time integral (TVI). AVA may be measured by planimetry of the AV via the midesophageal AV short axis view, with the imaging plane at approximately 30°. Another common method of calculating AVA is with the continuity equation, which states that the flow in one area must equal the flow in a second area if there are no shunts between the two areas. In practical terms, the flow from the left ventricular outflow tract (LVOT) is compared to the flow at the level of the aortic valve:

$$Aortic\ Valve\ Area\ \left(cm^2\right) = \frac{LVOT\ diameter^2 x\ 0.78540\ x\ LVOT\ TV1}{Aortic\ Valve\ TV1}$$

Where the CSA LVOT (cm^2) = 0.785 x LVOT Diameter2

TVI is an integral of instantaneous blood flow velocities during one cardiac cycle. To measure the LVOT TVI, the pulsed-Doppler sample volume is positioned just proximal to the aortic valve so that the location of the velocity recording matches the LVOT diameter measurement. When the sample volume is optimally positioned, the recording shows a smooth velocity curve with a well-defined peak and narrow band of velocities throughout systole. The TVI is measured by tracing the dense modal velocity throughout systole. The same is done for the AV TVI.

TEE assessment of cardiac and intrathoracic structures and function is a clinically established method that plays a critical role in the diagnosis and management of perioperative hemodynamic instability in many institutions [78]. However, its main disadvantage is that its use requires extensive training and a skilled operator [68]. Some measurements may be challenging to acquire and subject to methodical error or inability to obtain images adequately parallel to the ultrasound plane. Hemodynamic measurements obtained with TEE compared to TD with a PAC have resulted in agreements ranging from good [79] to possessing "accuracy limitations" [80]. A significant source of this inconsistency may result from interoperator variability. Further, in the instance of thoracic cases, proper contact with the stomach and esophagus in the lateral position can hinder the acquisition of adequate images. Other inconveniences include the expense of the equipment and the fact that an image cannot be easily fixed in order to provide continuous cardiac output readings without the presence of an expert user.

In summary, the physiologic and hemodynamic challenges inherent to thoracic surgery may require not only monitoring via an arterial wave pressure measurement, but possibly other modalities as well. PAC, lithium dilution, EDM, pulse contour cardiac output systems, partial CO_2 rebreathing, TEB, and TEE constitute such alternatives. While validation of these methods may be forthcoming, reasonable application of these modalities may improve perioperative management and overall patient outcomes.

3.4. Special operative scenarios and anesthetic considerations

3.4.1. VATS versus open thoracotomy

The decision as to whether a particular surgery can be performed using a video-assisted thoracoscopic or an open thoracotomy approach is a decision usually made by the surgeon. In 2007, at the International Society of Minimally Invasive Cardiothoracic Surgery conference, evidence revealed that VATS can be recommended to reduce overall postoperative complications, can reduce pain and overall functionality over the short term, improve delivery of adjuvant chemotherapy delivery, and can be recommended for lobectomy in clinical stage I and II non-small cell lung cancer patients. The recommendations were based on data derived from single and multiple randomized studies, but with conflicting evidence and/or divergence of opinion about the usefulness or efficacy of the procedure [81]. No general consensus using multiple randomized clinical trials has been done as to the preference of surgical technique. The bottom line is that with the learning curve for the VATS procedure, individual surgeons choose their own preferred method of surgical intervention. The role of an anesthesiologist is to be prepared for any lung surgery, both of which usually encompass one-lung ventilation, either through a double-lumen tube or a bronchial blocker as a general anesthetic. A minor VATS procedure such as pleural biopsy or thoracentesis can actually be done with local anesthesia +/- intravenous sedation [82]. These procedures are rare in the operating room however, and most VATS procedures are in actuality done under general anesthesia. An endobronchial ultrasound is done at our institute in the pulmonary lab as a general anesthetic with a laryngeal mask airway. Although a single-lumen endotracheal tube can be used under general anesthesia for open thoracotomy, the operative lung field would also undergo positive pressure ventilation, making it technically more difficult for the surgeon. In small infants, a balloon tipped bronchial blocker can be placed to isolate the lungmer[83] or placing ETT into the mainstem of the nonoperative lung are also other options if a double lumen tube is too large to be placed.

It is estimated that double lung tube placement has resulted in iatrogenic injury in 0.5-2 per 1000 cases of DLT placement[84], so care must be made to decrease these complications. One advantage of a double lumen tube above a bronchial blocker is the ability to suction out the operable lung if and when necessary, and increased intraoperative stability with the tube itself. The bronchial blocker is often difficult to obtain lung isolation in the right lung due to the takeoff of the right upper lobe being so close to the carina, but this technique is necessary to understand in case a double lumen is unable to be placed (in patients with abnormal anatomy) [85], or if a patient is already intubated with a single lumen tube with a difficult airway and needs lung isolation. There have been a number of cases where both are used successfully however. The key is having the lung isolated, and understanding physiology to understand how to utilize hypoxic pulmonary vasoconstriction to each patient's advantage.

In a thoracoscopic procedure, the surgeon does not have the ability to push the operative lung out of his/her way like an open thoracotomy. Thus, the importance of the lung being deflated is made apparent. Sometimes, a suction catheter can be placed in the operable lung to facilitate deflation of the lung. It is important to know if the surgeon is to insufflate with carbon dioxide, so that complications of insufflation can also be recognized. A VATS procedure is, although for the patient sometimes easier to manage postoperatively, for the surgeon and anesthesiologist comes with various difficulties. One of these difficulties has to do with not having enough access or visualization in cases where the pulmonary artery or another major vessel is inadvertently traumatized and the patient is bleeding. Therefore, it is always important to have blood available for a possible blood transfusion in both open thoracotomies and VATS procedures. An arterial line is necessary to keep a close eye on hemodynamics during both types of procedures. The positioning for both usually entails a lateral decubitus position, and pressure points must be checked. The postoperative pain level for patients with a thoracoscopic procedure is usually less than the open thoracotomy patient though this has been questioned. Chronic pain rates may be similar with VATS and open thoracotomies. A status post VATS procedure patient can achieve pain control with IV medications, while an epidural is usually recommended for thoracotomy patients. These methods of pain control will be discussed in a later chapter.

3.4.2. Airway disruptive surgeries

Airway disruptive surgeries require special communication between the surgeon and anesthesiologist as to what is going to be required intraoperatively. With surgical and anesthetic advances, now more than half the trachea can be safely excised in selected cases[86]. A tracheal resection is something done rarely, requiring the anesthesiologist and surgeon to share the airway. The type of anesthetic utilized depends on the skill of the anesthesiologist, and the experience within each independent institution as to the best way to carry out this surgical procedure. There have been many case reports depicting many different methods of maintaining oxygenation and ventilation for a patient while still undergoing a thoracic procedure that compromises the trachea or bronchus. The main anesthetic concern is always adequate ventilation and oxygenation when the airway is essentially open. It is also important to both the anesthesiologist and surgeon to protect the integrity of the new tracheal anastomosis postoperatively. Steroids are often given to help decrease airway edema. A high FiO_2 is necessary to help maintain oxygenation during periods of ventilatory pauses, but a close eye should be kept on electrocautery use. If indeed it is being used, then the lowest FiO_2 that the patient can tolerate should be kept to help prevent airway fire. An arterial line is a good monitor to check for innominate compression (such as in a medianstinoscopy) during surgical dissection.

A technique where a laryngeal mask airway is utilized with high-frequency jet ventilation for a patient with tracheal stenosis has also been reported. In this otherwise healthy patient with tracheal stenosis from prolonged intubation, an LMA was placed and the patient was put on positive pressure ventilation. A sterile 6-mm flexible tube was placed in the distal trachea and the patient adequately oxygenated/ventilated while the dissection and lesion was resected. Once the tracheal anastomosis started, a jet ventilator was placed in the distal trachea and the patient jet-ventilated for tracheal anastomosis. Once completed, the patient was once again placed on positive pressure ventilation through the LMA while the patient was awakened, found adequately spontaneously ventilating, and extubated successfully[87]. There are disadvantages to using high-frequency jet ventilation such as during exhalation there may be air trapping from the stenotic lesion, the catheter could become occluded by blood and displaced, and there might be distal aspiration of debris or blood[88].

More routinely, an endotracheal tube can be placed above the area of stenosis. Once surgical exposure is done, a separate tube can be placed distal to the stricture and the patient placed on the ventilator with sterility across the field. Once the trachea is resected, the primary endotracheal tube can be passed distal to the lesion and the anastomosis completed.

Another case has been reported in a patient with critical trachea stenosis. The patient underwent femoral-femoral extracorporeal bypass prior to induction. An endotracheal tube was placed after induction, and the patient was maintained on the endotracheal tube and positive pressure ventilation as he/she was weaned from the cardiopulmonary bypass machine[89].

A prospective study has been done in patients with upper tracheal stenosis that were managed with a cervical epidural anesthesia, local anesthesia and conscious sedation while maintaining spontaneous ventilation throughout the resection[90]. Although only twenty consecutive patients were enrolled, the outcome had a high level of patient satisfaction and immediate feedback from the patient throughout the procedure. This bypasses the need for jet ventilation or positive pressure ventilation, and enables communication with the patient throughout the surgical procedure.

Post resection, usually the patient is extubated with their neck in a flexed position to put less tension on the anastomosis. Not infrequently the patients chin is sutured to the manubrium sterni with a heavy stitch to maintain the flexion. A smooth extubation with minimal coughing/ bucking is preferred for the same reason. Extubation is important post operatively to reduce the positive pressure on the suture line as well. Pain control is often not an issue, a tracheal resection is not a very painful procedure, and intravenous narcotics and local anesthesia should be adequate for control.

3.4.3. Endotracheal tube exchange (Double to single lumen tube exchange)

These days, double lumen tubes are routinely used for surgeries requiring lung isolation. If extubation is unable to be accomplished at the conclusion of the surgery, the decision must be made to either keep the double lumen in place, or exchange it for a single lumen tube. Less than 1% of patients, however, require mechanical ventilation after surgery[91]. Exchanging the double lumen tube avoids the potential obstruction of the airway that can occur when secretions/blood get lodged in the bronchial tube. Also, the nursing staff that is to be taking care of the patient postoperatively might not understand how to troubleshoot a double lumen endobronchial tube, so misuse of the tube may occur including airway rupture.

Exchanging a double-lumen endobronchial tube to a single-lumen endotracheal tube has many considerations and should be approached with some trepidation. An airway that was initially easy to place the double lumen in might not be easyafter the surgery with volume shifts and edema. If it is thought the airway might be lost in the exchange, leaving the double lumen in overnight with the head of the bed elevated to help alleviate edema might be the safest option. It has been shown that the flow resistances of modern double lumen tubes are actually much lower than previously supposed, so the need to change them is not as important during spontaneous ventilation and weaning from the ventilator as previously thought[92]. The effective diameter of each lumen of an adult double lumen endobronchial tube is comparable to a 6.0-7.0 mm outside diameter ETT [93], so adequate oxygenation/ventilation is manageable without exchanging the tube. If an exchange is necessary, there are a few options described. The first option is using a tube exchanger to facilitate the exchange of the double lumen tube to a single lumen. First, adequate anesthesia and suctioning down both lumens of the double lumen should be done. FiO_2 should be 1.0. A tube exchanger is placed after being lubricated through the tracheal lumen, both cuffs are deflated, and the double lumen is removed over the stylet. A single lumen is then placed, sometimes while performing a direct laryngoscopy to facilitate the exchange. There are other scenarios described using the Eschmann stylet as a tube exchanger in various alternative ways [94]. The easiest and quickest method to exchanging the tube is just by performing a direct laryngoscopy after the patient is adequately anesthetized. If visualization of the cords is easy while the double lumen is still in place, it can be withdrawn and a single lumen placed under direct visualization.

Whichever technique is chosen, the safety of the patient comes first. If it is unsafe to change the tube out, an alternative is to just pull out the double lumen so the bronchial cuff is in the trachea, thus operating as a single lumen tube. Understanding that the airway anatomy and ease of visualization might not be the same as it was preoperatively is very important. Certainly it will not improve.

3.4.4. Post-operative need for bronchoscopy prior to emergence

Certain surgical scenarios may require fiberoptic bronchoscopic examination after completion of the surgical procedure, but prior to patient emergence (if extubation is planned). These scenarios include the examination of the integrity of anastomotic sites, the examination of anatomic structures (e.g.. the vocal cords) to ensure proper postoperative function, and the clearing of debris (tissue, secretions, and blood) from the proximal and distal airways. During fiberoptic bronchoscopic examination, the anesthesiologist must meticulously plan airway control techniques to ensure an optimal environment for bronchoscopy as well as adequate patient oxygenation and ventilation.

When a single-lumen endotracheal tube (SLT) is already in use, the procedure is usually straightforward. If a bronchial blocker is used in combination with an SLT for lung isolation, one simply removes the blocker from the SLT to facilitate fiberoptic bronchoscopy (bronchoscopy could also be performed with the blocker in place, if needed). However, one must keep in mind that the internal diameter of the indwelling SLT must be large enough to accommodate an appropriately sized bronchoscope, especially if adequate suction (provided by larger bronchoscopes) is required to clear debris.

When a double-lumen endotracheal tube (DLT) is used for lung isolation, the procedure is more complicated. Fiberoptic bronchoscopy with a DLT in place is difficult because of the specialized tube's design and required positioning. First, the internal diameters of the dual lumens of the DLT are small. This limits the size of bronchoscopes that may be used (3.6 - 4.9mm outer diameter)—smaller bronchoscopes do not provide the view or possess the suctioning capabilities of larger bronchoscopes. Second, DLTs are considerably longer and more invasive than conventional SLTs. DLTs are positioned (post intubation) so that the distal opening of the tracheal lumen closely abuts the primary carina with the distal bronchial end placed in the appropriate mainstem bronchi (for which the DLT was designed). Therefore, a properly placed DLT restricts direct bronchoscopic examination of a majority of the trachea and mainstem bronchi. Comprehensive bronchoscopic examination in this scenario requires removal of the DLT and subsequent replacement with an SLT or supraglottic airway device (e.g. Laryngeal Mask Airway™ - LMA North America, San Diego, CA, U.S.A.) in an anesthetized patient.

Supraglottic airway devices do not require endotracheal intubation and are preferred over reintubation with an SLT because they [1] reduce the possibility of trauma to fresh surgical anastomosis sites within the airways, [2] improve the visualization of proximal airway structures – vocal cords, proximal trachea – that would be otherwise obstructed by SLTs, [3] accommodate larger bronchoscopes for improved visualization and suctioning, and [4] are less complicated to place than SLTs and do not require neuromuscular blockade for easy placement. In patients with non-difficult airways, supraglottic airway devices may be immediately placed after deep extubation (in a blind fashion). In patients with difficult airways, supraglottic airway devices may be pre-positioned posterior to the DLT prior to extubation. This allows for fiberoptic visual confirmation of the device's proper positioning (by continuous visualization of the glottic opening) prior to, during, and after extubation. Once positioning of the supraglottic airway device and adequate ventilation are confirmed, fiberoptic examination of the airways may proceed. Upon completion of the bronchoscopic exam, the patient may be emerged from anesthesia with the device in place without the need for reintubation.

http://dx.doi.org/10.5772/56104

3.4.5. Pulmonary procedures in out-of-O.R. settings

A trend is growing toward performing pulmonary procedures in specialized non-O.R. pulmonary procedure suites, rather than the traditional operating room. These procedures may be performed for diagnostic or therapeutic purposes and include flexible/rigid bronchoscopy, pleuroscopy, tracheo-bronchial stent placement or dilation, and endobronchial ultrasound-guided lymph node sampling [95]. In these settings, special anesthetic considerations must be made regarding choice of agents, airway devices, and ventilatory modes.

a. Agents

A total intravenous anesthetic (TIVA) approach is the most practical mode of anesthetic delivery in these settings. A TIVA-based approach avoids volatile anesthetic agents that could be lost from airways in procedures that involve a breach of the airway (and/or the airway device). Loss of agent through a breach could result in inadequate anesthetic levels, exposure of personnel to volatile agents, combustion and airway fire (N2O), or production of toxic products after pyrolysis. Furthermore, special ventilatory modes (such as jet-ventilation) necessary for certain pulmonary procedures preclude the use of volatile anesthetics [96].

Two anesthetic challenges during pulmonary procedures are [1] providing adequate anesthesia during alternating periods of high and low stimulation (in which anesthetic requirements also fluctuate rapidly), and [2] rapid recovery post-procedure [96]. The intravenous agents propofol, remifentanil, and lidocaine have specific advantages in these situations, primarily as a result of their pharmacokinetic/pharmacodynamic profiles. The standard sedative-hypnotic for TIVA administration is propofol, and, in fact, propofol is the only sedative-hypnotic that is used on a standard basis for continuous infusion. Only propofol has the combination of quick onset, short half-life, rapid redistribution, amnesia, effective airway reflex depression, wide anesthetic depth range, and antiemetic properties. It does not, however, provide analgesia; therefore, narcotics are usually added to a TIVA regimen. Narcotics provide analgesia, reduce the propofol dosage needed, and also suppress the cough reflex. Remifentanil is an ultra-short acting narcotic (context sensitive half-life: 3-5 minutes) that is metabolized by nonspecific tissue and plasma esterases; therefore, it is ideal intraooperatively to manage moments of high stimulation while avoiding over-accumulation of narcotic when stimulation subsides [97]. In patients for whom post-procedure pain control or cough suppression is needed, a longer-acting narcotic may be coadministered with remifentanil. Lastly, intravenous lidocaine is a useful adjunct to propofol and remifentanil in TIVA. Lidocaine is an amide-type local anesthetic that reduces the need for both propofol and narcotics; it also suppresses airway reflexes and is an effective post-procedure anti-tussive [98].

b. Airway devices

Airway management for pulmonary procedures must address the need for adequate patient oxygenation/ventilation, permit complete examination of areas of interest of the airway, and accommodate the necessary diagnostic and/or interventional instruments needed for the procedure. In most cases, supraglottic airways (e.g., Laryngeal Mask Airway™) meet these requirements and are the airway devices of choice. They are easy to place without the need for specialized equipment, are an integral part of the standard difficult airway algorithm, may be used in spontaneously or mechanically ventilated patients, and provide limited airway protection from regurgitation. Furthermore, supraglottic airways may be easily used as a bridge in a case where definitive airway control will be managed via rigid bronchoscopy/jet-ventilation. In such a case, the supraglottic airway is placed as a temporary airway conduit during induction, is removed once the rigid bronchoscopy begins, and is replaced at the end of the procedure to serve as the airway conduit until emergence from anesthesia.

c. Ventilatory modes

Patient ventilation/oxygenation during pulmonary procedures may be spontaneous or mechanical, depending on the requirements of the procedure. Adequacy of oxygenation and ventilation is measured by pulse oximetry and end-tidal CO2 measurement. It is important to note that while end-tidal CO2 detection is vital in confirming adequate ventilation, it is often inconsistent due to airway breach and suctioning inherent during pulmonary procedures. Of the various mechanical ventilation modes, jet-ventilation deserves particular attention. Jet-ventilation is typically associated with rigid bronchoscopy. In this situation, total airway control will be in the hands of the interventionalist/surgeon, with the anesthesiologist controlling the jet-ventilator. Control of jet ventilation may be by automated jet delivery systems or manually by the anesthesiologist. Automated systems have several benefits over manual delivery, including greater control of delivered FiO2 and respiratory frequency, duration, and flow. Additionally, automation gives anesthesia personnel greater freedom to attend to other aspects of the anesthetic care.

3.4.6. Post anesthesia recovery considerations for patients undergoing thoracic procedures

The immediate post-operative care of the thoracic surgical patient is focused on ensuring conditions that optimize oxygenation/ventilation and recognizing possible post-operative complications inherent to thoracic surgery.

a. Extubation

If feasible, immediate post-operative extubation is favored to avoid unnecessary hemodynamic stress, the disruption of fresh surgical sites from continued intubation, positive-pressure ventilation, and/or coughing, and the development of ventilator-associated pneumonia [99]. However, the tentative respiratory condition of the typical thoracic surgery patient warrants careful consideration when making the decision to extubate (see preoperative anesthetic evaluation above). The physician must not only optimize routine respiratory criteria for extubation – pH ≥ 7.30, FiO2 ≤ 0.4-0.5, PaO2/FiO2 > 150-200, PEEP ≤ 5-8 cmH2O, RR ≤ 30 bpm, SpO2 ≥ 90%, PaO2 ≥ 60, PaCO2 ≤ 50, Vt > 5 ml/kg, VC >15 ml/kg, NIF > -20 cm H2O – but must also recognize the variable nature of emergence from anesthesia and consider the state of other important clinical variables [100]. These variables include the ability to follow commands, the return of airway protective reflexes, adequate reversal of neuromuscular blockade (with good motor strength), adequate pain control, normothermia, hemodynamic stability, and normal electrolyte values. Additionally, the rapid shallow breathing index (RSBI - the ratio of respiratory frequency to tidal volume (f/VT)) combines superior sensitivity (97%) and negative predictive value (95%) when predicting weaning success [101, 102].

http://dx.doi.org/10.5772/56104

Once extubation is achieved, the focus is on optimizing pulmonary physiology; three fundamental measures are essential. First, supplemental oxygen should be administered and adequate ventilation confirmed, because hypoxia and hypercarbia are well known to increase pulmonary vascular resistance [103]. Second, the patient should be positioned supine with the head of the bed elevated (semi-Fowler's position) to lessen the risk of aspiration and decrease the work of breathing. Third, pain control must be evaluated; pain increases sympathetic tone, elevating pulmonary artery pressures and pulmonary vascular resistance, and elicits respiratory splinting that limits ventilation and results in hypercapnea.

In some cases, continued intubation and mechanical ventilation is required postoperatively. Under these circumstances, it is important to achieve the transition from positive pressure to spontaneous ventilation as quickly as possible. In addition, extubation criteria should be assessed frequently so that extubation may be acheived as soon as possible.

b. Post-operative Complications

Operations involving vital thoracic structures place patients at higher risk of life-threatening post-operative complications. An in-depth discussion of these complications can be found in chapters detailing the post-operative course of these patients. This section focuses on select complications that may occur in the immediate post-operative recovery period: injuries in the conducting airways, pneumothorax, and cardiac herniation.

i. Injuries in the conducting airways

Advanced anesthetic airway management and surgical manipulation predispose the thoracic surgery patient to a variety of post-operative airway complications. Injuries range from erythema/edema (most commonly) to vocal cord injuries and tracheo-bronchial rupture (TBR) (rarely). Supportive therapy with supplemental humidified oxygen is adequate for mild symptoms of airway edema; however, constant monitoring for worsening respiratory obstruction is paramount. Iatrogenic vocal cord injuries resulting from intubation and/or damage to the recurrent laryngeal nerve may lead to airway compromise and increase risk of aspiration, if the damage is bilateral. Dyspnea, stridor, and inability to phonate are symptoms commonly associated with bilateral vocal cord injury/paralysis. If respiratory distress is present, the airway should be definitely controlled via intubation or tracheostomy. TBR caused by DLT intubation is extremely rare, with a reported incidence of less than 0.5 % [84]. Hemoptysis and subcutaneous crepitus (in the neck and upper chest area) are the most common presenting symptoms with respiratory distress and/or collapse occurring in advanced cases [104]. If TBR is suspected and surgical intervention planned, general anesthesia should be induced while preferably maintaining spontaneous ventilation to avoid worsening of the injury by barotrauma. Initial airway control with a supraglottic airway is preferred, when possible, to avoid further injury that can occur with endotracheal intubation. Further, a supraglottic airway allows for complete fiber-optic examination of the trachea, bronchi, and distal airways. Fiber-optic examination of the tracheobronchial tree is important to confirm the diagnosis of TBR and to locate the lesion. Once the location and extent of the injury is determined, the type and application of airway control may be chosen and surgical repair undertaken. In extreme situations, cardio-pulmonary bypass may be required to assure oxygenation and ventilation.

ii. Pneumothorax

Pneumothorax is a potentially grave immediate postoperative complication that may necessitate prompt intervention. The creation of a pneumothorax is inherent in any procedure involving the breach of the thoracic cavity. The severity of pneumothorax is determined by its magnitude and whether it is in communication externally with atmospheric pressure. A pneumothorax of small volume is usually well tolerated; however, with increased magnitude, it exerts considerable effects to the heart and vasculature in the confined space of the thoracic cavity. These may lead to hemodynamic collapse and respiratory compromise – a tension pneumothorax. Chest drainage tubes are used to decrease the magnitude of a pneumothorax by providing an avenue of escape for trapped air (and/or blood, secretions, etc.) from the thoracic cavity. Specialized "balanced" drainage systems have been developed for certain operations, such as pneumonectomy. Balanced systems provide a buffer to prevent excessive negative or positive intrathoracic pressures from developing, lowering the chance for both tension pneumothorax and cardiac herniation (see below) [105]. In circumstances where chest tubes are not placed or where the drainage system malfunctions, tension pneumothorax may develop. In this scenario, intrathoracic pressures must be relieved immediately via needle decompression and/or emergent chest tube insertion. One must recognize that contralateral pneumothorax is also a possibility from anesthetic (contralateral central venous catheters, epidural (paramedian) placement, barotrauma) as well as surgical (breach of the contralateral pleura) insult [106]. Care must be taken to avoid clamping chest tubes after thoracotomy to avoid formation of a pneumothorax.

iii. Cardiac herniation

Cardiac herniation, although rare, is a potentially fatal postoperative complication most commonly associated with disruption of the pericardium – most commonly during the course of or after a pneumonectomy. The usual presenting symptoms are generalized hypotension and tachycardia; however, right versus left sided cardiac herniation may present with additional distinct signs and symptoms inherent to the physiologic disruption unique to the direction of herniation [107, 108]. Leftward herniation places the heart at risk for myocardial ischemia and arrhythmias, because of the potential constriction of the ventricles by pericardial tissue during the course of the herniation [107, 108]. Rightward herniation predisposes the patient to superior vena cava (SVC) syndrome – head, neck and upper-extremity cyanosis, edema, etc. - secondary to torsion and obstruction of the SVC and inadequate cardiac preload because of impaired venous drainage [107, 108]. After assessing signs and symptoms, cardiac herniation may be confirmed via imaging - chest x-ray and/or echocardiography. Immediate surgical intervention to reduce the herniation and correct the pericardial defect is paramount to prevent further hemodynamic collapse [107, 108]. The gravity of cardiac herniation warrants recovery measures to help minimize its occurrence. Avoid patient positioning with the operative side dependent, to reduce gravitational effects favoring herniation. As discussed above, early extubation is favored to alleviate the effects of positive pressure ventilation and its tendency to instigate and worsen herniation. Lastly, avoid negative pressure via chest drainage tubes (preferably using balanced chest drainage systems in pneumonectomies) to minimize a vacuum effect that may predispose to herniation [107, 108].

4. Pain management for the thoracic surgical patient

4.1. Post-thoracotomy pain syndrome

Thoracotomies continue to cause substantial pain because of the degree of surgical injury. Insult to the intercostal nerves, soft tissue damage and inflammation, bone and joint disturbance, and visceral manipulation all contribute to the severity of pain[88]. The estimated incidence of chronic pain following thoracotomy is between 30-40%, with approximately 10% with severe disabling pain [109, 110]. Pain control is crucial after thoracic surgery not only for immediate pain relief, but also to prevent pulmonary complications.

"Pain that recurs or persists along a thoracotomy scar at least two months following the surgical procedure" [111] is the definition of post-thoracotomy pain syndrome (PTPS). Poor pain management after thoracotomy may contribute to PTPS [112]. The pain is largely described as aching, with tenderness and numbness at or around the surgical incision/scar [113]. In contrast to acute pain, which mostly affects respiratory function, PTPS may be responsible for inability to perform daily activities. Although PTPS likely plays a negative role in daily life, its impact is unclear because these subjective phenomena have not been reliably assessed [113, 114].

Although video assisted thoracic surgery (VATS) was anticipated to reduce pain when compared to traditional posterolateral thoracotomy, its smaller port sites do not necessarily avoid intercostal nerve injury owing to aggressive manipulation of the scopes and instruments. The pain associated with VATS is not significantly different to that of thoracotomy[115] and there are conflicting differences in the incidence of PTPS [113, 114]. It is unclear if patients with preventative analgesia by way of thoracic epidural analgesia have fewer propensities to develop PTPS [114]. Other regional techniques have not yet been studied in this capacity [114]. There is also conflicting evidence of the causality of acute pain on PTPS [114].

There are many modalities of postoperative pain control that will be briefly explained here.

4.2. Systemic analgesics

Opioids have a long-standing history of providing effective pain relief. It is the unwanted side-effects that discourage their use including: nausea, vomiting, respiratory depression, ileus, biliary spasms, urinary retention, sedation, and pruritis. Opioids can be given by many routes – oral, intravenous, intramuscular, transdermal, transmucosal. Intravenous patient controlled analgesia (PCA) allows for increased safety, less opioid use, ability to titrate to individual needs, and some increase in patient satisfaction [116]. Using opioids alone may lead to intolerable side effects, which has led to the concomitant use of other drug classes for their synergistic effects.

Ketamine is an *N*-methyl-D-aspartate (NMDA) antagonist that has direct spinal effects as well as depresses the thalamus and activates the limbic system. It acts at the phencyclidine binding site and has been used as an induction agent. At lower doses, it provides effective analgesia.

The use of low dose intraoperative ketamine offers decreased postoperative pain and morphine consumption [117, 118].

Nonsteroidal anti-inflammatory drugs (NSAIDs) inhibit conversion of arachidonic acid to prostaglandin E2 in inflamed areas via cyclooxygenase (COX). It is suggested that the maximum daily dose of NSAIDs should be given/ordered because small doses of NSAIDs are not useful in acute pain relief [118]. When given in conjunction with opioids, NSAIDs reduced the postoperative opioid utilization and decreased unwanted opioid side effects [118]. NSAIDs should be used cautiously in those susceptible to its side effects including risk of renal injury, bleeding and peptic ulcers, asthma and bronchospasm. COX-2 selective inhibitors were developed to avoid the unwanted side effects of NSAIDs and may play a role as an adjunct in postoperative pain control.

4.3. Thoracic epidural

Thoracic epidural refers to analgesic technique of injecting medication into the epidural space, the potential space that surrounds the spinal cord. A segmental block results with coverage both above and below the injection site. A single injection into the epidural space may be performed, or a catheter may be inserted for prolonged infusion. For post-thoracotomy pain relief, commonly a catheter is inserted via midline or paramedian technique in order to provide intermittent boluses as well as a continuous infusion for pain control. Infusions usually consist of a local anesthetic, an opioid, or a mixture of the two in order to optimize their synergistic effects [119] while reducing the individual doses and side effects [119, 120]. As the nerve roots leave the foramen and become peripheral nerves, they cross through the epidural space where they are bathed in the epidural solution.

The mechanism of action differs between local anesthetics and opioids. Local anesthetics block sodium channels ultimately leading to blocked nerve conduction. The density of local anesthetic blockade is primarily dependent on the concentration of local anesthetic present, and dermatomal spread of blockade is dependent on the volume infused. Also remember that the level of somatic block may be smaller than the sympathetic block because the somatic fibers are less sensitive [121]. Opioids bind to presynaptic and postsynaptic opioid receptors in the substantia gelatinosa, which inhibits the presynaptic release and postsynaptic response to neurotransmitters [121]. In a systemic review of randomized trials, Joshi et al. found that patients with thoracic epidural analgesia had a significantly lower pain scores and needed less supplemental analgesia compared to systemic opioid analgesia [122].

Adverse effects may be from various aspects of epidural placement. Those associated with needle and catheter placement include back pain, inadvertent dural puncture, post dural puncture headache, trauma to spinal cord or nerves, and neuropathy (usually transient). Dural puncture may lead to post dural puncture headache. The headache is usually characterized by severe fronto-occipital pain with head elevation that subsides, sometimes completely, upon return to the supine position [88]. The loss of CSF through the small puncture site may be enough to cause traction on the brain causing pain. Most patients' symptoms completely resolve after a few days to a week. Those that are not able or not willing to wait for spontaneous resolution may opt to undergo an epidural blood patch. Neurologic injury may be the most feared complication of epidural analgesia. Nerve injury is usually transient and may occur from direct trauma to the nerves or spinal cord during needle insertion. A more devastating nerve injury can result from an epidural hematoma or abscess. Spinal hematoma occurs very rarely, approximately less than 1 in 150,000 [88]. Although rare, if it is not detected and treated promptly, it leads to irreversible paraplegia. The occurrence of hematoma has been on the rise, whether it is from increased coexistence of anticoagulation and regional anesthesia technique or from increased reporting [123]. Infection can occur from ineffective sterile preparation, contaminated drugs, an underlying infection, or bacteremia. Any of these sources can cause an infection at the insertion site or lead to spread of infection from the skin along the indwelling catheter into the epidural space causing meningitis (if the dura was punctured) or abscess which could ultimately result in cord compression [123].

Effects related to epidural injection of local anesthetic are usually dose related and include hypotension, motor block, systemic toxicity, and urinary retention. Epidural opioid administration may result in adverse effects that are similar to their parenteral administration. These include pruritis, nausea, urinary retention, decreased arousability, ileus, and respiratory depression. Respiratory depression is the most concerning of the adverse effects and thus necessitates a monitored setting. After epidural injection, in the following 2-4 hours, early respiratory depression can occur which is likely due to the systemic absorption of the opioid [124]. Some opioids are more hydrophilic than others and have a tendency to remain in the CSF causing possible spread and delayed respiratory depression (usually occurs after 4 hours).

Relative contraindications to epidural include sepsis or bacteremia, infection at the insertion site, hypovolemia or shock, coagulopathy or thrombocytopenia, increased intracranial pressure (for risk of brain herniation if accidental dural puncture). One should use caution with patients who have underlying neurological diseases as not to confuse effects of the epidural versus pre-existing neurological deficits. The only absolute contraindication to epidural placement is patient refusal [88].

4.4. Thoracic paravertebral nerve block

TPVB involves injecting local anesthetic into the space adjacent to the thoracic vertebrae, which contains the spinal intercostal nerves. The boundaries of the space include the parietal pleura anterolaterally, the superior costotransverse ligament posteriorly, and medially by a portion of the vertebral body, intervertebral disc and intervertebral foramen [125]. The paravertebral space is continuous with the epidural space, intercostal space, and contralateral paravertebral space (by way of the prevertebral and epidural spaces). The caudal boundary of the space is at the origin of the psoas, while the cranial boundary is unknown. Cranially, radiographic dye has been noted after a thoracic paravertebral injection in the cervical area [126]. The intercostal nerves, dorsal rami, sympathetic chain and associated vessels lie within the fat of the paravertebral space [126]. A percutaneous technique is classically described whereby a needle is inserted into the space until a subtle loss of resistance is met followed by aspiration to ensure that the lung or pleura has not been breached before injecting small amounts of local anesthetic or insertion of a catheter [125]. The injection of local anesthetic can also be performed under direct visualization by the surgeon prior to the closure of the chest wall.

Injection of local anesthetic into the paravertebral space can give varying degrees of analgesia. The injection may remain localized to the area of injection producing a single level ipisilateral block, or it can spread to the above and below adjacent levels, as well as to the epidural space and contralateral paravertebral space. For example, Eason found that a single injection of 15ml of 0.375% bupivacaine spread over 4 spaces [125]. Similarly, 15ml of 0.5% bupivacaine injection led to a unilateral 5 level dermatome somatic block and 8 level sympathetic block [127].

Advantages of TPVB are many. TPVB is easy to learn and has a high success rate [126]. Successful placement of TPVB also can eliminate some unwanted effects of epidural analgesia such as spinal cord injury, spinal hematoma, excessive hypotension (owing to only a unilateral sympathetic blockade), and urinary retention [128]. Also, the nursing care required after TPVB is no different than normal post-surgical care [129]. A meta-analysis identified TPVB as having equivalent pain relief after thoracic surgery with less major side effects and decreased pulmonary complications to that of epidural analgesia [130].

Adverse effects of TPVB include accidental pleural puncture, which could lead to a pneumothorax. The incidence of puncture and pneumothorax are 0.8% and 0.5% respectively, which is similar to other anesthetic procedures with pneumothorax risk [128]. Other adverse effects include relative hypotension, failed block, and vascular puncture.

Contraindications to TPVB are similar to those of epidural placement including infection at the insertion site, bacteremia, epyema. Another relative contraindication would be if the patient has had a previous thoracotomy because the ipsilateral paravertebral space may have been altered or obliterated as a result of surgery [124]. With respect to anticoagulation, the paravertebral space is less vascular than the epidural space, and paravertebral vessel puncture is less common [128, 129].

4.5. Intercostal nerve block

The intercostal nerve provides sensory and motor innervation to chest wall and is found in the costal groove of each rib. Intercostal nerve blockade provides unilateral sensory and motor anesthesia to these areas. Local anesthetic is commonly injected 5 to 7 cm from the midline over several sections owing to the great deal of overlap between the intercostal nerves. There are different approaches to intercostal nerve blocks for thoracic procedures. The simplest is to inject local anesthetic around several intercostal nerves during thoracotomy when the chest wall is open. Cryotherapy, continuous infusion or successive boluses of local anesthetic are also options [131].

Direct intercostal nerve block is most easily done by direct visualization during thoracotomy, but can also be done percutaneously. Local is injected over multiple segments inferior to the rib with caution to avoid intravascular injection. Usually a small amount (2-5ml) of local is injected two to three spaces above and below the incision [131]. Cryoanalgesia interrupts nerve conduction for 1 to 3 months as a result of the freezing and subsequent damage of the myelin sheath [131] and is associated with long term intercostal neuralgia [132]. Extrapleural and interpleural infusion of local anesthetic are also techniques to block the intercostal nerves. Peeling back the pleura from the chest wall can create an extrapleural pocket, and a catheter can be introduced percutaneously into the space. After closure of the thoracotomy, an infusion of local anesthetic will fill the extrapleural space which leads to an intercostal block. Interpleural catheters can be inserted percutaneously to attain an intercostal nerve block, but one must keep in mind that a large volume of the anesthetic may be lost to the chest tubes. Interpleural anesthesia requires diffusion across the pleura and sub pleural space in order to attain an intercostal nerve blockade. Single shot direct intercostal nerve block appears to have the same or superior pain control compared to epidural on the day of surgery, but after the effects of the local anesthesia have been exhausted, epidural anesthesia is superior to intercostal nerve block [131-133] Detterbeck states that extrapleural infusion of local anesthetic is more effective than systemic narcotics, and at least as good as thoracic epidural. Extrapleural intercostal nerve block provides a unilateral blockade, so the amount of urinary retention and hypotension are decreased, and there is not a need for special monitoring because the risk of respiratory depression is minimal [131]. Pain relief from interpleural infusion is inconsistent [131].

Systemic absorption of local anesthetic is notoriously high for intercostal nerve block due to the vascularity of the area of injection. There are no specific absolute contraindications to intercostal nerve blocks. They should be avoided in patients in whom high systemic levels of local anesthetics will not be well tolerated such as those with seizure disorders.

4.6. Elastomeric pumps

Wound infiltration with local anesthetic targets the peripheral level of pain, and has been used widely in minor surgical procedures [134, 135]. The relatively short-term duration of the local infiltration limits the usefulness of one-time wound infiltration for more major thoracic surgery. An elastomeric pump connected to a multi orifice catheter allows for continuous local anesthetic incisional infusion. Implementation of this technique is quite simple, with a minimal technical failure incidence [116]. A catheter is threaded in or near the insult and connected to a reservoir pump of local anesthetic by way of a flow-limiting valve. The surrounding tissues are then continuously bathed in the local anesthetic at 4ml/hr. By providing anesthesia at the site of insult there may be less need for systemic narcotics, and avoid many systemic narcotic effects including postoperative nausea and vomiting. It is also believed that local anesthetic at the wound site can decrease the local inflammatory response which may in turn decrease pain and hyperalgesia [116]. Wheatley et al found that using an elastomeric pump is a safe and effective adjunct for post-thoracotomy pain relief. Also, patients had lower pain scores and decreased narcotic need when compared to thoracic epidural analgesia alone [136]. Although local anesthetic toxicity is always a concern with infusions, the incidence of systemic toxicity is low [116]. Wound infiltration is safe and not associated with increased acute wound-related complications or long-term effects on wound healing [137].

4.7. Anticoagulation

Hemorrhagic complications from neuraxial blockade are of great concern. Epidural analgesia is usually not initiated in patients who have a preexisting coagulopathy. The following are some consensus guidelines assembled by the American Society of Regional Anesthesia and Pain Medicine [138]:

1. Thrombolytic therapy

- Avoid thrombolytic for 10 days after neuraxial puncture,
- It is not clear how long to wait after thrombolytic therapy for safe performance of neuraxial anesthesia,
- If neuraxial block is at or near time of thrombolytic therapy neurologic checks should be none no less than every 2 hours,
- There is no recommendation for removal of neuraxial catheters in unexpected thrombolytic therapy

2. Subcutaneous unfractionated heparin

- Review of other medications that may affect clotting is advised
- There is little risk of spinal hematoma
- Placement of the block prior to therapy may be desirable although increased risk is not demonstrated in the presence of subcutaneous heparin
- In twice-daily doses – epidurals may be placed before the next scheduled dose, the catheter can coexist with regimen, and preferably the catheter can be removed one hour prior to next dose
- Thrice daily doses or more than 10,000units unfractionated heparin – there is no data published, but it is advised not to maintain an epidural catheter with this regimen
- If the patient has received more than four days of heparin, a platelet count should be obtained prior to block or removal of catheter in the instace of heparin induced thrombocytopenia
- After needle placement, wait one hour to administer heparin
- Wait 2-4 hours after heparin to remove cathers, resume therapy one hours after removal of catheter
- Bloody placement may increase risk of hematoma, but the case does not necessarily need to be cancelled.

3. Low-Molecular Weight Heparin

- A bloody placement does not mandate cancellation of the case, however LMWH should be delayed for 24 hours
- Epidural placement should happen 10-12 hours after last does
- If the patient is on higher dose LMWH, one should wait 24 hours to place epidural
- Do not place epidural at 2 hours after dose – peak anticoagulation activity

http://dx.doi.org/10.5772/56104

- Twice daily doses should not be initiated with an indwelling catheter, and must be removed before the first dose
- Once-daily dosing – may start 6-8 hours postoperatively, the catheter can be maintained, removal after 10-12 hours of last dose

4. Oral Anticoagulants – Warfarin

- INR should be normalized prior to neuraxial technique
- If initial does of warfarin is given more than 24 hours prior to surgery, INR should be checked prior to neuraxial block
- If low-dose warfarin therapy is ongoing during epidural anesthesia, neurological evaluations and daily INR checks are advised
- Catheters should be removed when INR is less than 1.5, and neurological assessment should be continued for 24 hours
- If $1.5 < INR < 3$, catheters should be cautiously removed
- If the INR is more than 3, the dose of warfarin should be held/reduced

5. Antiplatelet Medications

- NSAIDs have no specific concerns or added risk with epidural with or without catheter placement, unless concurrent medications affecting clotting
- The risk of bleeding with clopidogrel, ticlopidine, and GP IIB/IIIA inhibitors is not known.
- 7 and 14 days should elapse between discontinuation of ticlopidine and clopidogre, respectively, and placement of neuraxial block
- Platelet function normalization must occur before placement of neuraxial block if discontinued for only 5-7 days
- Epidural catheters should not be maintained while on GP IIB/IIIA inhibitor therapy

6. Herbals

- They do not create risk that impedes with neuraxial block
- Garlic inhibits platelet aggregation, increases fibrinolysis
- Ginko inhibits platelet-activating factor
- Ginseng has the potential to inhibit coagulation

7. Thrombin inhibitors

- Monitored by aPTTT
- Anticoagulation effect present for 1-3 hours
- There are no pharmacologic reversals

- Neuraxial techniques are best avoided

8. Fondaparinux

- Factor Xa inhibitor
- Unknown risk of spinal hematoma

5. Conclusion

The challenges of thoracic anesthesia are unique among all anesthetic subspecialties. Its practitioners must be well-versed in a wide range of anesthetic management principles, from advanced airway techniques to ventilations strategies and pain management. The two subspecialties of thoracic surgery and thoracic anesthesia continue to co-evolve to improve patient safety and surgical outcomes.

Author details

January Tsai, Teresa Moon, Shital Vachhani, Javier Lasala, Peter H Norman and Ronaldo Purugganan*

*Address all correspondence to: rpurugga@mdanderson.org

Department of Anesthesia and Perioperative Medicine, Division of Anesthesia and Critical Care, The University of Texas MD Anderson Cancer Center, Houston, Texas, USA

References

[1] BTS guidelines: guidelines on the selection of patients with lung cancer for surgery-Thorax. [Guideline Practice Guideline]. (2001). Feb;, 56(2), 89-108.

[2] Slinger, P. Update on anesthetic management for pneumonectomy. Curr Opin Anaesthesiol. [Review]. (2009). Feb;, 22(1), 31-7.

[3] Brunelli, A, & Rocco, G. Spirometry: predicting risk and outcome. Thorac Surg Clin. [Review]. (2008). Feb;, 18(1), 1-8.

[4] Nakahara, K, Ohno, K, Hashimoto, J, Miyoshi, S, Maeda, H, Matsumura, A, et al. Prediction of postoperative respiratory failure in patients undergoing lung resection for lung cancer. Ann Thorac Surg. (1988). Nov;, 46(5), 549-52.

[5] Beckles, M. A, Spiro, S. G, Colice, G. L, & Rudd, R. M. The physiologic evaluation of patients with lung cancer being considered for resectional surgery. Chest. [Guideline Practice Guideline]. (2003). Jan;123(1 Suppl):105S-14S.

[6] Olsen, G. N, Bolton, J. W, Weiman, D. S, & Hornung, C. A. Stair climbing as an exercise test to predict the postoperative complications of lung resection. Two years' experience. Chest. (1991). Mar;, 99(3), 587-90.

[7] Slinger, P, & Johnston, M. Preoperative assessment for lung cancer surgery. In: Slinger P, editor. Progress in thoracic anesthesia: a society of cardiovascular anesthesiologists monograph. 1st ed. Baltimore: Lippincott, Williams, and Wilkins; (2004)., 1-27.

[8] Ghaye, B, Szapiro, D, Fanchamps, J. M, & Dondelinger, R. F. Congenital bronchial abnormalities revisited. Radiographics. [Review]. (2001). Jan-Feb;, 21(1), 105-19.

[9] Slinger, P. Choosing the appropriate double-lumen tube: a glimmer of science comes to a dark art. J Cardiothorac Vasc Anesth. [Comment Editorial]. (1995). Apr;, 9(2), 117-8.

[10] Lohser, J. Managing hypoxemia during minimally invasive thoracic surgery. Anesthesiol Clin. (2012). Dec;, 30(4), 683-97.

[11] Narayanaswamy, M, Mcrae, K, Slinger, P, Dugas, G, Kanellakos, G. W, Roscoe, A, et al. Choosing a lung isolation device for thoracic surgery: a randomized trial of three bronchial blockers versus double-lumen tubes. Anesth Analg. [Comparative Study Randomized Controlled Trial]. (2009). Apr;, 108(4), 1097-101.

[12] Campos, J. H. Lung isolation techniques for patients with difficult airway. Curr Opin Anaesthesiol. [Review]. (2010). Feb;, 23(1), 12-7.

[13] Brodsky, J. B. Lung separation and the difficult airway. Br J Anaesth. [Review]. (2009). Dec;103 Suppl 1:i, 66-75.

[14] Purugganan, R. V, Jackson, T. A, Heir, J. S, Wang, H, & Cata, J. P. Video laryngoscopy versus direct laryngoscopy for double-lumen endotracheal tube intubation: a retrospective analysis. J Cardiothorac Vasc Anesth. (2012). Oct;, 26(5), 845-8.

[15] Benumof, J. L. The position of a double-lumen tube should be routinely determined by fiberoptic bronchoscopy. J Cardiothorac Vasc Anesth. [Editorial]. (1993). Oct;, 7(5), 513-4.

[16] Read, R. C, Friday, C. D, & Eason, C. N. Prospective study of the Robertshaw endobronchial catheter in thoracic surgery. Ann Thorac Surg. (1977). Aug;, 24(2), 156-61.

[17] Burton, N. A, Watson, D. C, Brodsky, J. B, & Mark, J. B. Advantages of a new polyvinyl chloride double-lumen tube in thoracic surgery. Ann Thorac Surg. (1983). Jul;, 36(1), 78-84.

[18] Alliaume, B, Coddens, J, & Deloof, T. Reliability of auscultation in positioning of double-lumen endobronchial tubes. Can J Anaesth. [Comparative Study]. (1992). Sep;, 39(7), 687-90.

[19] Fleischmann, K. E, Goldman, L, Young, B, & Lee, T. H. Association between cardiac and noncardiac complications in patients undergoing noncardiac surgery: outcomes and effects on length of stay. Am J Med. [Research Support, U.S. Gov't, P.H.S.]. (2003). Nov;, 115(7), 515-20.

[20] Law, S, Wong, K. H, Kwok, K. F, Chu, K. M, & Wong, J. Predictive factors for postoperative pulmonary complications and mortality after esophagectomy for cancer. Ann Surg. (2004). Nov;, 240(5), 791-800.

[21] Licker, M, De Perrot, M, Spiliopoulos, A, Robert, J, Diaper, J, Chevalley, C, et al. Risk factors for acute lung injury after thoracic surgery for lung cancer. Anesth Analg. [Research Support, Non-U.S. Gov't]. (2003). Dec;, 97(6), 1558-65.

[22] Kooguchi, K, Kobayashi, A, Kitamura, Y, Ueno, H, Urata, Y, Onodera, H, et al. Elevated expression of inducible nitric oxide synthase and inflammatory cytokines in the alveolar macrophages after esophagectomy. Crit Care Med. [Research Support, Non-U.S. Gov't]. (2002). Jan;, 30(1), 71-6.

[23] Misthos, P, Katsaragakis, S, Milingos, N, Kakaris, S, Sepsas, E, Athanassiadi, K, et al. Postresectional pulmonary oxidative stress in lung cancer patients. The role of one-lung ventilation. Eur J Cardiothorac Surg. (2005). Mar;discussion 82-3., 27(3), 379-82.

[24] Ng, J. M. Update on anesthetic management for esophagectomy. Curr Opin Anaesthesiol. [Review]. (2011). Feb;, 24(1), 37-43.

[25] Amato, M. B, Barbas, C. S, Medeiros, D. M, Magaldi, R. B, Schettino, G. P, Lorenzi-filho, G, et al. Effect of a protective-ventilation strategy on mortality in the acute respiratory distress syndrome. N Engl J Med. [Clinical Trial Comparative Study Randomized Controlled Trial Research Support, Non-U.S. Gov't]. (1998). Feb 5;, 338(6), 347-54.

[26] Lionetti, V, Recchia, F. A, & Ranieri, V. M. Overview of ventilator-induced lung injury mechanisms. Curr Opin Crit Care. [Research Support, Non-U.S. Gov't Review]. (2005). Feb;, 11(1), 82-6.

[27] Schilling, T, Kozian, A, Huth, C, Buhling, F, Kretzschmar, M, Welte, T, et al. The pulmonary immune effects of mechanical ventilation in patients undergoing thoracic surgery. Anesth Analg. [Clinical Trial Randomized Controlled Trial Research Support, Non-U.S. Gov't]. (2005). Oct;table of contents., 101(4), 957-65.

[28] Michelet, P, Journo, D, Roch, X. B, Doddoli, A, Marin, C, & Papazian, V. L, et al. Protective ventilation influences systemic inflammation after esophagectomy: a randomized controlled study. Anesthesiology. [Randomized Controlled Trial Research Support, Non-U.S. Gov't]. (2006). Nov;, 105(5), 911-9.

[29] Mols, G, Priebe, H. J, & Guttmann, J. Alveolar recruitment in acute lung injury. Br J Anaesth. [Review]. (2006). Feb;, 96(2), 156-66.

[30] Kilpatrick, B, & Slinger, P. Lung protective strategies in anaesthesia. Br J Anaesth. [Review]. (2010). Dec;105 Suppl 1:i, 108-16.

[31] Curley, G, Laffey, J. G, & Kavanagh, B. P. Bench-to-bedside review: carbon dioxide. Crit Care. [Research Support, Non-U.S. Gov't Review]. (2010).

[32] Tugrul, M, Camci, E, Karadeniz, H, Senturk, M, Pembeci, K, & Akpir, K. Comparison of volume controlled with pressure controlled ventilation during one-lung anaesthesia. Br J Anaesth. [Clinical Trial Comparative Study Randomized Controlled Trial]. (1997). Sep;, 79(3), 306-10.

[33] Sugasawa, Y, Yamaguchi, K, Kumakura, S, Murakami, T, Kugimiya, T, Suzuki, K, et al. The effect of one-lung ventilation upon pulmonary inflammatory responses during lung resection. J Anesth. (2011). Apr;, 25(2), 170-7.

[34] Zingg, U, Forberger, J, Frey, D. M, Esterman, A. J, Oertli, D, Beck-schimmer, B, et al. Inflammatory response in ventilated left and collapsed right lungs, serum and pleural fluid, in transthoracic esophagectomy for cancer. Eur Cytokine Netw. [Research Support, Non-U.S. Gov't]. (2010). Mar;, 21(1), 50-7.

[35] Komatsu, Y, Yamamoto, H, Tsushima, K, Furuya, S, Yoshikawa, S, Yasuo, M, et al. Increased Interleukin-8 in Epithelial Lining Fluid of Collapsed Lungs During One-Lung Ventilation for Thoracotomy. Inflammation. (2012). Jul 21.

[36] De Conno, E, Steurer, M. P, Wittlinger, M, Zalunardo, M. P, Weder, W, Schneiter, D, et al. Anesthetic-induced improvement of the inflammatory response to one-lung ventilation. Anesthesiology. [Randomized Controlled TrialResearch Support, Non-U.S. Gov't]. (2009). Jun;, 110(6), 1316-26.

[37] Schilling, T, Kozian, A, Kretzschmar, M, Huth, C, Welte, T, Buhling, F, et al. Effects of propofol and desflurane anaesthesia on the alveolar inflammatory response to one-lung ventilation. Br J Anaesth. [Randomized Controlled Trial]. (2007). Sep;, 99(3), 368-75.

[38] Sugasawa, Y, Yamaguchi, K, Kumakura, S, Murakami, T, Suzuki, K, Nagaoka, I, et al. Effects of sevoflurane and propofol on pulmonary inflammatory responses during lung resection. J Anesth. [Randomized Controlled Trial]. (2012). Feb;, 26(1), 62-9.

[39] Blumenthal, S, Borgeat, A, Pasch, T, Reyes, L, Booy, C, Lambert, M, et al. Ropivacaine decreases inflammation in experimental endotoxin-induced lung injury. Anesthesiology. [In Vitro Research Support, Non-U.S. Gov't]. (2006). May;, 104(5), 961-9.

[40] Nisanevich, V, Felsenstein, I, Almogy, G, Weissman, C, Einav, S, & Matot, I. Effect of intraoperative fluid management on outcome after intraabdominal surgery. Anesthesiology. [Clinical Trial Comparative Study Randomized Controlled Trial Research Support, Non-U.S. Gov't]. (2005). Jul;, 103(1), 25-32.

[41] Kita, T, Mammoto, T, & Kishi, Y. Fluid management and postoperative respiratory disturbances in patients with transthoracic esophagectomy for carcinoma. J Clin Anesth. (2002). Jun;, 14(4), 252-6.

[42] Marjanovic, G, Villain, C, & Timme, S. zur Hausen A, Hoeppner J, Makowiec F, et al. Colloid vs. crystalloid infusions in gastrointestinal surgery and their different impact on the healing of intestinal anastomoses. Int J Colorectal Dis. (2010). Apr;, 25(4), 491-8.

[43] Zeldin, R. A, Normandin, D, Landtwing, D, & Peters, R. M. Postpneumonectomy pulmonary edema. J Thorac Cardiovasc Surg. [Research Support, Non-U.S. Gov't Research Support, U.S. Gov't, P.H.S.]. (1984). Mar;, 87(3), 359-65.

[44] Patel, R. L, Townsend, E. R, & Fountain, S. W. Elective pneumonectomy: factors associated with morbidity and operative mortality. Ann Thorac Surg. (1992). Jul;, 54(1), 84-8.

[45] Slinger, P. D. Perioperative fluid management for thoracic surgery: the puzzle of postpneumonectomy pulmonary edema. J Cardiothorac Vasc Anesth. [Review]. (1995). Aug;, 9(4), 442-51.

[46] Zarins, C. K, Rice, C. L, Peters, R. M, & Virgilio, R. W. Lymph and pulmonary response to isobaric reduction in plasma oncotic pressure in baboons. Circ Res. [Research Support, U.S. Gov't, P.H.S.]. (1978). Dec;, 43(6), 925-30.

[47] Mayer, J, Boldt, J, Mengistu, A. M, Rohm, K. D, & Suttner, S. Goal-directed intraoperative therapy based on autocalibrated arterial pressure waveform analysis reduces hospital stay in high-risk surgical patients: a randomized, controlled trial. Crit Care. [Randomized Controlled Trial Research Support, Non-U.S. Gov't]. (2010). R18.

[48] Benes, J, Chytra, I, Altmann, P, Hluchy, M, Kasal, E, Svitak, R, et al. Intraoperative fluid optimization using stroke volume variation in high risk surgical patients: results of prospective randomized study. Crit Care. [Randomized Controlled Trial Research Support, Non-U.S. Gov't]. (2010). R118.

[49] Gan, T. J, Soppitt, A, Maroof, M, Moalem, H, Robertson, K. M, Moretti, E, et al. Goal-directed intraoperative fluid administration reduces length of hospital stay after major surgery. Anesthesiology. [Clinical Trial Randomized Controlled Trial Research Support, Non-U.S. Gov't]. (2002). Oct;, 97(4), 820-6.

[50] Bundgaard-nielsen, M, Holte, K, Secher, N. H, & Kehlet, H. Monitoring of peri-operative fluid administration by individualized goal-directed therapy. Acta Anaesthesiol Scand. [Review]. (2007). Mar;, 51(3), 331-40.

[51] Rivers, E, Nguyen, B, Havstad, S, Ressler, J, Muzzin, A, Knoblich, B, et al. Early goal-directed therapy in the treatment of severe sepsis and septic shock. N Engl J Med. [Clinical Trial Randomized Controlled Trial Research Support, Non-U.S. Gov't]. (2001). Nov 8;, 345(19), 1368-77.

[52] Haas, S, Eichhorn, V, Hasbach, T, Trepte, C, Kutup, A, Goetz, A. E, et al. Goal-directed fluid therapy using stroke volume variation does not result in pulmonary fluid overload in thoracic surgery requiring one-lung ventilation. Crit Care Res Pract. (2012).

[53] Daihua, Y, Wei, C, Xude, S, Linong, Y, Changjun, G, & Hui, Z. The effect of body position changes on stroke volume variation in 66 mechanically ventilated patients with sepsis. J Crit Care. (2012). Aug;27(4):416 e, 7-12.

[54] Kobayashi, M, Koh, M, Irinoda, T, Meguro, E, Hayakawa, Y, & Takagane, A. Stroke volume variation as a predictor of intravascular volume depression and possible hypotension during the early postoperative period after esophagectomy. Ann Surg Oncol. [Comparative Study Research Support, Non-U.S. Gov't]. (2009). May;, 16(5), 1371-7.

[55] De Waal, E. E, Rex, S, Kruitwagen, C. L, Kalkman, C. J, & Buhre, W. F. Dynamic preload indicators fail to predict fluid responsiveness in open-chest conditions. Crit Care Med. [Research Support, Non-U.S. Gov't]. (2009). Feb;, 37(2), 510-5.

[56] Denault, A. Y, Gasior, T. A, & Gorcsan, J. rd, Mandarino WA, Deneault LG, Pinsky MR. Determinants of aortic pressure variation during positive-pressure ventilation in man. Chest. [Research Support, U.S. Gov't, Non-P.H.S.]. (1999). Jul;, 116(1), 176-86.

[57] De Blasi, R. A, Palmisani, S, Cigognetti, L, Iasenzaniro, M, Arcioni, R, Mercieri, M, et al. Effects of sternotomy on heart-lung interaction in patients undergoing cardiac surgery receiving pressure-controlled mechanical ventilation. Acta Anaesthesiol Scand. (2007). Apr;, 51(4), 441-6.

[58] Suehiro, K, & Okutani, R. Influence of tidal volume for stroke volume variation to predict fluid responsiveness in patients undergoing one-lung ventilation. J Anesth. (2011). Oct;, 25(5), 777-80.

[59] Morisaki, H, Bloos, F, Keys, J, Martin, C, Neal, A, & Sibbald, W. J. Compared with crystalloid, colloid therapy slows progression of extrapulmonary tissue injury in septic sheep. J Appl Physiol. [Comparative Study Research Support, Non-U.S. Gov't]. (1994). Sep;, 77(3), 1507-18.

[60] Hiltebrand, L. B, Kimberger, O, Arnberger, M, Brandt, S, Kurz, A, & Sigurdsson, G. H. Crystalloids versus colloids for goal-directed fluid therapy in major surgery. Crit Care. [Research Support, Non-U.S. Gov't]. (2009). R40.

[61] Kimberger, O, Arnberger, M, Brandt, S, Plock, J, Sigurdsson, G. H, Kurz, A, et al. Goal-directed colloid administration improves the microcirculation of healthy and perianastomotic colon. Anesthesiology. [Comparative Study Research Support, Non-U.S. Gov't]. (2009). Mar;, 110(3), 496-504.

[62] Hotz, B, Hotz, H. G, Arndt, M, Holmer, C, Buhr, H. J, & Ritz, J. P. Fluid resuscitation with human albumin or hydroxyethyl starch--are there differences in the healing of

experimental intestinal anastomoses? Scand J Gastroenterol. [Comparative Study Research Support, Non-U.S. Gov't]. (2010). , 45(1), 106-14.

[63] Connors, A. F. Jr., Speroff T, Dawson NV, Thomas C, Harrell FE, Jr., Wagner D, et al. The effectiveness of right heart catheterization in the initial care of critically ill patients. SUPPORT Investigators. Jama. [Multicenter Study Research Support, Non-U.S. Gov't]. (1996). Sep 18;, 276(11), 889-97.

[64] Su, N. Y, Huang, C. J, Tsai, P, Hsu, Y. W, Hung, Y. C, & Cheng, C. R. Cardiac output measurement during cardiac surgery: esophageal Doppler versus pulmonary artery catheter. Acta Anaesthesiol Sin. [Clinical Trial Randomized Controlled Trial]. (2002). Sep;, 40(3), 127-33.

[65] Linton, R, Band, D, Brien, O, Jonas, T, & Leach, M. R. Lithium dilution cardiac output measurement: a comparison with thermodilution. Crit Care Med. [Clinical Trial Comparative Study Research Support, Non-U.S. Gov't]. (1997). Nov;, 25(11), 1796-800.

[66] Linton, R. A, Jonas, M. M, Tibby, S. M, Murdoch, I. A, Brien, O, & Linton, T. K. NW, et al. Cardiac output measured by lithium dilution and transpulmonary thermodilution in patients in a paediatric intensive care unit. Intensive Care Med. [Comparative Study Research Support, Non-U.S. Gov't Validation Studies]. (2000). Oct;, 26(10), 1507-11.

[67] Schober, P, Loer, S. A, & Schwarte, L. A. Perioperative hemodynamic monitoring with transesophageal Doppler technology. Anesth Analg. [Review]. (2009). Aug;, 109(2), 340-53.

[68] Lefrant, J. Y, Bruelle, P, Aya, A. G, Saissi, G, Dauzat, M, De La Coussaye, J. E, et al. Training is required to improve the reliability of esophageal Doppler to measure cardiac output in critically ill patients. Intensive Care Med. [Comparative Study]. (1998). Apr;, 24(4), 347-52.

[69] Takala, J, Ruokonen, E, Tenhunen, J. J, Parviainen, I, & Jakob, S. M. Early non-invasive cardiac output monitoring in hemodynamically unstable intensive care patients: a multi-center randomized controlled trial. Crit Care. [Multicenter Study Randomized Controlled Trial Research Support, Non-U.S. Gov't]. (2011). R148.

[70] Hadian, M, Kim, H. K, Severyn, D. A, & Pinsky, M. R. Cross-comparison of cardiac output trending accuracy of LiDCO, PiCCO, FloTrac and pulmonary artery catheters. Crit Care. [Comparative Study Research Support, N.I.H., Extramural]. (2010). R212.

[71] Chaney, J. C, & Derdak, S. Minimally invasive hemodynamic monitoring for the intensivist: current and emerging technology. Crit Care Med. [Review]. (2002). Oct;, 30(10), 2338-45.

[72] Ng, J. M, Chow, M. Y, Ip-yam, P. C, Goh, M. H, & Agasthian, T. Evaluation of partial carbon dioxide rebreathing cardiac output measurement during thoracic surgery. J

Cardiothorac Vasc Anesth. [Comparative Study Evaluation Studies Research Support, Non-U.S. Gov't]. (2007). Oct;, 21(5), 655-8.

[73] Rocco, M, Spadetta, G, & Morelli, A. Dell'Utri D, Porzi P, Conti G, et al. A comparative evaluation of thermodilution and partial CO2 rebreathing techniques for cardiac output assessment in critically ill patients during assisted ventilation. Intensive Care Med. [Comparative Study Research Support, Non-U.S. Gov't Validation Studies]. (2004). Jan;, 30(1), 82-7.

[74] Bernstein, D. Impedance cardiography: Pulsatile blood flow and the biophysical and electrodynamic basis for the stroke volume equations. Journal of electrical bioimpedance. (2010). , 1(1), 2-17.

[75] Spinale, F. G. (1988). Comparison of bioimpedance and thermodilution methods for determining cardiac output: experimental and clinical studies. Updated in 1995. Ann Thorac Surg. [Comparative Study]. 1995 Aug;, 60(2), 483-4.

[76] Wang, D. J, & Gottlieb, S. S. Impedance cardiography: more questions than answers. Curr Heart Fail Rep. [Review]. (2006). Sep;, 3(3), 107-13.

[77] Douglas, P. S, Garcia, M. J, Haines, D. E, Lai, W. W, Manning, W. J, Patel, A. R, et al. ACCF/ASE/AHA/ASNC/HFSA/HRS/SCAI/SCCM/SCCT/SCMR 2011 Appropriate Use Criteria for Echocardiography. A Report of the American College of Cardiology Foundation Appropriate Use Criteria Task Force, American Society of Echocardiography, American Heart Association, American Society of Nuclear Cardiology, Heart Failure Society of America, Heart Rhythm Society, Society for Cardiovascular Angiography and Interventions, Society of Critical Care Medicine, Society of Cardiovascular Computed Tomography, Society for Cardiovascular Magnetic Resonance American College of Chest Physicians. J Am Soc Echocardiogr. [Practice Guideline]. (2011). Mar;, 24(3), 229-67.

[78] Shillcutt, S. K, Markin, N. W, Montzingo, C. R, & Brakke, T. R. Use of rapid "rescue" perioperative echocardiography to improve outcomes after hemodynamic instability in noncardiac surgical patients. J Cardiothorac Vasc Anesth. [Evaluation Studies]. (2012). Jun;, 26(3), 362-70.

[79] Perrino, A. C. Jr., Harris SN, Luther MA. Intraoperative determination of cardiac output using multiplane transesophageal echocardiography: a comparison to thermodilution. Anesthesiology. [Clinical Trial]. (1998). Aug;, 89(2), 350-7.

[80] Brennan, J. M, Blair, J. E, Hampole, C, Goonewardena, S, Vasaiwala, S, Shah, D, et al. Radial artery pulse pressure variation correlates with brachial artery peak velocity variation in ventilated subjects when measured by internal medicine residents using hand-carried ultrasound devices. Chest. [Clinical Trial]. (2007). May;, 131(5), 1301-7.

[81] Downey, R. J, Cheng, D, Kernstine, K, Stanbridge, R, Shennib, H, Wolf, R, et al. Video-Assisted Thoracic Surgery for Lung Cancer Resection: A Consensus Statement of

the International Society of Minimally Invasive Cardiothoracic Surgery (ISMICS) 2007. Innovations (Phila). (2007). Nov;, 2(6), 293-302.

[82] Brodsky, J. B, & Cohen, E. Video-assisted thoracoscopic surgery. Curr Opin Anaesthesiol. (2000). Feb;, 13(1), 41-5.

[83] Hammer, G. B, Fitzmaurice, B. G, & Brodsky, J. B. Methods for single-lung ventilation in pediatric patients. Anesth Analg. [Review]. (1999). Dec;, 89(6), 1426-9.

[84] Massard, G, Rouge, C, Dabbagh, A, Kessler, R, Hentz, J. G, Roeslin, N, et al. Tracheobronchial lacerations after intubation and tracheostomy. Ann Thorac Surg. (1996). May;, 61(5), 1483-7.

[85] Slinger, P. Lung isolation in thoracic anesthesia, state of the art. Can J Anesth. (2001). RR5., 13.

[86] Pinsonneault, C, Fortier, J, & Donati, F. Tracheal resection and reconstruction. Can J Anaesth. [Review]. (1999). May;46(5 Pt 1):439-55.

[87] Adelsmayr, E, Keller, C, Erd, G, & Brimacombe, J. The laryngeal mask and high-frequency jet ventilation for resection of high tracheal stenosis. Anesth Analg. [Case Reports]. (1998). Apr;, 86(4), 907-8.

[88] Barash, P. G, Cullen, B. F, & Stoelting, R. K. Clinical anesthesia. Philadelphia: Lippincott; (1989).

[89] Zhou, Y. F, Zhu, S. J, Zhu, S. M, & An, X. X. Anesthetic management of emergent critical tracheal stenosis. J Zhejiang Univ Sci B. [Case Reports]. (2007). Jul;, 8(7), 522-5.

[90] Macchiarini, P, Rovira, I, & Ferrarello, S. Awake upper airway surgery. Ann Thorac Surg. (2010). Feb;discussion 90-1., 89(2), 387-90.

[91] Brodsky, J. B, & Lemmens, H. J. Left double-lumen tubes: clinical experience with 1,170 patients. J Cardiothorac Vasc Anesth. [Review]. (2003). Jun;, 17(3), 289-98.

[92] Slinger, P. D, & Lesiuk, L. Flow resistances of disposable double-lumen, single-lumen, and Univent tubes. J Cardiothorac Vasc Anesth. [Comparative Study]. (1998). Apr;, 12(2), 142-4.

[93] Hannallah, M. S, Miller, S. C, Kurzer, S. I, & Tefft, M. C. The effective diameter and airflow resistance of the individual lumens of left polyvinyl chloride double-lumen endobronchial tubes. Anesth Analg. (1996). Apr;, 82(4), 867-9.

[94] Rusch, V. W, Freund, P. R, & Bowdle, T. A. Exchanging double-lumen for single-lumen endotracheal tubes after thoracotomy. Ann Thorac Surg. (1991). Feb;, 51(2), 323-4.

[95] Ross, A. F, & Ferguson, J. S. Advances in interventional pulmonology. Curr Opin Anaesthesiol. [Review]. (2009). Feb;, 22(1), 11-7.

[96] Purugganan, R. V. Intravenous anesthesia for thoracic procedures. Curr Opin Anaesthesiol. [Review]. (2008). Feb;, 21(1), 1-7.

[97] Kapila, A, Glass, P. S, Jacobs, J. R, Muir, K. T, Hermann, D. J, Shiraishi, M, et al. Measured context-sensitive half-times of remifentanil and alfentanil. Anesthesiology. [Clinical Trial Comparative Study Randomized Controlled TrialResearch Support, Non-U.S. Gov't]. (1995). Nov;, 83(5), 968-75.

[98] Altermatt, F. R, Bugedo, D. A, Delfino, A. E, Solari, S, Guerra, I, Munoz, H. R, et al. Evaluation of the effect of intravenous lidocaine on propofol requirements during total intravenous anaesthesia as measured by bispectral index. Br J Anaesth. [Randomized Controlled Trial Research Support, Non-U.S. Gov't]. (2012). Jun;, 108(6), 979-83.

[99] Higgins, T. L. Postthoractomy Complications. In: Kaplan JA, Slinger P, editors. Thoracic Anesthesia. Third ed. Philadelphia: Elsevier; (2003).

[100] MacIntyre NRCook DJ, Ely EW, Jr., Epstein SK, Fink JB, Heffner JE, et al. Evidence-based guidelines for weaning and discontinuing ventilatory support: a collective task force facilitated by the American College of Chest Physicians; the American Association for Respiratory Care; and the American College of Critical Care Medicine. Chest. [Consensus Development Conference Guideline Practice Guideline Review]. (2001). Dec;120(6 Suppl):375S-95S.

[101] Meade, M, Guyatt, G, Cook, D, Griffith, L, Sinuff, T, Kergl, C, et al. Predicting success in weaning from mechanical ventilation. Chest. [Meta-Analysis Research Support, U.S. Gov't, P.H.S.]. (2001). Dec;120(6 Suppl):400S-24S.

[102] Epstein, S. K, & Ciubotaru, R. L. Independent effects of etiology of failure and time to reintubation on outcome for patients failing extubation. Am J Respir Crit Care Med. (1998). Aug;, 158(2), 489-93.

[103] Viitanen, A, Salmenpera, M, & Heinonen, J. Right ventricular response to hypercarbia after cardiac surgery. Anesthesiology. [Research Support, Non-U.S. Gov't]. (1990). Sep;, 73(3), 393-400.

[104] Hofmann, H. S, Rettig, G, Radke, J, Neef, H, & Silber, R. E. Iatrogenic ruptures of the tracheobronchial tree. Eur J Cardiothorac Surg. [Evaluation Studies]. (2002). Apr;, 21(4), 649-52.

[105] Deslauriers, J, & Gregoire, J. Techniques of pneumonectomy. Drainage after pneumonectomy. Chest Surg Clin N Am. [Historical Article Review]. (1999). May;xii., 9(2), 437-48.

[106] Venuta, F, Boehler, A, Rendina, E. A, De Giacomo, T, Speich, R, Schmid, R, et al. Complications in the native lung after single lung transplantation. Eur J Cardiothorac Surg. (1999). Jul;, 16(1), 54-8.

[107] Zellos, L, Jaklitsch, M. T, Al-mourgi, M. A, & Sugarbaker, D. J. Complications of extrapleural pneumonectomy. Semin Thorac Cardiovasc Surg. (2007). Winter;, 19(4), 355-9.

[108] Chambers, N, Walton, S, & Pearce, A. Cardiac herniation following pneumonectomy--an old complication revisited. Anaesth Intensive Care. [Case Reports Review]. (2005). Jun;, 33(3), 403-9.

[109] Gotoda, Y, Kambara, N, Sakai, T, Kishi, Y, Kodama, K, & Koyama, T. The morbidity, time course and predictive factors for persistent post-thoracotomy pain. Eur J Pain. (2001). , 5(1), 89-96.

[110] Kehlet, H, Jensen, T. S, & Woolf, C. J. Persistent postsurgical pain: risk factors and prevention. Lancet. [Research Support, N.I.H., Extramural Research Support, Non-U.S. Gov't Review]. (2006). May 13;, 367(9522), 1618-25.

[111] Merskey, H, & Bogduk, N. Classification of chronic pain : descriptions of chronic pain syndromes and definitions of pain terms. 2nd ed. ed. Seattle: IASP Press; (1994).

[112] Katz, J, Jackson, M, Kavanagh, B. P, & Sandler, A. N. Acute pain after thoracic surgery predicts long-term post-thoracotomy pain. Clin J Pain. [Clinical Trial Randomized Controlled Trial Research Support, Non-U.S. Gov't]. (1996). Mar;, 12(1), 50-5.

[113] Wildgaard, K, Ravn, J, & Kehlet, H. Chronic post-thoracotomy pain: a critical review of pathogenic mechanisms and strategies for prevention. Eur J Cardiothorac Surg. [Research Support, Non-U.S. Gov't Review]. (2009). Jul;, 36(1), 170-80.

[114] Wildgaard, K, & Kehlet, H. Chronic post-thoracotomy pain,ÄîWhat is new in pathogenic mechanisms and strategies for prevention? Techniques in Regional Anesthesia & Pain Management. (2011). , 15(3), 83-9.

[115] Landreneau, R. J, Mack, M. J, Hazelrigg, S. R, Naunheim, K, Dowling, R. D, Ritter, P, et al. Prevalence of chronic pain after pulmonary resection by thoracotomy or video-assisted thoracic surgery. J Thorac Cardiovasc Surg. [Comparative Study]. (1994). Apr;discussion 85-6., 107(4), 1079-85.

[116] Liu, S. S, Richman, J. M, Thirlby, R. C, & Wu, C. L. Efficacy of continuous wound catheters delivering local anesthetic for postoperative analgesia: a quantitative and qualitative systematic review of randomized controlled trials. J Am Coll Surg. [Meta-Analysis Review]. (2006). Dec;, 203(6), 914-32.

[117] Roytblat, L, Korotkoruchko, A, Katz, J, Glazer, M, Greemberg, L, & Fisher, A. Postoperative pain: the effect of low-dose ketamine in addition to general anesthesia. Anesth Analg. [Clinical Trial Randomized Controlled Trial Research Support, Non-U.S. Gov't]. (1993). Dec;, 77(6), 1161-5.

[118] Camu, F, & Vanlersberghe, C. Pharmacology of systemic analgesics. Best Pract Res Clin Anaesthesiol. [Review]. (2002). Dec;, 16(4), 475-88.

[119] Kaneko, M, Saito, Y, Kirihara, Y, Collins, J. G, & Kosaka, Y. Synergistic antinociceptive interaction after epidural coadministration of morphine and lidocaine in rats. Anesthesiology. (1994). Jan;, 80(1), 137-50.

[120] Scott, D. A, Blake, D, Buckland, M, Etches, R, Halliwell, R, Marsland, C, et al. A comparison of epidural ropivacaine infusion alone and in combination with 1, 2, and 4 microg/mL fentanyl for seventy-two hours of postoperative analgesia after major abdominal surgery. Anesth Analg. [Clinical Trial Comparative Study Randomized Controlled Trial Research Support, Non-U.S. Gov't]. (1999). Apr;, 88(4), 857-64.

[121] Morgan, G. E, Mikhail, M. S, & Murray, M. J. Clinical anesthesiology. 4th ed. ed. New York: Lange Medical Books/McGraw Hill ; London : McGraw-Hill [distributor]; (2006).

[122] Joshi, G. P, Bonnet, F, Shah, R, Wilkinson, R. C, Camu, F, Fischer, B, et al. A systematic review of randomized trials evaluating regional techniques for postthoracotomy analgesia. Anesth Analg. [Research Support, Non-U.S. Gov't Review]. (2008). Sep;, 107(3), 1026-40.

[123] Wheatley, R. G, Schug, S. A, & Watson, D. Safety and efficacy of postoperative epidural analgesia. Br J Anaesth. [Review]. (2001). Jul;, 87(1), 47-61.

[124] Norman, P. H, & Kowalski, M. D. A. Postoperative analgesia for thoracotomy patients: A current review. In: Franco KL, Putnam JB, editors. Advanced therapy in thoracic surgery. 2nd ed. ed. Hamilton, Ont.; London: B.C. Decker; (2005). , 1-31.

[125] Eason, M. J, & Wyatt, R. Paravertebral thoracic block-a reappraisal. Anaesthesia. [Case Reports]. (1979). Jul-Aug;, 34(7), 638-42.

[126] Karmakar, M. K. Thoracic paravertebral block. Anesthesiology. [Review]. (2001). Sep;, 95(3), 771-80.

[127] Cheema, S. P, Ilsley, D, Richardson, J, & Sabanathan, S. A thermographic study of paravertebral analgesia. Anaesthesia. [Research Support, Non-U.S. Gov't]. (1995). Feb;, 50(2), 118-21.

[128] Naja, Z, & Lonnqvist, P. A. Somatic paravertebral nerve blockade. Incidence of failed block and complications. Anaesthesia. [Clinical Trial]. (2001). Dec;, 56(12), 1184-8.

[129] Richardson, J, & Sabanathan, S. Thoracic paravertebral analgesia. Acta Anaesthesiol Scand. [Review]. (1995). Nov;, 39(8), 1005-15.

[130] Davies, R. G, Myles, P. S, & Graham, J. M. A comparison of the analgesic efficacy and side-effects of paravertebral vs epidural blockade for thoracotomy--a systematic review and meta-analysis of randomized trials. Br J Anaesth. [Comparative Study Meta-AnalysisResearch Support, Non-U.S. Gov't Review]. (2006). Apr;, 96(4), 418-26.

[131] Detterbeck, F. C. Efficacy of methods of intercostal nerve blockade for pain relief after thoracotomy. Ann Thorac Surg. [Research Support, Non-U.S. Gov't Review]. (2005). Oct;, 80(4), 1550-9.

[132] Wurnig, P. N, Lackner, H, Teiner, C, Hollaus, P. H, Pospisil, M, Fohsl-grande, B, et al. Is intercostal block for pain management in thoracic surgery more successful than epidural anaesthesia? Eur J Cardiothorac Surg. [Clinical Trial Comparative Study-Randomized Controlled Trial]. (2002). Jun;, 21(6), 1115-9.

[133] Meierhenrich, R, Hock, D, Kuhn, S, Baltes, E, Muehling, B, Muche, R, et al. Analgesia and pulmonary function after lung surgery: is a single intercostal nerve block plus patient-controlled intravenous morphine as effective as patient-controlled epidural anaesthesia? A randomized non-inferiority clinical trial. Br J Anaesth. [Comparative Study Randomized Controlled Trial]. (2011). Apr;, 106(4), 580-9.

[134] Dahl, J. B, Moiniche, S, & Kehlet, H. Wound infiltration with local anaesthetics for postoperative pain relief. Acta Anaesthesiol Scand. [Research Support, Non-U.S. Gov't Review]. (1994). Jan;, 38(1), 7-14.

[135] Kehlet, H, & Dahl, J. B. Anaesthesia, surgery, and challenges in postoperative recovery. Lancet. [Review]. (2003). Dec 6;, 362(9399), 1921-8.

[136] Wheatley, G. H. rd, Rosenbaum DH, Paul MC, Dine AP, Wait MA, Meyer DM, et al. Improved pain management outcomes with continuous infusion of a local anesthetic after thoracotomy. J Thorac Cardiovasc Surg. [Comparative Study Research Support, N.I.H., Extramural Research Support, Non-U.S. Gov't Research Support, U.S. Gov't, P.H.S.]. (2005). Aug;, 130(2), 464-8.

[137] Baig, M. K, Zmora, O, Derdemezi, J, Weiss, E. G, Nogueras, J. J, & Wexner, S. D. Use of the ON-Q pain management system is associated with decreased postoperative analgesic requirement: double blind randomized placebo pilot study. J Am Coll Surg. [Randomized Controlled Trial Research Support, Non-U.S. Gov't]. (2006). Feb;, 202(2), 297-305.

[138] Horlocker, T. T, Wedel, D. J, Rowlingson, J. C, Enneking, F. K, Kopp, S. L, Benzon, H. T, et al. Regional anesthesia in the patient receiving antithrombotic or thrombolytic therapy: American Society of Regional Anesthesia and Pain Medicine Evidence-Based Guidelines (Third Edition). Reg Anesth Pain Med. [Practice Guideline]. (2010). Jan-Feb;, 35(1), 64-101.

Chapter 2

Evolution of Surgical Approaches for Lung Resection

Trevor Williams and Wickii T. Vigneswaran

Additional information is available at the end of the chapter

http://dx.doi.org/10.5772/56641

1. Introduction

Early surgical interventions were highly morbid, painful and deadly. Understanding of antisepsis, after Lister's first report in 1867 and development of anesthetic techniques, in particular chloroform and ether made way for early successful surgical intervention. Thoracic surgery and lung resection, however, proved more difficult to advance than other surgical specialties due to the problem of pneumothorax. The principles of intra-thoracic and intra-pleural surgery developed during the early 20th century with significant progress in a short time.

Lung surgery prior to the late 1800's was largely rare reports of draining deep abscesses, resecting prolapsing gangrenous tissue after trauma and resecting portions of the chest wall with small segments of accompanying lung. Tuffier performed the first partial lung resection that consisted of placing a ligature on the lung, excising and suturing the lung to the periosteum.[1], [2] Initial works demonstrating the feasibility of lung resection came from extensive animal experimentation. Block of Danzig described many lung resections in rabbits and dogs. The animals survived surgery and returned to health. The problem of pneumothorax however plagued the operative and the post-operative period. Positive pressure ventilation was not immediately seen as a solution to advance intra-thoracic surgery and those who did use it were divided between the use of face-masks, intra-pharyngeal and endotracheal insufflation. Sauerbruch, in Germany, with the support of the internationally acclaimed Von Mikulicz, persisted for many years operating in expensive negative pressure chambers. He pioneered the first tank ventilator in 1907, allowing surgeons to operate on an open thorax with the patient's head and anesthesiologist literally in another room. Surgery in the US, less hindered by the negative pressure camp, was quicker to adopt endotracheal intubation, the use of bellows and ultimately endobronchial lung isolation ventilation. Negative pressure was used extensively however and persisted through the polio epidemic until the late 1930's.[2], [3]

Lung surgery developed and progressed because of chronic infections of the lung and pleura particularly tuberculosis and bronchiectasis. Lilienthal described the plight of his patients in 1922[4]:

Occasionally an individual coughs his way through life - never a long one - and manages to exist as a semi-invalid, with copious foul expectoration no medicine can control, being a handicap difficult to bear. Patients have even threatened suicide if refused the chance for cure by operation, though they knew the danger was great.

The stethoscope existed from the early 1800's making some diagnosis possible. Higher level of precision and certainty regarding surgical intervention became possible with the advent X-Ray by Röentgen's in 1895. This was quickly taken up by the medical field and the first chest X-ray was performed in 1896.

Gluck from Germany is credited with the first lobectomy in 1907. Morriston Davies reported a landmark lobectomy in 1912 describing individual vessel and bronchial ligation much like we do today but his technique was not followed for some twenty years. It was believed at that time that bronchial stump healing was dependent on the amount of peribronchial tissue remaining after resection and mass ligation was the preferred method.[1] The lung resection was performed in stages as illustrated. The first operation consisted of rib resection without entering the pleura, as done by Robinson at the Massachusetts General Hospital in 1917. Abrading the pleura during the first operation was common to help adhesions form and prevent a pneumothorax during the second operation. A week later the pleura is entered and the lobe resected if the patient tolerated. The bronchus and vasculature were clamped en-mass, transfixed with a suture or left with a clamp in place to be removed a week later. Peri-operative mortality was about 50%. Getting out of the operating room was often an urgency given cyanosis from large amounts of purulent sputum. The diseased lung could be left in place and allowed to slough. The diseased bronchial stump would likely open regardless. Infection was expected post-operatively, packs were left in the chest and wounds granulated in over months.

Samuel Robinson's presidential address to the American Association of Thoracic surgery in 1923 was very telling:

The danger of pneumothorax in wide operation on the human thorax has been dispelled...since the development of the differential pressure apparatus...(regarding bronchiectasis) The patient is placed on the operating table...There may be cyanosis...evacuation of large amounts of pungent, purulent sputum...the pleura is no sooner opened... the need for general anesthesia is obvious...The lower lobe obstinately resists being delivered, the pleural adhesions are strong and widespread... ropelike and tenacious... work with a knife and scissors is blind... the patient's condition may become distressing...then the difficulties multiply. The complete liberating at one setting may have to be abandoned. Tight closure of the chest without drainage seems inadvisable under such conditions, and yet necessary to avoid the ills of post-operative pneumothorax. Suddenly it seems time to return the patient to his bed. Not much has been accomplished... The intra-thoracic pressure has been so altered; the lung expansion is further minimized. Then come the dangers of pleural infection, later in convalescence. There is more operating to do... Nevertheless, we have obtained cures.[1]

Brunn published a landmark paper in 1929 on one stage lobectomy. He described the concept of early lung expansion using closed suction drainage. Local anesthesia was used, phrenicotomy, cautery for lung and air testing. He emphasized an airtight closure to allow lung expansion but used a clamp on the pedicle, which caused necrosis and ultimately a bronchopleural fistula with empyema. The argument at the time was that the expanded lung restricted the space into which the empyema would fill allowing it and the subsequent fistula to more easily be controlled and permit an easier recovery.[3],[5]

Nissen performed his first pneumonectomy in 1931 using a staged technique. In 1932 Shenstone & Janes published an article delineating their experience with 14 operations, five fistula and three deaths. They emphasized not crushing the hilum to preserve the bronchial blood supply, catgut (not silk which could harbor infection) to close the bronchus and suturing the stump to the undersurface of the remaining lobe. The phrenic nerve was crushed and an underwater drain used. Tourniquets and snares were subsequently developed and became common operating equipment.[1], [2], [6] Evarts Graham performed the first single stage pneumonectomy for lung cancer in 1933. He used cautery liberally during his operations reporting somewhat lower mortality in the 20% range.

By the end of the 1930's dissection technique was established. Kent and Blades and Belsey and Churchill delineated the anatomy for lobar and segmental resection. A landmark article in 1940 by Kent and Blades is said to have set the stage for the future of thoracic surgery and the segment, rather than the lobe, was proposed to be the new unit of the lung.[3], [7] Overholt described the intersegmental vein for a plane of dissection and he emphasized the utility of suction over simply underwater drainage.[3] Tumors involving or approaching major airways precluded lesser resections. The lower lobe would be sacrificed for large upper lobe tumors or bronchial tumors. Price-Thomas performed the first sleeve lobectomy in 1947. Since that time all matter of bronchial and arterial reconstructions evolved to preserve lung tissue.[8] Regarding completeness of cancer treatment, now we know sleeve lobectomy has 5-year survival rates better than pneumonectomy with improved quality adjusted life years as determined by decision analysis.[9]

The use of the surgical stapler became common in the 1950's and 60's. Initially, a Russian stapler with a single row of staples oriented parallel to the bronchus was replaced with two rows of staggered staples oriented perpendicularly to the bronchus. Though not eliminating bronchial fistula, stapling was found to be superior to suture techniques in closure of bronchus. It also permitted less sacrifice of lung parenchyma and decreased blood loss.[10]

2. Current practice

The classic postero-lateral thoracotomy, as practiced until recently, provides excellent access to the thoracic cavity but involves transecting the latissimus and serratus muscles and subperiosteal rib resection. With increasing application of thoracic surgery, younger more active patients and improved peri-operative pain control, reduced morbidity became increasingly important.[11] With improved survival, improving quality of life and early return to full activity became very important. Post-thoracotomy syndrome, defined as post-operative pain lasting greater than two months, occurred in 50% of thoracotomies. Interventions to reduce this in the immediate post-operative period include modifications in surgical technique and, among others, the use of epidural catheters, which has shown improvement in long-term pain relief. Early post-operative pain control helps clear secretions, maintain lung function and reduce complication.[12]

A myriad of thoracic incisions developed, the widely used posterolateral thoracotomy has been modified to decrease the length, reduce the amount of muscle disrupted and protect the intercostal nerves all with varying amounts of patient benefit in terms of improved pain control, lung function and shoulder strength.[13], [14] Alternative incisions include the sternotomy, the clamshell incision, axillary and anterior thoracotomies. Median sternotomy allows access to the majority of both thoracic cavities. Proposed by Cooper, they discovered during cadaver dissection that after division of the pulmonary ligament the vast majority of the lung can be resected. This was ideal for the increasing numbers of patients found to have resectable pulmonary metastasis bilaterally. Only the left lower lobe was felt to be a less ideal operative field because of the need for retracting the heart. Post-sternotomy patients recovered peak airflow and vital capacity significantly sooner when compared to posterolateral thoracotomy patients.[15]

The clamshell incision was championed by Bains. Bilateral submammary anterior thoracotomies and a transverse sternotomy performed in the supine position are referred to as the clamshell incision. This is useful for bilateral pulmonary disease, extensive lung tumors involving the mediastinum and large mediastinal tumors. Sternotomy is felt to be more limiting for centrally and posteriorly located tumors that are accessible by clamshell. The hemiclamshell involves a unilateral anterior thoracotomy with sternal extension. The inner half of the clavicle can be removed with extension of the incision laterally for a trapdoor incision.[16]

Distortion of normal anatomy and division of muscles was thought to be an important contributor to post-operative morbidity and therefor muscle sparing techniques were developed. Bethencourt & Holmes developed the muscle sparing posterolateral thoracotomy. The incision begins 2cm anterior to the latissimus and ends 2 cm posterior and inferior to the tip of the scapula. The latissimus is dissected from the subcutaneous tissues and the serratus. The posterior boarder of the serratus is divided from its fascia and underlying tissues. The serratus is retracted forward, the latissimus posteriorly and the fourth to the seventh interspace may be chosen for entry into the chest cavity (Figure 1). Excessive subcutaneous flap elevation leads to seromas which caused these authors to place drains routinely. It is anecdotally reported that patients had less pain, improved arm motion and earlier ambulation.[17] Ginsberg preferred a vertical incision, or vertical axillary throacotomy, which requires no creation of subcutaneous flaps and is made in the midaxillary line. The latissimus and serratus are similarly elevated and retracted. The exposure takes the shape of a square rather than a parallelogram, which can cause some difficulty inserting staplers or suturing. Patients are said to be pain free and the cosmetic outcome superior.[18]

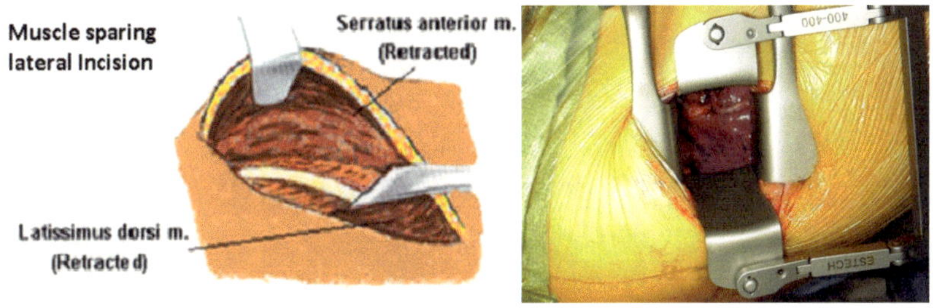

Figure 1. Muscle sparing lateral thoracotomy. The cartoon illustrates the preservation and retraction of the serratus anterior muscle and lattissimus dorsi muscle, exposing the intercostal space. The incision provides excellent exposure to hilar structures and allows complex lung resections.

Physiologic studies demonstrate improvements in maximal inspiratory/expiratory pressure at three months, lesser degrees of intercostal nerve impairment and improved shoulder function with muscle sparing techniques.[14], [19], [20] Prospective studies comparing muscle sparing and muscle splitting thoracotomies did not find differences in immediate or longer term post-operative pain or physical function.[19], [21] Notably adequate epidural anesthesia was provided in these trials. It is postulated that the intercostal nerves are the primary source of pain related to thoracotomy and efforts to spare these nerves the intercostal sutures has been rigorously studied. This is done by dissection of the intercostal neurovascular bundle or the entire muscle off of the undersurface of the superior rib to be closed and or drilling/suturing through the ribs, to avoid any nerve compression/trauma. With these steps pain scores and analgesic requirements were reported to be significantly less compared to conventional methods.[13], [14]

Building on the concept improving patient outcomes, surgery in general has moved towards less invasive with the help of video technology. Video assisted thoracoscopic surgery (VATS) is the thoracic variant. Much smaller incisions through which a camera and longer instruments enter allow surgeons to perform lung resections of the same quality as open techniques. Thoracoscopy has its roots in the early 20th century when Jacobaeus in Stockholm used a modified cystoscope for a tuberculosis effusion. He used a two port technique to perform adhesiolysis - primarily to allow collapse therapy for tuberculosis treatment.[3] With high resolution video equipment for endoscopic viewing in combination with single lung ventilation and endoscopic stapling VATS exploded in the 1990s. Two to four 5-10 mm incisions are placed in a 180 degree arc with the surgical site of interest at the apex of a baseball diamond, triangulated. One of these ports is enlarged to extract a specimen. The larger "utlility port" is usually placed anterior to the latissimus high on the chest wall (Figure 2). Currently close to 40% of lung resections are performed in the US using VATS technique[22], [23] A recent analysis of the Society of Thoracic Surgery database from 2000-2010 found that 35% (4531/12970) of all lobectomies registered are performed by VATS techniques. This has increased from 20% in a previous analysis in 2006.[24], [25] Additionally, they found that respiratory complication increased significantly after thoracotomy compared to VATS in patients with decreased pulmonary function (FEV1 < 60%). A randomized trial found VATS techniques have less complications overall (18% vs. 50%)[26]. Less narcotic requirements are universal and there were lower incidences of pneumonia and atrial fibrillation, improved shoulder range of motion and pulmonary function, less hospital stay and need for nursing home transfers.[22]

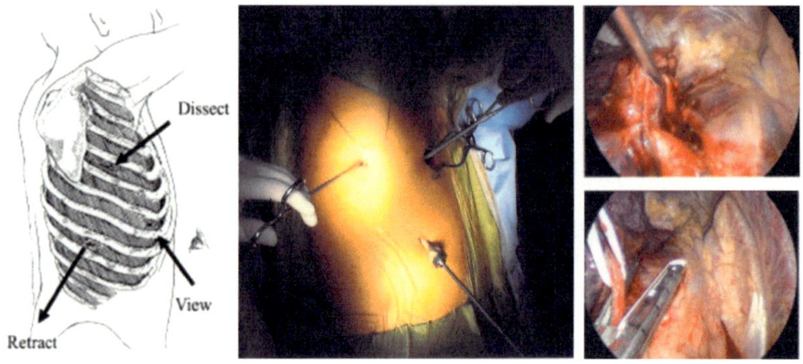

Figure 2. Video assisted thracoscopic surgical (VATS) approach for lung resection. The anterior utility incision provides access to majority of the dissection. Endoscopic stapling device make this surgical approach for lung resection safe and feasible.

The late 1990's saw the development of robotic surgical systems with Intuitive's da Vinci system. The technique utilizes instruments that hinge on a chest wall fulcrum and operate within a cone. The da Vinci system uses multiarticulated instruments that provide seven degrees of rotational freedom, akin to a surgeon's wrist and can be placed exactly where dissection is needed with three-dimensional optics. The skin incisions and trocars are not appreciably different from VATS but the mobility at the end of the instrument is. Da Vinci can be used to retract, grasp, cut, ligate and suture. There is however absence of haptic feedback and therefore tension of tissues is determined solely from visual input (Figure 3).

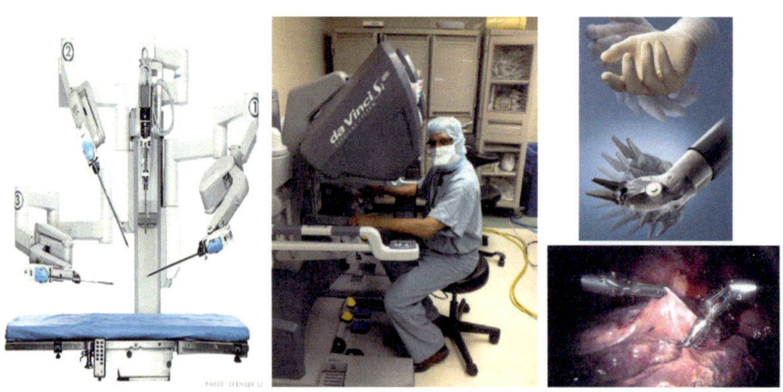

Figure 3. Robotic approach to lung resection is the latest evolution in lung resection. The surgeon operates from a remote location using the console to control the robot that is 'docked' to the patient. The instrument articulations are such, it is more versatile than the human hand, allowing detail dissection in small spaces, however lacks the tactile sensation.

Many centers are pushing the envelope to investigate the merits of robotic lobectomy and finding good outcomes.[27] True investigation determining the benefits of robotic surgery over VATS are lacking. It is questioned whether we should be spending our efforts promoting robotic surgery when VATS, with it's clear benefits, is not widely adopted.[28] Cost analysis finds robotic lobectomy is cheaper than open thoracotomy principally because of length of hospital stay.

Surgery for lung resection evolved through the twentieth century from a highly morbid procedure with upwards of 50% mortality to a streamlined <2% mortality and 2-3 day admission procedure.[29] Refinements in anesthesia, anatomic dissection and minimal access techniques continue to benefit patients. The current trend in high technology application remains to be proven for lung resection but the surgery for lung is continuing to evolve.

Author details

Trevor Williams and Wickii T. Vigneswaran*

*Address all correspondence to: wvignesw@surgery.bsd.uchicago.edu

Department of Surgery, University Of Chicago Medicine, Chicago, IL, USA

References

[1] Meade R. A History of Thoracic Surgery. Springfield, IL: Charles Thomas, 1961.

[2] Mountain K, Pomerantz. Thoracic Surgery Clinics: History of Thoracic Surgery, Feb 2000.

[3] Hurt R. The History of Cardiothoracic Surgery: From Early Times: Parthenon Publishing Group, 1996.

[4] Lilienthal H. Resection of the lung for suppurative cases with a report based on 31 operative cases in which resection was done or intended. *Ann Surg* 1922; 75(3): 257-320.

[5] HB B. Surgical principles underlying one-stage lobectomy. *Arch Surg* 1929; 18:490-6.

[6] Shenstone NS, Janes RM. Experiences in pulmonary lobectomy. *Can Med Assoc J* 1932; 27(2):138-45.

[7] Faber LP. Individual ligation technique for lower lobe lobectomy. *Ann Thorac Surg* 1990; 49(6):1016-8.

[8] Thomas CP. The present position relating to cancer of the lung. Lobectomy with sleeve resection. *Thorax* 1960; 15:9-11.

[9] Ferguson MK, Lehman AG. Sleeve lobectomy or pneumonectomy: optimal management strategy using decision analysis techniques. *Ann Thorac Surg* 2003; 76(6):1782-8.

[10] Betts RH, Takaro T. Use of a lung stapler in pulmonary resection. *Ann Thorac Surg* 1965; 24:197-202.

[11] Kittle CF. Which way in?--The thoracotomy incision. *Ann Thorac Surg* 1988; 45(3):234.

[12] Soto RG, Fu ES. Acute pain management for patients undergoing thoracotomy. *Ann Thorac Surg* 2003; 75(4):1349-57.

[13] Cerfolio RJ, Bryant AS, Maniscalco LM. A nondivided intercostal muscle flap further reduces pain of thoracotomy: a prospective randomized trial. *Ann Thorac Surg* 2008; 85(6):1901-6; discussion 1906-7.

[14] Ziyade S, Baskent A, Tanju S, et al. Isokinetic muscle strength after thoracotomy: standard vs. muscle-sparing posterolateral thoracotomy. *Thorac Cardiovasc Surg* 2010; 58(5):295-8.

[15] Cooper JD, Nelems JM, Pearson FG. Extended indications for median sternotomy in patients requiring pulmonary resection. *Ann Thorac Surg* 1978; 26(5):413-20.

[16] Bains MS, Ginsberg RJ, Jones WG, et al. The clamshell incision: an improved approach to bilateral pulmonary and mediastinal tumor. *Ann Thorac Surg* 1994; 58(1): 30-2; discussion 33.

[17] Bethencourt DM, Holmes EC. Muscle-sparing posterolateral thoracotomy. *Ann Thorac Surg* 1988; 45(3):337-9.

[18] Ginsberg RJ. Alternative (muscle-sparing) incisions in thoracic surgery. *Ann Thorac Surg* 1993; 56(3):752-4.

[19] Nosotti M, Baisi A, Mendogni P, et al. Muscle sparing versus posterolateral thoracotomy for pulmonary lobectomy: randomised controlled trial. *Interact Cardiovasc Thorac Surg* 2010; 11(4):415-9.

[20] Benedetti F, Vighetti S, Ricco C, et al. Neurophysiologic assessment of nerve impairment in posterolateral and muscle-sparing thoracotomy. *J Thorac Cardiovasc Surg* 1998; 115(4):841-7.

[21] Athanassiadi K, Kakaris S, Theakos N, et al. Muscle-sparing versus posterolateral thoracotomy: a prospective study. *Eur J Cardiothorac Surg* 2007; 31(3):496-9; discussion 499-500.

[22] de Hoyos A, Kerstein Kea, Mahtabifard A. General Thoracic Surgery. Shields, T ed. Ch 33-35. 7th ed. Philidelphia, PA: Lippincott, 2009.

[23] Brunelli A, Xiume F, Refai M, et al. Bilateral staged uniportal VATS for synchronous lung cancers. *Interact Cardiovasc Thorac Surg* 2006; 5(5):658-9.

[24] Ceppa DP, Kosinski AS, Berry MF, et al. Thoracoscopic lobectomy has increasing benefit in patients with poor pulmonary function: a society of thoracic surgeons database analysis. *Ann Surg* 2012; 256(3):487-93.

[25] Boffa DJ, Allen MS, Grab JD, et al. Data from The Society of Thoracic Surgeons General Thoracic Surgery database: the surgical management of primary lung tumors. *J Thorac Cardiovasc Surg* 2008; 135(2):247-54.

[26] Hoksch B, Ablassmaier B, Walter M, et al. [Complication rate after thoracoscopic and conventional lobectomy]. *Zentralbl Chir* 2003; 128(2):106-10.

[27] Park BJ, Melfi F, Mussi A, et al. Robotic lobectomy for non-small cell lung cancer (NSCLC): long-term oncologic results. *J Thorac Cardiovasc Surg* 2012; 143(2):383-9.

[28] Swanson SJ. Robotic pulmonary lobectomy--the future and probably should remain so. *J Thorac Cardiovasc Surg* 2010; 140(5):954.

[29] Tovar EA, Roethe RA, Weissig MD, et al. One-day admission for lung lobectomy: an incidental result of a clinical pathway. *Ann Thorac Surg* 1998; 65(3):803-6.

Chapter 3

Postoperative Care and Complications After Thoracic Surgery

Anand Iyer and Sumit Yadav

Additional information is available at the end of the chapter

http://dx.doi.org/10.5772/55351

1. Introduction

Postoperative care of thoracic surgical patients is a very important part of patient recovery and can be very challenging. Pulmonary complications are responsible for significant numbers of deaths and morbidity of patients undergoing thoracotomy. Thoracic surgery impairs postoperative respiratory function resulting in a relatively high risk of developing postoperative pulmonary complications. The incidence (19-59%) is much higher than following upper (16-17%) or lower abdominal surgery (0-5%). The overall incidence of complications following thoracic surgery varies from 15% to 37.5%, primarily due to the type of pulmonary complications studied, the clinical criteria used in the definition and the type of surgery included. The clinical and potential economic impact of these complications is marked, with significantly longer hospital and high Dependency unit stay, frequency of ICU admission and number of deaths.

A centre can achieve excellent results by concentrating on the basics of postoperative care like pulmonary hygiene and physiotherapy, fluid and pain management and management of pleural spaces. Risk factors for complications following thoracic surgery have been identified from numerous clinical studies using a variety of research designs and definitions. The most frequent risk factors include age, preoperative pulmonary function tests, cardiovascular co morbidity, smoking status and chronic obstructive pulmonary disease (COPD). [1]- [4] In the current era there has to be more emphasis on postoperative care due to the complexity of referrals with the thoracic units doing more patients with multiple risk factors for post operative complications. This gets more challenging with cost containment.

High-risk patients can be optimised with preoperative and postoperative cardiopulmonary rehabilitation to reduce their operative risk, frequency of complications and hospital stay and improve postoperative outcomes including postoperative lung function. [5], [6] In addition, preoperative pulmonary rehabilitation may improve preoperative exercise capacity and so operability. [7], [8] The future development and adoption of innovative strategies is required to reduce the impact of post operative complications in an ageing co morbid population.

In this section will cover the routine care of a postoperative thoracic patient with specific emphasis on prevention and management of common complications.

2. Preoperative optimisation of specific risk factors

The outcome of surgical procedures is not measured only by clinical end points but also shorter stays and lower costs [9]. Patients' discharge is delayed commonly due to inadequate pain relief, infection, arrhythmias, prolonged air leak and debility [9]. Many complications that occur from thoracic operations can be anticipated. An aggressive preoperative work up mitigates morbidity and shortens convalescence.

2.1. Smoking

Preoperative cessation of smoking prevents postoperative complications to a large extent.

Support groups, counselling and nicotine replacement therapy should be used [10]. Historically, 6 weeks of smoking cessation before surgery is recommended to avoid the copious bronchorrhea that accompanies regeneration of the cilia that clear mucus between 2 and 4 weeks after smoking cessation [11].there are few studies which challenge this challenge this notion of timing of smoking cessation. Even 3-5 days of stopping could improve clearance and decrease of secretions. Vaporciyan el al showed that patients who quit smoking 4 weeks or more before surgery had a lower incidence of pulmonary complications than patients who continued to smoke or quit fewer than 4 weeks before pneumonectomy [12]. However, Barrera and co-workers found no difference in the incidence of pulmonary complications between patients who were still smoking at the time of surgery and those who had quit fewer than 2 months before thoracotomy for lung resection [13]. In many centres including ours the recommendation is to stop smoking at any time and provide support services to help out with the same.

2.2. Preoperative education and physiotherapy

Preoperative physiotherapy and education is done in many centres as part of work up for thoracotomy. Physiotherapists and thoracic ward medical and other staff perform a variety of care for patients undergoing surgery both pre and post operatively. All these are done to prevent postoperative complications like atelectasis, pneumonia, effusions and empyema. Various manoeuvres include education, deep breathing and coughing manoeuvres, chest physiotherapy and early mobilization education post sugery [14]. According to few studies this has led to an improvement in the prevention of atelectasis, collapse and consolidation. Many other interventions like incentive spirometry and respiratory muscle strengthening have been shown to reduce the incidence of these complications. During the work up assessment of the pulmonary functions are done and bronchodilators optimised.

In the education session instructions may be given for deep breathing and splinted coughing exercises, prophylaxis exercises for deep vein thrombosis, and shoulder exercises [15]. There studies which question the benefit of preoperative education and physiotherapy and few studies have shown them to be non-beneficial16 but we continue to follow preoperative education as well as physiotherapy prior to thoracic surgery.

Patients are also investigated for cardiac ailments if there are symptoms, signs or significant cardiac history prior to performing elective thoracic surgery. Investigations may include echocardiography, cardiac viability study or angiogram. Patients who are on antiplatelets should have their medications withheld 7 days prior to surgery is possible. If patients are on warfarin then it is stopped 3 days prior to surgery and are covered with heparin

Patients are given a single dose of antibiotics for elective cases and they are continued for infected cased or restarted postoperatively if needed. If surgical intervention is elective, we advocate a short period of preparation may be beneficial if directed at improving the patient's physical status and specifically at pulmonary preparation, conditioning exercises, and nutrition.

3. Operative factors

3.1. VATS vs. OPEN

Video assisted Thoracoscopic procedures are done with increasing frequency for many indications. The incidence of postoperative complications is 9% after VATS and they include haemorrhage, empyema, air leak, pneumonia and surgical emphysema [17] commonly but most of the complications which happen in thoracotomy could potentially happen with video assisted Thoracoscopic procedures.

Most importantly the incidence of postoperative pain is much less in VATS than open procedures and they have shorter hospital stay. The proponents of VATS have published many series about the feasibility, lesser complication rate, reduced pain, early mobility and discharge [18], [19]. There are groups who did not find any statistical benefit in performing VATS and have quoted a higher bleeding and intraoperative complication rate [20]. In our unit we perform VATS for all kinds of thoracic procedures if patients are suitable for it. VATS lobectomy is a safe procedure, which reduces peri operative pain and improves postoperative physical status. The results obtained with early stage lung cancer are excellent and may reflect inherent oncologic advantageous consequent upon reduced operative trauma. Detection of early stage lung cancer is potentially rewarding and will become a practical imperative if survival results are to be improved. Thus the scope for VATS resection may increase significantly. In our view VATS lobectomy is the procedure of choice for early stage lung cancer and multicentre prospective randomised trials comparing this therapy against conventional open resection are overdue.

3.2. Use of staplers and glues to reduce and seal air leaks

Various procedures like wedge resections, lobectomies, excision of bullae may cause prolonged air leaks especially if patients have COAD. Traditionally diathermy dissection and ligation was used and later staplers were used for parenchymal resections. Although certain studies pointed towards improved results with regards to air leaks using staplers [21] and reported that surgical morbidity due to air leaks decreased with this technique other studies have not shown any particular reduction in duration of air leaks using staplers alone. [22]

The air leaks caused by the holes of the suture needles are of the same magnitude as that caused by the surface tension between the parallel staple lines when the lung inflates. Nevertheless staplers are quicker to use and they have a big role in minimally invasive Thoracoscopic procedures

Polyglycolic acid fabric, polydioxan ribbon, bovine pericardial strips, bovine collagen, and recently, expanded polytetrafluoroethylene have been employed in an attempt to reinforce the staple lines, especially for resections performed in emphysematous lungs [23]- [27]. Other techniques like the electrothermal bipolar sealing have shown good results in lung parenchymal surgery.

Air leaks are common after pulmonary resections. They can be inspiratory, expiratory, continuous and forced expiratory. Most of the leaks are expiratory or forced expiratory. Inspiratory leaks happen on positive pressure ventilation. If there is no pleural space then they are managed by underwater seal. If there is a space negative suctions is applied to the underwater seal. If the leak persists beyond a particular time frame then TALC or reopening should be considered.

4. Post operative care

4.1. Pain management

Pain management is of paramount importance post operatively as it is essential for patients to comply for chest physiotherapy and ambulation and they will be unable to do so if they have severe pain. There are various ways by which pain is managed. They include epidural catheters preoperatively, paravertebral methods pre or intraoperatively or intravenous patient controlled analgesia. On withdrawing these agents patients will need oral analgesics for duration of time till they are pain free. These include paracetamol, NSAID and narcotic agents.

4.1.1. Epidural analgesia

The catheter is placed approximately with the midpoint of the dermatomal distribution of the skin incision. Epidural local anaesthetics increase segmental bioavailability of opioids in the cerebrospinal fluid and increase the binding of opioids to m receptors and the blocking of the release of substance P in the substantia gelatinosa of the dorsal horn of the spinal cord [28]. The thoracic segmental effects of local anaesthetic and opioid combinations is the only way to minimize motor and sympathetic blockade maintain conscious level and cough reflex and reliably produce increased analgesia with movement and increased respiratory function after thoracotomy [29]. Generally the most popular regimens are fentanyl or diamorphine combined with levobupivacaine [29]. The regimens can be administered as an infusion, patient controlled analgesia or both.

Potential issues include failure, technical difficulty and hypotension. It can also reduce the effectiveness of coughing, especially in patients who already have a low FEV1. It is not offered when there is local or systemic sepsis.

Paravertebral block is an effective modality to provide pain relief. It can be done by the anaesthesiologist before the start of surgery or by the surgeon before closure. It offers several technical and clinical advantages and is indicated for anaesthesia and analgesia when the afferent pain input is predominantly unilateral from the chest and/or abdomen. We prefer placing the catheter under direct vision during thoracic surgery and give pain relief as a continuous infusion. The chest drain loss of local anaesthetic is four times lower than that of interapleural block [30].

4.1.2 Systemic analgesics

Opioids remain the mainstay of postoperative analgesia and have demonstrated their efficacy in the management of severe pain. The side effects include nausea, vomiting, ileus, biliary spasms and respiratory depression, Opioids can be administered IM, subcutaneously, or IV.

A very efficient method of delivery of opioids is via PCA (Patient Controlled Analgesia) devices. Numerous studies have demonstrated the safety and opioid-sparing effect of PCA. After thoracic surgery PCA is often combined with other modalities to offer adequate pain relief.

4.1.3. Intrapleural

Intrapleural local anaesthetics produce a multi-level intercostal block. However, the analgesia is extremely dependent on patient position, infusion volume, and the type of surgery. With the drains insitu most of the anaesthetic is drained out and hence the efficacy of the procedure is less. In spite of occasional successes most clinicians have not found the reliability of intrapleural techniques adequate to justify their use on a routine basis. [31]

4.1.4. Other techniques

Cryoanalgesia is the application of a -600ºC probe to the exposed intercostal nerves intra-operatively produces an intercostal block that can persist for up to six months. This can be moderately efficient to decrease post-operative pain, but is associated with an incidence of chronic neuralgia that has lead many centres to abandon the technique [32]. Transcutaneous electrical nerve stimulation (TENS) may be useful in mild to moderate pain but is ineffective when pain is severe. [33]

4.2. Management of fluid electrolytes

Patients are managed generally in a high dependency unit post surgery or the wards if it is a dedicated thoracic unit. Post thoracic surgery especially in resections intravenous fluids are given in reduced amounts to prevent pulmonary insufficiency. Care is taken not to overhydrate the patient and oral feeding in encouraged as soon as possible. Intravenous fluids should be used judiciously and a conservative strategy of administration of maintenance fluids is recommended at 1–2 ml/kg/h in the intra- and post-operative periods and that a positive fluid balance of 1.5 l should not be exceeded, to mitigate the risk of multifactorial post operative acute lung injury/ARDS. Caution should be exercised with regard to silent hypovolaemia, impaired oxygen delivery and acute kidney injury. A high index of suspicion for pulmonary insufficiency should be adopted if there is volume overload. If a patient develops signs of hypo perfusion after these thresholds are exceeded, inotropic/vasopressor support should be considered. [34]

4.3. Intercostal catheter

Intercostal catheter is watched for drainage and air leak. If the postoperative chest X-ray shows expanded lung fields the no suction is applied even if there is bubbling. If there is airspace the suction is applied. It is preferable to use a balanced drainage system in all patients. In pneumonectomy patients no suction is applied after surgery and the balanced drainage system is filled with 1cm of liquid unlike routine thoracic cases where it is filled with 2 cm of fluid. In pneumonectomy patients the drains are removed the next day and in lobectomy patients as soon as possible. Suction is also applied in cases of pleurodesis with talc so that the visceral and parietal pleurae are approximated. If the drains have to stay due to persistent minimal bubbling and if the parenchyma is expanded without any suction a Heimlich valve container is attached for earlier complete ambulation or discharge.

4.4. Physiotherapy and early mobilisation.

Postoperative insufficiency occurs because of infection, inability to clear secretions or oedema around day 2 or 3, to prevent these from happening attention should be given to physiotherapy, bronchodilators, restriction of intravenous fluids and tracheal toilet. Chest physiotherapy includes deep breathing and coughing exercises and incentive spirometry. Pulmonary insufficiency is more common in patients have low FEV1. If there is inability to do so then endotracheal suctioning or mini tracheostomy should be used for clearing secretions. Diuretics are used if necessary and antibiotics are started if clinically indicated without waiting for radiological deterioration.

Early postoperative ambulation and physiotherapy reduces complications like atelectasis, pneumonia, empyema and DVT.

Aspiration should be prevented postoperatively as it can result in multiorgan dysfunction and sepsis. Patients should be allowed to eat only when they are fully alert and sitting up. If there is a tendency to aspirate patients are kept nil by mouth and nasogastric feeding initiated as required. If there is damage to the vocal cords then a speech pathology is sought for and patients are initially kept on nasogastric feeds and based on recovery are put on graded diet beginning from thickened fluids.

4.5. Deep Venous thrombosis prophylaxis

The prophylaxis should start when the patients are admitted in the hospital. Everyone should be given a prophylactic dose of heparin subcutaneously if not contraindicated at a dose 5000 IU twice daily and this is continued in the postoperative period till discharge. All patients should have stockings and the high-risk patients should be on compression stockings. If there are signs of DVT then a Doppler in arranged and patients put in treatment dose of heparin infusion and an IVC filter put in if necessary.

5. Complications

5.1. Postoperative haemorrhage

Immediate postoperative bleeding can be caused due to surgical bleeding or coagulopathy, surgical bleeding being more common. A set of standard coagulation tests are performed and coagulopathy is corrected accordingly. Depending on the coagulation profile factors like FFP, Platelets, cryoprecipitate or factor 7 is given if the patient is bleeding due to profound coagulopathy.The threshold for taking back a patient for re-exploration should be low, as a surgical cause of bleeding should be ruled out. Bleeding after thoracic surgery is rare. It occurs in less than 2% of video assisted Thoracoscopic procedures (VATS) and around 01% to 3% of open procedures. [35]- [38] Generally postoperative bleeding results from technical complications, but certain co morbidities may predispose a patient to bleeding. A chest tube output of 1000 ml in 1 hour necessitates an immediate return to the operating room with concurrent correction of coagulopathy. Serial drainage exceeding 200 ml per hour for 2 to 4 hours after correction of a coagulopathy also indicates surgical bleeding and dictates re-exploration. If the patient is hemodynamic ally stable but the chest output is high, checking the haematocrit on the chest tube drainage can be helpful in distinguishing active bleeding from a lymphatic leak. If a patient in the immediate postoperative period is hemodynamically unstable but the chest tube output does not suggest active haemorrhage, a chest radiograph may show radiopacity of the operative side with thrombosed chest tubes. [40]

Medications like aspirin, other antiplatelet agents' warfarin could cause increased bleeding tendencies. Several herbs like garlic, ginseng etc. effect a prolonged bleeding time, which can result in peri operative haemorrhage. [39] The effect of herbal medications in thoracic surgery specifically is lacking, but discontinuing herbs 2 weeks before a lung resection is recommended. [40]

Recommendation for perioperative antiplatelet the current recommendations aim at providing the best option for patients. There are issues regarding continuing or discontinuing these medications. These recommendations are mainly form observational data. [41], [42], [43]

In the current era Aspirin is a lifelong therapy and it is not necessary to stop it for surgery when there are specific indications like prevention after stroke, acute coronary syndrome, MI, or coronary revascularization, regardless of the time since the event that led to the recommendation of aspirin. [44]

Dual antiplatelet therapy is recommended during the two weeks after simple dilatation, six weeks after bare-metal stents, and at least 12 months after drug-eluting stents. [41], [42], [43] Elective operations should be postponed beyond these delays but most of the thoracic procedures have to be done as soon as possible as a bulk of cases are due to malignancy hence unless the hemorrhagic risk is excessive, dual antiplatelet therapy should not be interrupted before surgery.

Even if clopidogrel treatment must be interrupted in high-risk surgical situations, aspirin must be continued without interruption.41,42,43 Heparin has no antiplatelet activity and therefore is not an adequate substitution for aspirin or clopidogrel treatment because stent thrombosis is a platelet-mediated phenomenon. [42] Although not proven by any randomised controlled trials bridging therapy with a short-acting platelet glycoprotein IIb/IIIa inhibitor like tirofiban is a possible substitution for clopidogrel while aspirin is being maintained. [46] After the operation, antiplatelet therapy is resumed within the first 12 to 24 hours; clopidogrel therapy is reinitiated with a 300-mg loading dose, which reduces the time to achieve maximal platelet inhibition to four to six hours and decreases the risk of hyporesponsiveness from competition of other drugs with hepatic cytochromes.

Ticagrelor is used more often these days and should be stopped 36 to 48 hours prior to a planned procedure. It is reversible $P2Y_{12}$ adenosine disphosphate receptor binder with shorter duration of action unlike clopidogrel which is irreversibly binds to it. The perioperative management for it is similar to the clopidogrel.

Warfarin should be discontinued 3 days preoperatively, the INR checked. It should be substituted with heparin and APTT checked.

Conversion to an open thoracotomy for control of bleeding is done in case of bleeding due to VATS. Intraoperative bleeding can be massive from injury to the pulmonary artery or vein. Proximal control of the pulmonary artery before dissection of its branches is a safe preventive measure in open lobectomies. Rarely vascular stapler on a pulmonary vessel can cause bleeding and so can its used in the parenchyma. Suturing of the lung is done to control bleeding. Bleeding can also happen from peribronchial tissue, parenchyma, adhesions, intercostal vessels, and muscles.

In some patients, postoperative bleeding develops that is not hemodynamically significant enough to indicate re-exploration but results in a residual clotted hemothorax. As is true for a posttraumatic clotted hemothorax, treatment options include VATS or open exploration and evacuation of the hematoma to prevent development of a trapped lung, respiratory compromise, and empyema.

5.2. Cardiac complications

Arrhythmia, more particularly atrial fibrillation (AF), is by far the most common cardiac complication after thoracic surgery, with an incidence ranging from 10% to 20% after lobectomy and as much as 40% after pneumonectomy [46]- [47]

Risk factors for tachyarrhythmias include [48], patient related (pre-existing cardiovascular disease, postural change, limited pulmonary reserve), surgery related (extensive procedure, intrapericardial pneumonectomy, extra pleural pneumonectomy, anaesthetic agents, major bleeding), treatment related (previous thoracic irradiation) or older age [47], [49]. The most common arrhythmia encountered is supraventricular tachycardia.

If patients have atrial fibrillation with haemodynamic compromise then electrical cardioversion should be carries out immediately. If patients have sympromatic AF chemical cardioversion should be attempted first followed by electrical cardioversion if necessary. New-onset postoperative AF is often transient and self-limiting and it is generally accepted that rate comtrolling agents be given first. Rate control resolves AF in most cases in thoracic surgery. AF generally resolves within 1 day of hospital discharge with rate control alone. [50]

A selective Beta 1-blocking agent is recommended as the initial drug for rate control in the absence of moderate-severe chronic obstructive pulmonary disease or active bronchospasms and Diltiazem should be the first agent used in the presence of moderate-severe chronic obstructive pulmonary disease or active bronchospasm. [51]

Digoxin as a single agent should not be used for rate control, although it may be effective in combination with a beta1-blocker or diltiazem. Beta blockers are considered better than calcium channel blockers and digoxin for treating AF in thoracic surgery. The only concern is COPD where it may cause bronchospasms specific beta 1 blockers such as metoprolol are considered safer in this regard. [52]

When chemical cardioversion is employed in the setting of continuous or recurrent paroxysmal postoperative AF, the most reasonable initial drugs are intravenous followed by oral amiodarone or oral flecainide. [51]

Amiodarone is not given if the patient has severe lung disease or if the patient as undergone pneumonectomy The incidence of ARDS was 11% in the patients treated with amiodarone and 1.8% in the nonamiodarone group [53]. Flecainide is not given if there is organic cardiac disease. Other drugs include disopyramide, ibutilide, procainamide, propafenone, quinidine, and sotalol. Patients who received flecainide had an approximately doubled rate of mortality or cardiac arrest, likely due to a proarrhythmic effect on the ventricle possibly due to structural heart disease. Side effect of amiodarone relevant to thoracic surgery is its pulmonary toxicity [51].

Both amiodarone and flecainide are highly effective and relatively safe drugs, but the specific contraindications to their use must be kept in mind antiarrhythmic therapy is given usually from 1 to 6 weeks. The only study that has evaluated optimal length of therapy with antiarrhythmic drugs, once initiated, for postoperative AF (after coronary artery bypass graft surgery) found that there was no difference in the rate of recurrent AF whether the treatment was continued for 1, 3, or 6 weeks after discharge. [54]

Anticoagulation Therapy For patients with two or more risk factors for stroke (age >75 years, hypertension, impaired left ventricular function, prior stroke or transient ischemic attack) who have postoperative AF that recurs or persists for more than 48 hours, anticoagulation therapy is reasonable if not otherwise contraindicated. [51]

For patients with fewer than two risk factors for stroke and patients considered not suitable for warfarin who have postoperative AF that recurs or persists for more than 48 hours, aspirin, 325 mg daily is recommended. [51]

Oral metoprolol initiated preoperatively and continued postoperatively decreased the incidence of atrial fibrillation from 40% to 6.7% ($p < 0.05$). [55] In another trial, administration of magnesium sulphate starting the day of operative resection also resulted in a decrease in the incidence of atrial fibrillation from 26.7% to 10.7. [56]

5.3. Ischemia

In a large series the incidence of ischemic electrocardiographic changes was 3.8% and myocardial infarction in 1.2%. According to this study hypotension and abnormal exercise testing were the strongest predictors for ischemic events. [57]

Patients are monitored invasively, base line medication was continued, and peri operative fluid administration was minimalized. We recommend continuous monitoring for at least 2 days in high-risk patient.

The American College of Cardiology and the American Heart Association guidelines [58] for peri operative cardiovascular evaluation for no cardiac surgery remain the best available method for risk assessment in noncardiac thoracic surgery. Thoracic surgery is categorized as a high-risk surgical procedure in this matter. Coronary angiography is advocated in case of major clinical predictors such as unstable angina, decompensated heart failure, significant arrhythmias, or severe valvular disease. In cases of intermediate or minor clinical predictors the decision whether to perform an angiography is based on non-invasive testing [59].

As adenosine and dipyridamole should be avoided in patients with clinical bronchospasms, dobutamine stress echocardiography is the evaluation of choice for patients with cardiac ischemia referred for thoracic surgery [60]. In general the indications for coronary angiography are similar to those in the nonoperative setting. No prospective randomized data exists on the role of prophylactic coronary bypass surgery. Whether percutaneous coronary intervention is superior to bypass surgery is uncertain, but in cases of angioplasty with stenting it is probably safer to postpone surgery for 2 to 4 weeks. In conclusion, the preoperative cardiac assessment of thoracic surgery patients is of great importance, although prospectively controlled data for this type of surgery are lacking. [59]

5.4. Right-to-left shunt

It is estimated that 20% of the general population may have a persistently patent foramen ovale (PFO). With the increased right-sided pressures associated with pulmonary resection, these patients can develop a right-to-left shunt with refractory hypoxia in the post-operative period. This shunting increases most dramatically after a right pneumonectomy. In some patients, symptoms may not present until after 1 to 5 months, particularly after a right pneumonectomy. [61] Patients often present with dyspnoea (platypnea) and hypoxia (orthodexia) in the upright position, which resolves upon recumbence. This is because of nediastinal shift, which modifies the relationship between the right and left atrium and distorts the foramen ovale. Cardiac rotation and compression of the right atrium by pleural fluid causes preferential flow of the inferior caval vein into the left atrium. Hemodynamic factors may also have a role, such as reversal of the interatrial pressure gradient. A decrease in right ventricular compliance and the hydrostatic pressures in the left lateral decubitus or orthostatic positions increase the shunt. Lastly, factors such as pulmonary emboli, right ventricular infarction, increased intrathoracic pressure, chronic obstructive pulmonary disease, and positive pressure ventilation may drive shunt physiology. [62] The aetiology of this complication is unclear.

The diagnosis is made with arterial blood gas analysis, nuclear lung perfusion scanning, echocardiography, MRI, and cardiac catheterization or a combination thereof. Standard treatment is surgical repair, although several cases of successful intravascular occlusion of the septal defect have been performed.

Other causes of dyspnoea must be evaluated, including but not limited to pulmonary embolism, airway narrowing, and post resection pulmonary oedema.

5.5. Cardiac herniation

Cardiac herniation is a rare complication and happens in the early postoperative period. Cardiovascular collapse is the presenting feature Jugular pulse is elevated and there can be cyanosis in the drainage area of superior venacava. Ventricular fibrillation may occur [63]. Treatment is emergency thoracotomy with reposition of the herniated heart into the pericardial sac and repairing the defect of the pericardium [64]. Most documented cases of cardiac herniation have occurred through surgically created defects as a result of intrapericardial pneumonectomy or lobectomy with partial pericardectomy [65]. Combination of a sudden superior vena cava syndrome and heart sounds in the right side of the chest should alert the physician to the possibility of cardiac herniation. Surgical defects of the pericardium as a result of right intrapericardial pneumonectomy should be closed. This can be accomplished either by suturing the cut edges of the pericardium to the epicardium or by patching the defect with bovine pericardial patch, PTFE patch or parietal pleura. In cases of left pneumonectomy, it may be sufficient to enlarge the pericardial defect in order to prevent strangulation, should herniation occur [66].

5.6. Heart failure

Few studies have addressed the problem of postoperative right ventricular dysfunction, which is because of changes in right ventricular afterload and contractility [67]- [71]. Although right ventricular end-diastolic volume remains stable in the early postoperative hours, significant increases may be observed on the first and second postoperative days. Although many authors [69]- [71] claim that afterload alteration is the major determinant of RV dysfunction. Pulmonary artery pressure and pulmonary vascular resistance only rose modestly in a study [66], suggesting that the rise in afterload is not the only causing factor. Another argument favouring afterload augmentation as the cause of RV dysfunction is the fact that postoperative pulmonary artery pressure, pulmonary vascular resistance, and central venous pressure only change significantly during exercise [70]. Changes in RV function are able to compensate for the increased RV end-diastolic volume at rest, but not during exercise, with a resultant increase in pulmonary artery pressure and pulmonary vascular resistance. [59] One study used serially performed transthoracic echocardiography to assess the effects of pulmonary resection [71]. Only pneumonectomy patients had mild postoperative pulmonary hypertension without significant RV systolic dysfunction. Pulmonary embolism and cardiac herniation are rare mechanisms that may cause RV dysfunction.

Left heart failure is generally a consequence of impaired right heart function, either by decreasing left ventricular preload or by shifting the intraventricular septum resulting in a decreased left ventricular volume. Other causes of left ventricular dysfunction are acute myocardial infarction, pre-existing valvular disorders or cardiac herniation. [59]

5.7. Pulmonary oedema

Respiratory complications occur in 5-14% of patients [72]- [74]. The risk factors include age of the patient, extent of resection, preoperative lung function and other co morbidities.

However, a number of case studies have described what appears to be a specific syndrome of post pulmonary resection lung injury, which has been called post-pneumonectomy pulmonary edema (PPO). [75], [76], [77] The syndrome consisted of the onset of severe respiratory failure, within 48 h of operation, associated with diffuse radiographic changes on plain chest films consistent with pulmonary oedema. However, central pressure measurements showed no evidence of left ventricular failure or cardiogenic pulmonary oedema. Its incidence is approximately 2.5% to 4% [78]- [83].

The mechanisms of injury are that ischaemia–reperfusion injury and [84] reactive oxygen species. [85] Pulmonary capillary stress failure occurs when the pulmonary microvascular bed is subjected to increased pressure and could produce capillary injury. [86]

Following are the recommendations and statements concerning fluid administration: (1) there is no "third space" in the thorax, (2) total positive fluid balance in the first 24 hours should not exceed 20 mL/kg, (3) a urinary output greater than 0.5 mL/kg/h is unnecessary, (4) the use of invasive monitoring techniques is advisable if increased tissue perfusion is necessary postoperatively, (5) factors that contribute to increased pulmonary venous pressures should be minimized postoperatively, (6) hyperinflation of the residual lung should be avoided, (7) regular chest roentgenograms should be obtained postoperatively, (8) prolonged periods with the residual lung in the dependent position should be avoided, and (9) prophylactic digitalization has not been shown to reduce the incidence of post resection supraventricular arrhythmias or of postpneumonectomy pulmonary edema. [59]

Therapy [59] consists of administration of diuretics, restriction of fluid, nutritional support, and maintenance of adequate oxygenation, even with mechanical ventilation if necessary. Despite aggressive treatment, the clinical outcome is poor with mortality exceeding 50%. Nitric oxide ventilation and extracorporeal membrane oxygenation were tried as possible therapies. In particular the use of inhaled nitric oxide, in doses of 10 to 20 ppm, was able to lower mortality rates to 30% in a small series of patients. In the same report early intubation (at first signs of ARDS), aspiration, bronchoscopy, and postural changes are also advocated.

Pulmonary hypertension is a major concern for patients undergoing general thoracic surgery and often contraindicates pulmonary resection. Multiple aetiologies exist, such as cardiomyopathy or intrinsic cardiac valvular disease, as well as destructive pulmonary parenchymal processes resulting in cor pulmonale. The presence of pulmonary hypertension puts patients at increased risk for anaesthesia and surgical morbidity.

5.8. Postpneumonectomy syndrome

Postpneumonectomy syndrome refers to bronchial compression occurring as a result of massive mediastinal shift following pneumonectomy [87]- [89]. Incidence is approximately one in 640 cases [90]. This syndrome is much more common after right pneumonectomy: the mediastinum undergoes counterclockwise rotation as it shifts toward the pneumonectomy space [87], [88], [90], [91], [92]. This results in stretching, distortion, and compression of the left main bronchus between the pulmonary artery anteriorly and the aorta and vertebral column posteriorly. The syndrome has also been described after left pneumonectomy, both in patients with and without an aberrant right aortic arch [92], [94], [95], [96], [99]

Risk factors include young age and female sex [88], [97], [98]. These patients have more elastic mediastinal tissues (thus prone to shifting) and a softer, more compliant airway (thus subject to compression). [77] Patients typically present with exertional dyspnoea, stridor, and recurrent pulmonary infection] within one year of pneumonectomy. The onset is usually gradual, but acute obstruction may ensue in children. [99]

Airway stenting has been used in the treatment of inoperable patients and as a bridge to surgery in cases of acute obstruction [95], [98]. Definitive treatment involves surgical repositioning of the mediastinum in the midline. The mediastinum is then maintained in position by a saline-filled silicone prosthesis which is inserted into the pneumonectomy space. [99]

5.9. Lobar torsion and gangrene

Lobar torsion represents a rotation of the bronchovascular pedicle with resultant airway obstruction and vascular compromise. This disorder has been described in 3 different circumstances: as a complication of thoracic surgery, after blunt trauma, and spontaneously [100]

The overall incidence of lung torsion has been reported as 0.089%–0.2%, and is equally rare after thoracic surgery. [100], [101]. The pathophysiological mechanisms of torsion development were previously postulated as an airless lobe, incision of the inferior pulmonary ligament, pleural effusion, a long slim lobar pedicle, and lack of pleural adhesions. [100]

Patient's condition manifests as high fever, severe chest pain, massive haemoptysis, bronchorrhea, and sepsis, seen radiographically as abrupt consolidation and abnormal location of the collapsed lung. Only meticulous observations of both clinical and radiological manifestations, although uncharacteristic, can provide an indication of torsion development. [102]. Thereafter, bronchoscopy, contrast chest computed tomography, or angiography can be diagnostic in finding the distorted or occluded bronchi or tapered pulmonary artery. [100], [102]. Subsequent manoeuvres, such as contrast computed tomography, would have been diagnostic and prompted reoperation. Intrathoracic bleeding was suspected considering the history of extensive mediastinal adhesions, voluminous drainage, and blood loss. The distinguishing features were: the chest opacity appeared hypertensive, and the resultant huge tension markedly shifted the mediastinum; the serous fluid drainage, albeit a large amount, was inconsistent with the severity of the anaemia; and radiographically, there was a convex pulmonary margin around the chest tube. Wagner and Nesbitt stated that lobar torsion after right upper lobe resections accounted for 70% of the cases in the literature, whereas 15% followed resection of the left upper lobe. Torsion could happen in any lobe [103]

Options for surgical intervention include simple detorsion or resection of the involved pulmonary segments. Detorsion alone is advocated only in patients who undergo re-intervention within a few hours of the primary procedure; while in the majority of patients, pulmonary resection is mandatory due to pulmonary gangrene. Embolisms to other vital organs are the main complications after surgery, which should therefore be carefully monitored. [102]

It seems reasonable to staple or suture the middle lobe to the lower lobe after a right upper lobectomy if the oblique fissure is complete to prevent middle lobe torsion. Postoperatively, the possibility of a lobar torsion after lobectomy should be considered when an infiltrate or complete atelectasis persists or worsens; bronchoscopic intervention should be performed promptly.

5.10. Cardiac tamponade

Pericardial tamponade, though rare after open lobectomy, should be considered along with other complications when a patient repeatedly develops hypotension with therapies that causes venodilation. A rising CVP and its equalization with pulmonary artery diastolic pressure indicate cardiac tamponade. Symptoms include those related to cardiac tamponade: low cardiac output and Beck's triad (hypotension, muffled heart sounds, and increased central venous pressure). Diagnosis of this complication again requires a high index of suspicion. Echocardiography is the diagnostic study of choice to visualize impaired filling of the right ventricle because of increased pericardial pressure from the pericardial effusion.

Treatment include an urgent pericardiocentesis as a temporizing measure followed by reopening of the thoracotomy or a formal median sternotomy, which allows full inspection of the interior of the pericardium and provides adequate access for definite management of the cause. Minor injuries during retraction and dissection can produce life-threatening conditions like pericardial tamponade. Episodes of unexplained hypotension suggest a cardiac aetiology; a high index of suspicion and urgent surgical intervention can prevent adverse outcome.

5.11. Chylothorax

The thoracic duct can be injured during any thoracic procedure. Pleuro-pulmonary procedures, esophageal resection, intrapericardial and mediastinal procedures, and even less invasive procedures like subclavian puncture may lead to thoracic duct injury and subsequent chylothorax [104]- [108]. The incidence of chylothorax after pulmonary resection is between 0.7% and 2%. [109]- [110] This complication typically occurs at the time of resection. Aetiologies in thoracic surgery include aggressive mediastinal lymph node dissection with incomplete ligation of lymphatic channels or direct injury to the thoracic duct either during extra pleural pneumonectomy or division of the pulmonary ligament. There will be loss of calories, fluids, and proteins cause nutritional deficiency, dehydration, and immunologic dysfunction and if not drained can cause respiratory compromise.

Chylothorax can compress the lung resulting in shortness of breath and respiratory distress. Empyema is a rare complication due to the bacteriostatic nature of lecithin and fatty acids. Sterile chyle does not cause pleuritic pain or a fibrotic inflammatory reaction. Loss of proteins and vitamins, more than fat, leads to metabolic and nutritional defects, immunodeficiency, coagulopathy, malnutrition and death. A prompt diagnosis and an accurate early treatment are therefore essential. Analysis of the effusion demonstrates a triglyceride level >110 mg/dL and a lymphocyte count >90%, gram, Sudan 3 stain, chylomicrins on electrophoresis. The total protein concentration in the effusion is near or equal to the plasma protein concentration.

Leads to cardiopulmonary abnormalities and metabolic and immunologic

Mostly, it occurs from 2 days to 4 weeks postoperatively and varies from slight to severe forms determined by the volume and rate of chyle loss. Conservative treatment initially involves replacing the nutrients lost in the chyle and draining large chylothoraces using chest drain insertion if necessary, to ensure complete lung expansion, nil by mouth or the administration of low fat medium chain triglycerides by mouth. Medium chain triglycerides are directly absorbed in to the portal system, bypassing the intestinal lymph system. This reduces the flow of chyle in the thoracic duct allowing it the opportunity to heal. [111] If the chyle leak does not stop following the use of medium chain triglycerides, then total parenteral feeding to reduce the chyle flow even further should be considered. [111]- [112] Somatostatin and octreotide have proved to be useful in the conservative treatment of chylothorax. These agents reduce intestinal chyle production, thereby reducing the volume flowing through the injured thoracic duct. [113]- [115]

Chemical pleurodesis with TALC is an alternative option in the majority of patients that are too unwell for surgical closure of the chyle leak. A cannulation and embolisation technique prospectively to treat chylothorax was curative in patients' with demonstratable duct leakage [115] however reproducibility and success have varied in different centres. Surgical therapy [115] is recommended in cases where despite conservative management the patient drains more than 1.5 l/day in an adult or >100 ml/kg body weight per day in a child, leaks chyle at a rate of >1 l/day for5 days or has persistent chyle flow for more than 2 weeks. Surgery is also recommended if there has been a rapid decline in nutritional status despite conservative management. Thoracic duct ligation can be performed during thoracotomy or by thoracoscopic intervention. [116], [117] The main problem is identifying the chyle leak. Ligation of the thoracic duct is successful in 90% of patients when performed just above the right hemidiaphragm. [118] Ligating here, also has the advantage of halting flow from any unidentified accessory ducts. Collateral circulation redirects the chyle around the ligation point ensuring that the chyle still completes its journey to the circulation. In cases of loculated or complicated chylothorax pleural decortication with pleurodesis may be performed. [115]

5.12. Prolonged air leak

One of the common problems after thoracic surgery is prolonged postoperative air leak. Not all patients have an air leak after pulmonary resection. However, many patients having a lobectomy, segmentectomy, or a complicated wedge resection will leave the operating room with a leak

The vast majority of postoperative air leaks, however, are alveolar air leaks, and therefore initial management should be aimed at treating this entity. The management of bronchopleural fistulas is substantially different than that of alveolar air leaks, often requiring early surgical intervention. [119]

Air leaks that persist beyond a certain point may prolong the hospital length of stay. The Society of Thoracic Surgeons database mentions air leaks are those which are typically present when the patient could otherwise be discharged were it not for a continued air leak. The STS Thoracic Surgery Database defined prolonged air leak as lasting >5 days. Prolonged air leak may be associated with an increased complication rate and certainly may increase length of stay. Okereke et al. [120] found complications in up to 30% for patients with any air leak but only 18% in patients without, but this may have been a marker of extent of surgery or disease. Varela and colleagues [121] found that air leak lasting at least 5 days was associated with greater pulmonary morbidity, such as atelectasis, pneumonia, and empyema. They also found that the length of stay was extended by 6 days. Most leaks will stop within 2 to 3 weeks

By far the most common treatment of airleaks is watchful waiting with continuous drainage through a tube thoracostomy. More than 90% of air leaks seemed to stop within several weeks after operation with this form of management alone, with only rare development of an empyema. [119]A valved, outpatient system, such as a Heimlich, can only be considered in patients who have no more than a small, stable, asymptomatic pneumothorax on water seal. [119]

Blood patch or chemical pleurodesis may be considered as the next step. Experience with these techniques is variable. The instillation of sclerosing materials into the pleural space through the thoracostomy tube promotes symphysis of visceral and parietal pleura and may produce leak closure. Given the low rate of infection reported in published series, it remains unclear whether antibiotics should routinely be used. [119]

Autologous blood patch is another nonsurgical option to treat PAL after the operation or spontaneous pneumothorax [122]- [127]. To summarize, blood-patch pleurodesis involves the instillation of autologous blood into the pleural space through a chest catheter. It is simple, relatively painless, and often effective, but some information suggests that blood-patch pleurodesis may also carry an increased risk of intrathoracic infection. Although there are six articles on this subject, it is difficult to draw definitive conclusions due to the variable study sizes (from 2 patients to 32 patients), quantity of blood injected (50 to 150 mL), and endpoint definitions.

Pneumoperitoneum instilled through a transabdominal catheter has been reported to be effective in some cases [128], [129]. Surgical options to accomplish pleural symphysis or control the source of an alveolar air leak, or both, include video-assisted thoracic surgery (VATS) with parenchymal stapling, VATS with chemical pleurodesis, VATS with pleural abrasion [130], [131], VATS with application of topical sealants [132], [133], and the less well-supported use of VATS with laser sealing of the site of leak [134]. Omental or muscle flaps placed at re-thoracotomy can also be used successfully to obliterate the pleural space in patients with incomplete lung expansion and residual air leaks [135].

6. Injuries to surrounding structures

Injuries can happen to the oesophagus, phrenic nerve, recurrent laryngeal nerve, dural lacerations and spinal cord injury and peripheral embolisation of tumour.

6.1. Injury to the phrenic nerve

Thoracic surgical procedures can produce phrenic nerve injury. It happens when there are adhesions or in redo surgeries. Surgeries like anterior mediastinal tumor excision, resection of superior sulcus tumours, repair of thoracic outlet syndrome, or right-sided mediastinal lymph node dissection could all cause phrenic nerve injury. Such injuries may be temporary or permanent. Presenting features are shortness of breath on exertion and impaired exercise tolerance [136]. If patients are on a ventilator then there may be difficulty in weaning of ventilator. X-ray shows elevation of the affected hemi diaphragm. This is confirmed by ultrasound or fluoroscopy, which is the diagnostic study of choice in evaluation of these injuries. The best method of management of unilateral palsy is diaphragmatic plication [136].

6.2. Injury to the recurrent laryngeal nerve

Injury to the recurrent laryngeal nerve generally present in the postoperative phase with a weak hoarse and whispery voice. They nay describe a voice, which gets weaker as the day progresses, which may cause aspiration or impaired physiotherapy due to inability to cough effectively. A laryngoscopy is done to confirm the diagnosis and adduction of the affected vocal cord or sluggish motion will be absent. Treatment depends on whether the injury is temporary or permanent. A fibre optic evaluation is necessary to test swallowing and sensation. To assist with pulmonary physiotherapy and decrease the risk of aspiration, medialization laryngoplasty may be suggested [136]. This can be done as an office procedure with the aid of autologous fat, Gel foam, collagen, or polytetrafluoroethylene. [136]

7. Infections

Infectious complications after pulmonary surgery include operative wound infection, empyema, and nosocomial pneumonia. Antibiotic prophylaxis should therefore be guided against these three entities. The incidence varies from 5% to 24.4%. They are responsible for increased hospital mortality to up to 19% as well as increased costs and length of hospital stay. In one study 53.6% of the germs identified were gram-negative bacteria, 39.3% gram-positive bacteria, and 7.1% were fungi [137]. These infections should be aggressively treated with appropriate antibiotics after culture. Chest physiotherapy, pain control, bronchodilators, and early ambulation should be done for all patients but regardless of these pneumonia develops. Postoperative atelectasis after pulmonary surgery should be aggressively managed before it deteriorates into pneumonia. Our policy is to give Ticarcillin Sodium and Potassium Clavulanate 3.1 g four times a day in divided doses till a positive culture is obtained.

The incidence of empyema is dropping but could happen if there is prolonged air leak. Generally they are managed with antibiotics but may necessitate thoracotomy and wash out.

Other complications include pulmonary embolism, deep venous thrombosis, renal failure, strokes, major gastrointestinal bleed and late empyema. These complications should be recognised very early and aggressive management should be instituted if they are to be tackled successfully.

Thus postoperative care and management of postoperative complications is a team approach and good preoperative and intraoperative measures minimize the incidence of postoperative complications and early recognition and treatment is essential for successful outcomes.

Author details

Anand Iyer and Sumit Yadav

Department of Cardiothoracic surgery, Townsville Hospital, Queensland, Australia

References

[1] Stéphan F, Boucheseiche S, Hollande J, et al. Pulmonary complications following lung resection: a comprehensive analysis of incidence and possible risk factors. Chest 2000;118:1263e70.

[2] Brunelli A, Al Refai M, Monteverde M, et al. Stair climbing test predicts cardiopulmonary complications after lung resection. Chest 2002;121:1106e10.

[3] Bernard A, Deschamps C, Allen MS, et al. Pneumonectomy for malignant disease: factors affecting early morbidity andmortality. J Thorac Cardiovasc Surg 2001; 121:1076e82.

[4] Licker MJ, Widikker I, Robert J, et al. Operative mortality and respiratory complications after lung resection for cancer: impact of chronic obstructive pulmonary disease and time trends. Ann Thorac Surg 2006; 81:1830e7.

[5] Sekine Y, Chiyo M, Iwata T, et al. Perioperative rehabilitation and physiotherapy for lung cancer patients with chronic obstructive pulmonary disease. Jpn J Thorac Cardiovasc Surg 2005;53:237e43.

[6] Weiner P, Man A, Weiner M, et al. The effect of incentive spirometry and inspiratory muscle training on pulmonary function after lung resection. J Thorac Cardiovasc Surg 1997;113:552e7.

[7] Jones L, Peddle CJ, Eves N, et al. Effects of presurgical exercise training on cardiorespiratory fitness among patients undergoing thoracic surgery for malignant lung lesions. Cancer 2007;110:590e8.

[8] Bobbio A, Chetta A, Ampollini L, et al. Preoperative pulmonary rehabilitation in patients undergoing lung resection

[9] Wright CD, et al. Pulmonary lobectomy patient care pathway: a model to control cost and maintain quality. Ann Thorac Surg 1997;64:299.

[10] Karnath B. Smoking cessation. Am J Med 2002;112:399-405.

[11] Camu F, Beckers S. The anesthetic risk of tobacco smoking. Acta Anaesthesiol Belg 1991;42:45-56.

[12] Vaporciyan AA, Merriman KW, Ece F, Roth JA, Smythe WR, Swisher SG, et al. Incidence of major pulmonary morbidity after pneumonectomy: association with timing of smoking cessation. Ann Thorac Surg 2002;73:420-6.

[13] Barrera R, Shi W, Amar D, et al. Smoking and timing of cessation: impact on pulmonary complications after thoracotomy. Chest 2005;127:1977-83.

[14] Reeve J, Denehy L, Stiller K. The physiotherapy management of patients undergoing thoracic surgery: a survey of current practice in Australia and New Zealand. Physiother Res Int. 2007;12:59–71

[15] Brasher PA, McClelland KH, Denehy L, Story I. Does removal of deep breathing exercises from a physiotherapy program including pre-operative education and early mobilisation after cardiac surgery alter patient outcomes? Aust J Physiother. 2003;49:165–73

[16] Julie C. Reid, Anne Jamieson, Jennifer Bond, Bashir M. Versi, Arpit Nagar, Bernard H.K. Ng, and Julie D. Moreland. A Pilot Study of the Incidence of Post-thoracotomy Pulmonary Complications and the Effectiveness of Pre-thoracotomy Physiotherapy Patient Education. Physiother Can. 2010 Winter; 62(1): 66–74.

[17] Mason AC, Miller BH, Krasna MJ, White CS. Accuracy of CT for detection of pleural adhesions: correlation with video-assisted thoracoscopic surgery. Chest 1999; 115:423-427.

[18] R.J. McKenna Jr. VATS lobectomy with mediastinal lymph node sampling or dissection. Chest Surg Clin North Am, 4 (1995), p. 223

[19] Todd L. Demmy , Chukwumere Nwogu. Is Video-Assisted Thoracic Surgery Lobectomy Better? Quality of Life Considerations. The Annals of Thoracic Surgery, Volume 85, Issue 2, February 2008, Pages S719–S728

[20] Gopaldas RR, Bakaeen FG, Dao TK, Walsh GL, Swisher SG, Chu D. Video-assisted thoracoscopic versus open thoracotomy lobectomy in a cohort of 13,619 patients. Ann Thorac Surg 2010;89:1563-70

[21] Temes RT, Willms CD, Endara SA, Wernly JA. Fissureless lobectomy. Ann Thorac Surg 1998;65:282–4

[22] Ufuk Cagirici, Semra Bilaceroglu, Mustafa Cikirikçioglu, Hakan Posacioglu, Yüksel Atay, Tahir Yagdi, Önol Bilkay. Parenchymal Stapling in Pulmonary Lobectomies: Is it Really Necessary? Asian Cardiovasc Thorac Ann 1999;7:225-227

[23] Nakamura T, Shimizu Y, Mizuno H, Hitomi S, Kitano M, Matsunobe S. Clinical study of bioabsorbable PGA sheets for suture reinforcement and use as artificial pleura. Jpn Lung Surg J 1992;40:1828–31.

[24] Juettner F-M, Kohek P, Pinter H, Klepp G, Friehs G. Reinforced staple line in severely emphysematous lungs. J Thorac Cardiovasc Surg 1989;97:362–3.

[25] Cooper JD. Technique to reduce air leaks after resection of emphysematous lung. Ann Thorac Surg 1994;57:1038–9.

[26] Fischel RJ, McKenna RJ. Bovine pericardium versus bovine collagen to buttress staples for lung reduction operations. Ann Thorac Surg 1998;65:217–9.

[27] Vaughn CC, Wolner E, Dahan M, Grunenwald D, Vaughn CC III, Klepetko W, et al. Prevention of air leaks after pulmonary wedge resection. Ann Thorac Surg 1997;63:864–6.

[28] Hansdottir V, Woestenborghs R, Nordberg G. The pharmacokinetics of continuous epidural sufentanil and bupivacaine infusion after thoracotomy. Anesth Analg 1996; 83: 401–6

[29] Richard Hughes MB ChB, FRCA Fang Gao FRCA MPhil. Pain control for thoracotomy. Continuing Education in Anaesthesia, Critical Care & Pain | Volume 5 Number 2 2005, 56-60

[30] Karmakar MK. Thoracic paravertebral block . Anesthesiology. 2001 Sep;95(3):771- 80

[31] Schnieder RF, Villamena PC, Harvey J, et al., Lack of efficacy of intrapleural bupivacaine for post-operative analgesia following thoracotomy, Chest, 1993;103:414–6.

[32] Muller LC, Salzer GM, Ransmayr G, Neiss A, Intraoperative cryoanalgesia for postthoracotomy pain relief, Ann Thor Surg,1989;48(1):15–8.

[33] Benedetti F, Amazanio M, Casadio C, Control of postoperative pain by transcutaneous electrical nerve stimulation after thoracic operations, Ann Thorac Surg, 1997;63:773–6.

[34] Evans RG ,Naidu B. Does a conservative fluid management strategy in the perioperative management of lung resection patients reduce the risk of acute lung injury? Interactive Cardio Vascular and Thoracic Surgery Advance Access published May 22, 2012 0 (2012) 1–7

[35] A. Peterffy, A. Henze. Haemorrhagic complications during pulmonary resection: a retrospective review of 1428 resections with 113 haemorrhagic episodes. Scand J Thorac Cardiovasc Surg, 17 (3) (1983), pp. 283–287

[36] H. Sirbu, T. Busch, I. Aleksic et al. Chest re-exploration for complications after lung surgery Thorac Cardiovasc Surg, 47 (2) (1999), pp. 73–76

[37] M.J. Krasna, S. Deshmukh, J.S. McLaughlin. Complications of thoracoscopy. Ann Thor Surg, 61 (4) (1996), pp. 1066–1069

[38] A.P. Yim, H.P. Liu. Complications and failures of video-assisted thoracic surgery: experience from two centers in Asia. Ann Thorac Surg, 61 (2) (1996), pp. 538–541

[39] M.K. Ang-Lee, J. Moss, C.S. Yuan. Herbal medications and perioperative care JAMA, 286 (2) (2001), pp. 208–216

[40] Virginia R. Litle, Scott J. Swanson. Postoperative Bleeding: Coagulopathy, Bleeding, Hemothorax. Thoracic Surgery Clinics Volume 16, Issue 3, August 2006, Pages 203–207

[41] Fleisher LA, Beckman JA, Brown KA, et al.; American College of Cardiology/American Heart Association Task Force on Practice Guidelines (Writing Committee to Re-

vise the 2002 Guidelines on Perioperative Cardiovascular Evaluation for Noncardiac Surgery); American Society of Echocardiography; American Society of Nuclear Cardiology; Heart Rhythm Society; Society of Cardiovascular Anesthesiologists; Society for Cardiovascular Angiography and Interventions; Society for Vascular Medicine and Biology; Society for Vascular Surgery. ACC/AHA 2007 guidelines on perioperative cardiovascular evaluation and care for noncardiac surgery: executive summary: a report of the American College of Cardiology/American Heart Association Task Force on Practice Guidelines (Writing Committee to Revise the 2002 Guidelines on Perioperative Cardiovascular Evaluation for Noncardiac Surgery). Anesth Analg. 2008;106(3):685–712.

[42] American Society of Anesthesiologists Committee on Standards and Practice Parameters. Practice alert for the perioperative management of patients with coronary artery stents: a report by the American Society of Anesthesiologists Committee on Standards and Practice Parameters. Anesthesiology. 2009;110(1):22–23.

[43] Douketis JD, Berger PB, Dunn AS, et al. The perioperative management of antithrombotic therapy: American College of Chest Physicians Evidence-Based Clinical Practice Guidelines (8th Edition). Chest. 2008;133(6 suppl):299S–339S.

[44] Biondi-Zoccai GG, Lotrionte M, Agostoni P, et al. A systematic review and meta-analysis on the hazards of discontinuing or not adhering to aspirin among 50,279 patients at risk for coronary artery disease. Eur Heart J. 2006;27(22):2667–2674.

[45] King SB, 3rd, Smith SC, Jr., Hirshfeld JW, Jr., Jacobs AK, Morrison DA, Williams DO, et al. 2007 focused update of the ACC/AHA/SCAI 2005 guideline update for percutaneous coronary intervention: a report of the American College of Cardiology/American Heart Association Task Force on Practice guidelines. J Am Coll Cardiol. 2008 Jan 15;51(2):172-209.

[46] Asamura H., Naruke T., Tsuchiya R., Goya T., Kondo H., Suemasu K. What are the risk factors for arrhythmias after thoracic operations?. J Thorac Cardiovasc Surg 1993;106:1104-1110

[47] Amar D. Cardiac arrhythmias. Chest Surg Clin North Am 1998;8:479-493

[48] Amar D., Zhang H., Roistacher N. The incidence and outcome of ventricular arrhythmias after noncardiac thoracic surgery. Anesth Analg 2002;95:537-543

[49] Asamura H. Early complications; cardiac complications. Chest Surg Clin North Am 1999;9:527-541

[50] Rena O, Papalia E, Oliaro A, et al. Supraventricular arrhythmias after resection surgery of the lung. Eur J Cardiothorac Surg 2001;20:688 –93.

[51] Hiran C. Fernando, Michael T. Jaklitsch, Garrett L. Walsh, James E. Tisdale, Charles D. Bridges, John D. Mitchell, and Joseph B. Shrager. The Society of Thoracic Surgeons Practice Guideline on the Prophylaxis and Management of Atrial Fibrillation Associ-

ated With General Thoracic Surgery: Executive Summary. Ann Thorac Surg 2011;92:1144–52

[52] van der Woude HJ, Zaagsma J, Postma DS, Winter TH, vannHulst M, Aalbers R. Detrimental effects of beta-blockers in COPD: a concern for nonselective beta-blockers. Chest 2005;127:818 –24.

[53] Van Mieghem W., Coolen L., Malysse I., Lacquet L.M., Deneffe G.J.D., Demedts M.G.P. Amiodarone and the development of ARDS after lung surgery. Chest 1994;105:1642-1645

[54] Izhar U, Ad N, Rudis E, et al. When should we discontinue antiarrhythmic therapy for atrial fibrillation after coronary artery bypass grafting? A prospective randomized study. J Thorac Cardiovasc Surg 2005;129:401– 6.

[55] Jakobsen CJ, Bille S, Ahlburg P, et al. Perioperative metoprolol reduces the frequency of atrial fibrillation after thoracotomy for lung resection. J Cardiothorac Vasc Anesth 1997;11:746–751

[56] Terazi A, Furlan G, Chiavacci P, et al. Prevention of atrial tachyarrhythmias after non-cardiac thoracic surgery by infusion of magnesium sulfate. Thorac Cardiovasc Surg 1996;44:300–303

[57] von Knorring J., Lepantalo M., Lindgren L., Lindfors O. Cardiac arrhythmias and myocardial ischemia after thoracotomy for lung cancer. Ann Thorac Surg 1992;53:642-647

[58] Eagle K.A., Berger P.B., Calkins H., Chaitman B.R., Ewy G.A., et al. ACC/AHA guideline update for perioperative cardiovascular evaluation for noncardiac surgery. Circulation 2002;105:1257-1267

[59] Koen De Decker, Philippe G Jorens, Paul Van Schil. Cardiac complications after noncardiac thoracic surgery: an evidence-based current review. Ann Thor Surg. Volume 75, Issue 4, April 2003, Pages 1340–1348.

[60] M.H. Kim, K.A. Eagle. Cardiac risk assessment in noncardiac thoracic surgery Semin Thorac Cardiovasc Surg, 13 (2001), pp. 137–146

[61] Bakris NC, Siddiqi AJ, Fraser CD Jr, Mehta AC. Right-to-left interatrial shunt after pneumonectomy. Ann Thorac Surg 1997; 63:198–210

[62] John M. Karamichalis, Joe B. Putnam Jr., Eric S. Lambright. Cardiovascular Complications After Lung Surgery. Thoracic Surgery Clinics Volume 16, Issue 3, August 2006, Pages 253–260

[63] C.A. Montero, J.M. Gimferrer, G. Fita, M. Serra, M. Catalán, E. Canalís. Unexpected postoperative course after right pneumonectomy Chest, 117 (2000), pp. 1184–118

[64] M.H. Yacoub, W.G. Williams, A. Ahmad. Strangulation of the heart following intrapericardial pneumonectomy. Thorax, 23 (1968), pp. 261–265

[65] A.K. Deiraniya, Cardiac herniation following intrapericardial pneumonectomy Thorax, 29 (1974), pp. 545–552

[66] B.C. Papsin, L.A. Gorenstein, M. Goldberg. Delayed myocardial laceration after intrapericardial pneumonectomy. Ann Thorac Surg, 55 (1993), pp. 756–757

[67] Reed C.E., Spinale F.G., Crawford F.A. Effect of pulmonary resection on right ventricular function. Ann Thorac Surg 1992;53:578-582.

[68] Reed C.E., Dorman B.H., Spinale F.G. Mechanisms of right ventricular dysfunction after pulmonary resection. Ann Thorac Surg 1996;62:225-232

[69] Reed C.E., Dorman B.H., Spinale F.G. Assessment of right ventricular contractile performance after pulmonary resection. Ann Thorac Surg 1993;56:426-432.

[70] Okada M., Ota T., Okada M., Matsuda H., Okada K., Ishii N. Right ventricular dysfunction after major pulmonary resection. J Thorac Cardiovasc Surg 1994;108:503-511.

[71] Amar D., Burt M.E., Roistacher N., Reinsel R.A., Ginsberg R.J., Wilson R.S. Value of perioperative doppler echocardiography in patients undergoing major lung resection. Ann Thorac Surg 1996;61:516-520.

[72] Nagasaki F, Flehinger BJ, Martini N. Complications of surgery in the treatment of carcinoma of the lung. Chest 1982; 82: 25–9

[73] Deslauriers J, Ginsberg RJ, Dubois P, Beaulieu M, Goldberg M, Piraux M. Current operative morbidity associated with elective surgical resection for lung cancer. Can J Surg 1989; 32: 335–9

[74] Tedder M, Anstadt MP, Tedder SD, Lowe JE. Current morbidity, mortality, and survival after bronchoplastic procedures for malignancy. Ann Thorac Surg 1992; 54: 387–91

[75] Jordan S, Mitchell JA, Quinlan GJ, Goldstraw P, Evans TW. The pathogenesis of lung injury following pulmonary resection. Eur Respir J 2000; 15: 790–9

[76] Bauer P. Postpneumonectomy pulmonary oedema revisited. Eur Respir J 2000; 15: 629–30

[77] Zeldin RA, Normandin D, Landtwing D, Peters RM. Postpneumonectomy pulmonary edema. J Thorac Cardiovasc Surg 1984; 87: 359–65

[78] van der Werff Y.D., van der Houwen H.K., Heijmans P.J.M., et al. Postpneumonectomy pulmonary edema: a retrospective analysis of incidence and possible risk factors. Chest 1997;111:1278-1284.

[79] Deslauriers J., Aucoin A., Grégoire J. Postpneumonectomy pulmonary edema. Chest Surg Clin North Am 1998;8:611-631.

[80] Waller A., Keavey P., Woodfine L., Dark J.H. Pulmonary endothelial permeability changes after major lung resection. Ann Thorac Surg 1996;61:1435-1440.

[81] Waller D.A., Gebitekin C., Saunders N.R., Walker D.R. Noncardiogenic pulmonary edema complicating lung resection. Ann Thorac Surg 1993;55:140-143.

[82] Jordan S., Mitchell J.A., Quinlan G.J., Goldstraw P., Evans T.W. The pathogenesis of lung injury following pulmonary resection. Eur Respir J 2000;15:790-799.

[83] Turnage W.S., Lunn J.J. Postpneumonectomy pulmonary edema: a retrospective analysis of associated variables. Chest 1993;103:1646-1650.

[84] Hamvas A, Palazzo R, Kaiser L, et al. Inflammation and oxygen free radical formation during pulmonary ischemia–reperfusion injury. J Appl Physiol 1992; 72: 621–8

[85] Halliwell B. Reactive oxygen species in living systems: source, biochemistry, and role in human disease. Am J Med 1991; 91: 14S–22

[86] West JB. Invited review: pulmonary capillary stress failure. J Appl Physiol 2000; 89: 2483–9

[87] RodefeldMD, Wile FD, Whyte RI, Pitlick PT, Black MD. Pulmonary vascular compromise in a child with postpneumonectomy syndrome. J Thorac Cardiovasc Surg2000; 11910733780: 851–853.

[88] Macaré van MaurikAF, Stubenitsky BM, van Swieten HA, Duurkens VA, Laban E, Kon M. Use of tissue expanders in adult postpneumonectomy syndrome. J Thorac Cardiovasc Surg2007; 134: 608–612.

[89] PodevinG, Larroquet M, Camby C, Audry G, Plattner V, Heloury Y. Postpneumonectomy syndrome in children: advantages and long-term follow-up of expandable prosthesis. J Pediatr Surg2001; 36: 1425–1427.

[90] JansenJP, Brutel de la Rivière A, Alting MP, Westermann CJ, Bergstein PG, Duurkens VA. Postpneumonectomy syndrome in adulthood. Surgical correction using an expandable prosthesis. Chest1992; 101: 1167–1170.

[91] OzcelikC, Onat S, Askar I, Topal E. Surgical correction of postpneumonectomy syndrome by intrapleural expandable prosthesis in a child. Interact CardioVasc Thorac Surg2004; 3: 390–392.

[92] MehranRJ, Deslauriers J. Late complications: postpneumonectomy syndrome. Chest Surg Clin N Am1999; 9: 655–673.

[93] GrilloHC, Shepard JA, Mathisen DJ, Kanarek DJ. Postpneumonectomy syndrome: diagnosis, management, and results. Ann Thorac Surg1992; 54: 638–650.

[94] KellyRF, Hunter DW, Maddaus MA. Postpneumonectomy syndrome after left pneumonectomy. Ann Thorac Surg2001; 71: 701–703.

[95] CordovaFC, Travaline JM, O'Brien GM, Ball DS, Lippmann M. Treatment of left pneumonectomy syndrome with an expandable endobronchial prosthesis. Chest1996; 109: 567–570. yama T

[96] UyamaT, Monden Y, Sakiyama S, Fukumoto T, Sumitomo M, Harada K. Management of postpneumonectomy syndrome by intrapleural injection of sulfur hexafluoride. Case report. Scand J Thorac Cardiovasc Surg1993; 27: 179–181.

[97] ReedMF, Lewis JD. Thoracoscopic mediastinal repositioning for postpneumonectomy syndrome. J Thorac Cardiovasc Surg2007; 133: 264–265.

[98] RégnardJF, Pouliquen E, Magdeleinat P, Sohier L, Gourden P, Gharbi N, Bourcereau J, Levasseur P. Postpneumonectomy syndrome in adults: description and therapeutic propositions apropos of 8 cases. Rev Mal Respir1999; 16: 1113–1119

[99] George Rakovich, Jean Bussières, Eric Fréchette. Postpneumonectomy syndrome. Multimedia Manual of Cardiothoracic Surgery / doi:10.1510/mmcts.2008.003475

[100] Cable DG, Deschamps C, Allen MS, Miller DL, Nichols FC, Trastek VF, et al. Lobar torsion after pulmonary resection: presentation and outcome. J Thorac Cardiovasc Surg 2001; 122:1091–3

[101] Larsson S, Lepore V, Dernevik L, Nilsson F, Selin K. Torsion of a lung lobe: diagnosis and treatment. Thorac Cardiovasc Surg 1988;36:281–3

[102] Chang C. Hui Z. et al. Complete Lobar Torsion Simulating Hemorrhagic Shock After Left Upper Lobectomy. Asian Cardiovasc Thorac Ann 2009; 17:191-193

[103] Wagner RB, Nesbitt JC. Pulmonary torsion and gangrene. Chest Surg Clin North Am. 1992;2:839-52

[104] Ceves P.G., Vecchioni R., D'Amico D.F., et al. Postoperative chylothorax. J Thorac Cardiovasc Surg 1975;69:966-971.

[105] Joyce L.D., Lindsy W.G., Nicolott D.M. Chylothorax after median sternotomy for intrapericardial surgery. J Thorac Cardiovasc Surgery 1976;71:476-480.

[106] Van Mulders A., Lacquet L.M., Van Meghem W., Deneffe G. Chylothorax complicating pneumonectomy. Thorax 1984; 38:954-955.

[107] Lam H., Lim S.T.K., Wong J., Ong G.B. Chylothorax following resection of the oesophagus. Br J Surg 1979;66:105-109.

[108] Hertzog P., Toty L., Personne C., Rotten D. Chylothorax apre's chirurgie pleuro-pulmonaire. à propos de 12 cas personnels. Ann Chir 1975; 14:159-171.

[109] Kutlu CA, Sayar A, Olgac G, et al. Chylothorax: a complication following lung resection in patients with NSCLC: chylothorax following lung resection. Thorac Cardiovasc Surg 2003;51:342–345

[110] Suemitsu R, Ondo K, Fukuyama S, Ueda H. Late-period-onset chylothorax after a pulmonary resection for lung cancer: a case report. Ann Thorac Cardiovasc Surg 2007;13:345–348

[111] de Beer HG, Mol MJ, Janssen JP. Chylothorax. Neth J Med 2000; 56(1):25e31.

[112] Fernandez Alvarez JR, Kalache KD, Grauel EL. Management of spontaneous congenital chylothorax: oral medium-chain triglycerides versus total parenteral nutrition. Am J Perinatol 1999;16(8):415e20.

[113] Markham KM, et al. Octreotide in the treatment of thoracic duct injuries. Am Surg 2000;66(12):1165e7.

[114] Rimensberger PC, et al. Treatment of a persistent postoperative chylothorax with somatostatin. Ann Thorac Surg 1998;66(1):253e4.

[115] Emmet E. M, Zoe B, Paul B. A. Chylothorax: Aetiology, diagnosis and therapeutic options. Respiratory Medicine (2010) 104, 1-8

[116] Graham DD, et al. Use of video-assisted thoracic surgery in the treatment of chylothorax. Ann Thorac Surg 1994;57(6): 1507e11 [discussion 1511e2].

[117] Kent 3rd RB, Pinson TW. Thoracoscopic ligation of the thoracic duct. SurgEndosc 1993;7(1):52e3.

[118] Paes ML, Powell H. Chylothorax: an update. Br J Hosp Med 1994;51(9):482e90.

[119] Sunil S, Victor A. F, Charles R. B, Ellen R. C, John D. M, Hiran C. F, Joseph B. S. Management of Alveolar Air Leaks After Pulmonary Resection. Ann Thorac Surg 2010;89:1327-1335

[120] Okereke I, Murthy SC, Alster JM, et al. Characterization and importance of air leak after lobectomy. Ann Thorac Surg 2005;79:1167–1173

[121] Varela G, Jimenez MF, Novoa N, Aranda JL. Estimating hospital costs attributable to prolonged air leak in pulmonary lobectomy. Eur J Cardiothorac Surg 2005;27:329–333

[122] Droghetti A, Schiavini A, Muriana P, et al. Autologous blood patch in persistent air leaks after pulmonary resection J Thorac Cardiovasc Surg 2006;132:556-559.

[123] Shackcloth MJ, Poullis M, Jackson M, Soorae A, Page RD. Intrapleural instillation of autologous blood in the treatment of prolonged air leak after lobectomy: a prospective randomized controlled trial Ann Thorac Surg 2006;82:1052-1056.

[124] Yokomise H, Satoh K, Ohno N, Tamura K. Autoblood plus OK432 pleurodesis with open drainage for persistent air leak after lobectomy Ann Thorac Surg 1998;65:563-565.

[125] Dumire R, Crabbe MM, Mappin FG, Fontenelle LJ. Autologous "blood patch" pleurodesis for persistent pulmonary air leak Chest 1992;101:64-66.

[126] Cagirici U, Sahin B, Cakan A, Kayabas H, Buduneli T. Autologous blood patch pleurodesis in spontaneous pneumothorax with persistent air leak Scand Cardiovasc J 1998;32:75-78.

[127] Lang-Lazdunski L, Coonar AS. A prospective study of autologous 'blood patch' pleurodesis for persistent air leak after pulmonary resection Eur J Cardiothorac Surg 2004;26:897-900.

[128] De Giacomo T, Rendina EA, Venuta F, et al. Pneumoperitoneum for the management of pleural air space problems associated with major pulmonary resections Ann Thorac Surg 2001;72:1716-1719.

[129] Handy Jr JR, Judson MA, Zellner JL. Pneumoperitoneum to treat air leaks and spaces after a lung volume reduction operation Ann Thorac Surg 1997;64:1803-1805.

[130] Suter M, Bettschart V, Vandoni RE, Cuttat JF. Thoracoscopic pleurodesis for prolonged (or intractable) air leak after lung resection Eur J Cardiothorac Surg 1997;12:160-161.

[131] Torre M, Grassi M, Nerli FP, Maioli M, Belloni PA. Nd-YAG laser pleurodesis via thoracoscopy. Endoscopic therapy in spontaneous pneumothorax Nd-YAG laser pleurodesis. Chest 1994;106:338-341.

[132] Thistlethwaite PA, Luketich JD, Ferson PF, Keenan RJ, Jamieson SW. Ablation of persistent air leaks after thoracic procedures with fibrin sealant Ann Thorac Surg 1999;67:575-577.

[133] Carrillo EH, Kozloff M, Saridakis A, Bragg S, Levy J. Thoracoscopic application of a topical sealant for the management of persistent posttraumatic pneumothorax J Trauma 2006;60:111-114.

[134] Sharpe DA, Dixon C, Moghissi K. Thoracoscopic use of laser in intractable pneumothorax Eur J Cardiothorac Surg 1994;8:34-36.

[135] Nonami Y, Ogoshi S. Omentopexy for empyema due to lung fistula following lobectomy. A case report. J Cardiovasc Surg (Torino) 1998;39:695-696.

[136] Haithcock, Benjamin E.; Feins, Richard H Complications of Pulmonary Resection. Shields, MD, Thomas W.; LoCicero, Joseph; Reed, Carolyn E.; Feins, Richard H. General Thoracic Surgery. 7th Edition 2009, page 558

[137] Radu DM, Jauréguy F, Seguin A, et al. Postoperative pneumonia after major pulmonary resections: an unsolved problem in thoracic surgery Ann Thorac Surg 2007;84:1669-1674

Chapter 4

Management of Malignant Pleural Effusion

Hidir Esme and Mustafa Calik

Additional information is available at the end of the chapter

http://dx.doi.org/10.5772/54441

1. Introduction

Pleural effusions can form basing on the disease of the pleural membranes themselves or thoracic or abdominal organs [1]. The pleura is also important to maintain local fluid homeostasis. The exact mechanisms of pleural fluid production and absorption are complex and not fully understood [2, 3].

The normal pleural space is approximately 18 to 20 μm in width, although it widens at its most dependent areas. It has been shown that the pleural membranes do not touch each other and that the pleural space is a real gap, not a potential space [1].

Classically described; pleural effusion is the accumulation of fluid in the pleural gap that may be caused by any reason [4]. If there is an evidence of invasion by the tumor or any malignant cells detected in this fluid, it is described as malignant pleural effusion. Although there has been no epidemiologic study with respect to pleural effusion yet, it is a common clinic problem which is estimated to be a million cases in the United States of America every year. Malignant diseases account for over 22% of all cases that means; approximately 220 000 new patients in the United States and 40 000 in the United Kingdom [5].

Primary tumours of the pleural space are less common [6]. Pleural metastasis may be caused by any organ. Malignant pleural effusions (MPE) are most frequently produced by carcinomas of the lung (37%), breast (25%), and ovary (10%). Other reasons include malignancies of the genitourinary (7%) or gastrointestinal tract (9%) and lymphoma (10%) [7]. Even today, in up to 10% of the malignant pleural effusions, the origin of tumour is not identified [8].

The incidence and prevalence of mesothelioma may vary from region to region. Interestingly, despite its grim reputation, mesothelioma whose curative treatments are not yet available, offers better survival than does metastatic pleural disease, with a median survival of less than 12 months [6].

Asymptomatic patients with either a malignant or a paramalignant effusion need not be treated initially [9]. Malignant pleural effusion will eventually develop into cancer in the majority of patients. It often recurs challenging the physicians, patients and the patient's family in balancing the benefits of symptomatic improvement with the risk and inconvenience of therapy [10, 11].

2. Pathogenesis

Pathophysiology of MPE has not been fully understood yet and is still on debate. There are many hypotheses on the pathogenesis of MPE in cancer. It commonly results from disruption of normal starling forces regulating pleural fluid absorption by obstruction of mediastinal lymphatics, which drain the pleural space [9]. There is a strong relationship between mediastinal metastasis and development of MPE [12, 13]. Other causes of MPE include direct invasion (e.g. lung cancer, breast cancer, chest wall neoplasms), hematogenous spread of tumor to the pleura (eg, metastasis, non-Hodgkin's lymphoma), or increased capillary permeability caused by tumor invasion-related local inflammatory changes or vascular endothelial growth factor production [14]. Just the presence of metastasis does not seem sufficient to explain the pathogenesis of pleural effusions. In fact, only about 60% of patients with proven pleural metastases develop pleural effusions [15, 16].

Indeed, the accumulation of excess pleural fluid associated with cancer may be the result of a number of separate factors in an individual patient [16]. Postmortem studies have demonstrated a strong relationship between carcinomatous infiltration of the mediastinal lymph nodes and the occurrence of pleural effusion [11,15]. This finding suggests an important role of the impaired lymphatic drainage in the pathogenesis of MPE. However, if this was to be the only mechanism, one would expect MPEs to be transudative, but instead, the majority of these effusions are exudates [16].

Local effects of tumor	Systemic effects of tumor
Lymphatic	Pulmonary embolism
Bronchial obstruction with pneumonia	Hypoalbuminemia
Bronchial obstruction with atelectasis	
Trapped lung	Complications of therapy
Chylothorax	Radiation therapy (Early or late)
Superior vena cava syndrome	Chemotherapy

Table 1. The Causes of paramalignant Effusion [17]

All fluids of pleura may not be malignant in patients with malignancy. The effusion caused by a neoplasm without the evidence of malignant cells in the pleural effusion as well as surrounding tissues is called as "paramalignant" effusion. Presence of paramalignant effusion is not a contraindication for the surgery. Obstructive pneumonia or atelectasia, lymphatic obstruction, cheilothorax caused by the invasion of thoracic duct, trapped lung, pulmonary embolism, hypoalbuminemia, cachexia, radiotherapy and, chemotherapeutics such as bleomycin, methotrexate and cyclophosphamide are the well known causes of para-malignant effusion [17].

3. Clinical presentations

The first and most common presenting symptom is dyspnea (96%) [12, 18]. The pathogenesis of dyspnea caused by a large pleural effusion has not been clearly elucidated, but several factors may be involved including a decrease in the compliance of the chest wall, contralateral shifting of the mediastinum, a decrease in the ipsilateral lung volume, and reflex stimulation from the lungs and chest wall [19]. After other causes of dyspnea have been excluded; detailed anamnesis, physical examination and radiological monitoring are required. As many as a third of patients with malignant pleural effusions present with weight loss and cachexia and appear debilitated by chronic illness [20]. Malignant causes should be excluded firstly in the list of differential diagnosis in patients diagnosed as exudates. A complete medical history and physical examination should be done considering any potential causes or risk factors of malignancy.

Other bothersome symptoms are cough [44%) and chest pain (56%) [18]. The majority of patients with MPE are symptomatic while less than 25% have no respiratory complaints [12]. Other symptoms include sharp pleuritic pain, dull ache with a feeling of pressure, and heaviness in the chest. A physical examination can reveal decreased breath sounds, and dullness to percussion [12].

4. Imaging techniques

Although standard chest radiographs can detect as little as 50 mL of PF on a lateral view,[21] it provides only suggestive findings for the diagnosis of MPE. A massive effusion increases the probability of a malignant aetiology and commonly produces a meniscus sign with fluid tracking up the lateral chest wall, a shift of the mediastinum to the contralateral side, and an inversion of the diaphragm. Radiographic signs of an MPE include circumferential lobulated pleural thickening, crowding of ribs, and elevation of the hemidiaphragm or ipsilateral mediastinal shift consistent with lung atelectasis due to airway obstruction by a tumor [22]. Due to resembling the other causes of pleural effusion other imaging studies may be necessary such as ultrasound and computed tomography (CT) scan [23].

Ultrasound is an important device during evaluating the presence of an effusion and may be used as a guide during thoracentesis. Ultrasound also may aid in distinguishing an exudates (echogenic) from a transudate (anechoic) although this finding is not definitive [24]. Ultrasound is, in fact, more sensitive than radiography and can detect as little as 5 mL of pleural fluid and is superior to CT for characterization of collections for the presence of septations and loculations [25].

Computed tomography (CT) scanning is even more accurate in detecting small effusions, including as little as 2 mL of fluid. The volume of the fluid presence can be best determined radiographically by using three-dimensional reconstruction [26]. Currently, the most useful radiographic study is a chest CT scan. CT scans help to establish the presence of a loculated pleural effusion, allow the evaluation of the pulmonary parenchyma if there is not complete lung compression, and distinguish pleural thickening from effusion. It also provides an excellent way to evaluate the mediastinum for the presence of masses or lymphadenopathy and permits detection of pleural-based nodules [27].

The role of magnetic resonance imaging (MRI) in the evaluation of pleural effusions is limited; however, it may be beneficial in better characterizing possible tumour involvement of the chest wall or diaphragm [28]. Neither MRI nor CT scan can distinguish transudates from exudates accurately although both can be helpful in evaluating the pleural contents for masses, nodules, and pleural based thickening once the fluid is removed [29].

Positron emission tomography (PET scan) with 18F-fluorodeoxyglucose provides less anatomic information but has the potential advantage of providing diagnostic information about the effusion. This information may prove useful [30]. The true value of a PET scan would be to provide additional information about disease elsewhere, not to give a diagnosis of malignancy. In addition, diagnosis or treatment of a malignant effusion will depend on the type of cancer, and this cannot be determined with a PET scan [31].

5. Pleura and fluid characteristics

Once a pleural effusion is documented, diagnostic or therapeutic thoracentesis should be performed to establish the nature of the effusion. For adequate separation of transudates and exudates in pleural fluid, protein and LDH levels are determined and also the following tests on pleural fluid are recommended: description of the fluid; cell count and differential; glucose; pH particularly if the patient has a parapneumonic effusion; cytology; smears and cultures for bacteria, mycobacteria, and fungi; and adenosine deaminase (ADA) if tuberculous pleuritis is in the differential [32].

Effusions are classified as either exudative or transudative basing on established criteria and now commonly known as Light's criteria: [33]

1. Ratio of pleural fluid protein to serum protein concentration is greater than 0.5
2. Ratio of pleural fluid lactate dehydrogenase (LDH) to its serum concentration is greater than 0.6
3. LDH concentration in pleural effusion is greater than two thirds of the upper normal value for the serum LDH

This defines an exudate if any one of three criteria are met. The overall accuracy of these criteria is 93% to 95% [34, 35]. Light criteria have commonly misclassify effusions when any one of three criteria has a value close to its cutoff point [36]. Although the majority of malignant pleural effusions are exudates, it is important to keep in mind that a few are transudates [37, 38]. These circumstances result from the defective implementation of diagnostic rules that classify pleural effusions or coexisting conditions with transudates, such as hypoalbuminemia, cirrhosis with ascites, or chronic heart failure [39]. This does not suggest that every individual with a transudative pleural effusion should have pleural fluid cytological examination. However, in the appropriate clinical setting and the absence of congestive heart failure or a pleural fluid LDH level close to the exudative range, determination of pleural fluid cytology is suggested [17].

The primary problem with the Light criteria is that they identify 15% to 20% of transudative effusions as exudative effusions [40]. A re-evaluation of Light's criteria demonstrates that Light's criteria have an overall sensitivity for an exudate of near 100%, but a specificity of only approximately 80% [41]. In the search for the ideal test or improvement of Light's criteria; from the first day of Light criteria that were published the most widely accepted and so far have stood the test of time. Based on a meta-analysis of study in order to find the ideal diagnostic criteria, including 1448 patients, an updated version of Light's criteria, the original light studies a slightly modified by the addition of cholesterol as a marker, recommended as the best way to determine exudate. Judged by these criteria, a patient with any of the following criteria is provided, said to be exudates [42]:

- Pleural fluid protein greater than 2.9 g/dL
- Pleural fluid cholesterol greater than 45 mg/dL
- Ratio of pleural fluid LDH to serum LDH greater than 0.6

The appearance of the pleural fluid obtained by thoracentesis, its consistency and color should be noted. In patients with a known underlying malignancy, it is daily practice not only to obtain the usual tests to differentiate a transudate from an exudate (total protein and lactate dehydrogenase both in the fluid and in the serum) but also to obtain total and differential cell count, pH, glucose level, cholesterol and triglycerides, cytological analysis, hematocrit (if fluid is grossly bloody), and cultures. [37, 38].

Malignant pleural effusions may be serous, serosanguineous, or bloody, and usually are exudative in nature [21]. There are four characteristics features of pleural effusion; suggesting malignancy in patients with undiagnosed pleural effusion: that is to say, [1] a symptomatic period of more than a month, [2] absence of fever, [3] blood-tinged or bloody pleural fluid, or [4] CT findings suggestive of malignancy (pulmonary or pleural masses, pulmonary atelectasis, or lymphadenopathy) [43].

Despite all the progress in the imaging of the chest, for the diagnosis of MPE cytologic or tissue biopsy is required for approval. Cytology is the simplest definitive and most accurate method to diagnose malignant pleural effusion. Recent data suggests that at least 50 mL of pleural fluid should be studied in order to provide optimal cytological analysis [44, 45].

Diagnostic success of cytology can improve with repeated thoracentesis [46]. Fluids should be concentrated first for optimal detection of malignancy. There is a large variation in diagnostic yields of pleural fluid cytology ranging from 62 to 90% [47, 48]. The sensitivity depends on the type of malignancy, extent of disease, and experience of the cytopathologist [49].

Cytology of MPE in breast cancer has a sensitivity of 47% [50]. The diagnosis of adenocarcinomas can be established in nearly all patients whereas patients with pleural effusions secondary to Hodgkin's disease, have a positive cytologic examination in less than 25% of cases [51, 52]. Cytology is superior to blind percutaneous pleural biopsy in the diagnosis of malignant pleural effusion. Blind percutaneous pleural biopsy carries an 8% risk of pneumothorax, and has limited contribution to the diagnosis of patient with suspected malignancy. In a series of 118 patients with pleural effusions and negative cytology, closed pleural biopsy established the diagnosis of malignant pleural effusion in only 17% of the cases [53].

Low diagnostic value of pleural biopsy depends on costal pleural involvement of cancer cells in only half of patients with MPE since initial metastatic disease most commonly occurs on the visceral, mediastinal, and diaphragmatic pleurae [54].

After thoracentesis, pleural biopsy might be indicated in cases with cytological examination undiagnosed or suspected. Diagnostic value of conventional closed pleural biopsy with Abrams or Cope needles is lower when compared with image-guided and thoracoscopic biopsy techniques. The specificity of closed needle biopsy for MPE is high, but case series report sensitivities that range from 7% to 72% [53, 55-57]. However, closed pleural biopsy adds little to the cytological diagnosis in most cases and this is related to the scarce and irregular distribution of the tumour lesions in the pleural cavity when cytology is negative [54]. The yield of blind needle biopsy is higher when the pleural lesions are diffuse, as in tuberculosis and advanced neoplastic disease. In contrast, thoracoscopy has a very high yield in malignant effusions. It can be performed with local anesthesia and a single port of entry, and it has a little more complications than needle biopsy [47]. Contraindications to pleural biopsy include bleeding diathesis, anticoagulation, chest wall infection, and lack of patient cooperation. Important complications include pneumothorax, haemothorax, and vasovagal reactions. A rapid clinical deterioration or increased postprocedure effusion should alert the clinician to a possible haemothorax [58]. Nevertheless, pleural needle biopsy can be performed on outpatient basis [59] whereas thoracoscopy is much more complex and always requires hospitalization.

Normal pleural fluid pH ranges from 7.60 to 7.64. When a diagnostic thoracentesis is performed, pleural fluid pH is measured at any time. Analysis should be via a blood gas machine, not on litmus paper, because the latter is unreliable and not an acceptable alternative [60]. Approximately one-third of malignant effusions have a pleural fluid pH of <7.30 at presentation [61, 62]; this low pH is associated with glucose values of <60 mg/dL [63]. The cause of these low-glucose, low-pH malignant effusion appears to be an increased tumour mass within the pleural space compared with those with a higher pH effusion, resulting in decreased glucose transfer into the pleural space and decreased efflux of the acidic by-products of glucose metabolism, carbon dioxide (CO2], and lactic acid, due to an abnormal pleural membrane [64, 65]. Clinicians should keep in mind that parapneumonic effusions have pH less than 7.3 or puslike looking.

In general, cell counts obtained from the pleural fluid is rarely useful or pathognomonic. Because most cells are normally neutrophils or monocytes, a predominance of lymphocytes (>50%) should make one more seriously entertain the idea of a carcinomatous pleural effusion, and greater than 85% lymphocytes should make one entertain the diagnosis of lymphoma, sarcoidosis, chylothorax, rheumatoid pleurisy, or yellow nail syndrome [66, 67]. An increase in pleural fluid eosinophilia (>10% of nucleated cells) might be associated with benign disease (hemo- or pneumothorax), but also can be associated with all types of malignancy [68]. The presence of mesothelial cells is not helpful in terms of diagnosis [67, 69]

Several tumor markers have been used in diagnosing of MPE, but their clinical role has not been firmly established [70]. Higher levels of CEA are seen in squamous cell cancer and adenocarcinoma of lung while higher levels of CA 15-3 are observed in breast cancer [71]. The addition of any tumor marker assay would improve the diagnostic value of cytology [70].

Chromosome analysis has low sensitivity and specificity in diagnosing of MPE [71]. It may be helpful particularly with MPE secondary to lymphoma and leukaemia [72]

The molecular biology of pleural effusions has begun to be understood, with vascular endothelial growth factor (VEGF) emerging as a major role player [73]. Because it induces endothelial vasodilatation and enhances the permeability of the mesothelium 50,000 times more potently than histamine, VEGF is thought to be a major, if not the most important, cytokine in the etiology of effusions [74]. VEGF may be a part of the diagnosis of effusion in the future.

6. Diagnosis

MPE has a wide variety of diagnostic methods. Diagnostic methods are often chosen according to health care provider's medical facilities, the clinician's ability and most importantly the patient. In spite of all the advances in today's thoracic imaging confirmation of suspected malignant pleural effusion done by cytological methods or a pleural biopsy, a diagnostic thoracentesis is recommended for any unilateral effusion or bilateral effusion in an individual without obvious evidence of congestive heart failure [75]. Diagnostic thoracentesis is a useful initial approach for patients with MPEs. Thoracentesis takes place in diagnosis of MPE as well as reducing the symptoms. Thoracentesis also helps us in evaluation of the expansion capacity of the lung and relieving acute symptoms.

Traditionally, land selection for thoracentesis is determined by radiographic and physical examination findings [76]. There is no absolute contraindication for thoracentesis. Relative contraindications include a minimal effusion < 1 cm in thickness from the fluid level to the chest wall on a lateral decubitus view, bleeding diathesis, anticoagulation, and mechanical ventilation. There is no increased bleeding in patients with mild-to moderate coagulopathy or thrombocytopenia (prothrombin time or partial thromboplastin time >1.8 times normal, platelets <25,000/mm^3, or creatinine >6 mg/dL) [77]. Although it does not seem to increase the risk of pneumothorax in patients undergoing mechanical ventilation; if a pneumothorax occurs, the development of tension pneumothorax may be higher. Although the risk of pneumothorax rate is 10% in experienced hands, this risk increases in novices.

Important complications of thoracentesis include pneumothorax, bleeding, infection, and spleen or liver laceration. The amount of fluid drained during thoracentesis should be sufficient to obtain a diagnosis, relieve symptoms of dyspnea, and to avoid re-expansion pulmonary oedema or pneumothorax. The general belief and the guidelines proposed removal of more than 1500 ml in one hemithorax during a single transaction. However, this random number does not consider each patient's height and weight. As a general rule, the amount of fluid discharged from thoracentesis is 20 ml per kilogram of body weight [78]. On the other hand in recent studies, the risk of re-expansion pulmonary oedema was shown to be unrelated to the amount of drained fluid and it has been suggested that no upper limit is required [79].

Diagnostic thoracentesis is also useful in determining a patient's respiratory complaints that can be connected with effusion: Improvement in the patient's symptoms after thoracentesis indicates that the patient can take advantage of more invasive procedures and improve the quality of life. Persistence of respiratory symptoms in patients after thoracentesis, other causes should be investigated and before proceeding, more invasive diagnostic options should be considered twice.

The use of ultrasound guidance is preferred in thoracentesis. Ultrasound guidance, at the time of determining the location of the pleural fluids reduces accidental injury, and this technique to remove the liquid used to assess the degree of lung reexpansion [80].

Thoracoscopy should only be done in patients not diagnosed by less invasive procedures. Actual thoracoscopic techniques include video-assisted thoracoscopic surgery (VATS) [81] and medical thoracoscopy with either a rigid thoracoscope [82] or a semirigid pleuroscope [83, 84]. The advantages of thoracoscopy include visually directed and selective biopsies of parietal, mediastinal, and visceral pleura, direct visualization and examination of the entire hemithorax, and simultaneous lung or lymph node biopsy if required. The procedure is well tolerated with less than 1% mortality [85, 86].

Medical thoracoscopy when compared with surgical thoracoscopy (which is more precisely known as video-assisted thoracic surgery (VATS) has the advantage that it can be performed under local anaesthesia or conscious sedation, in an endoscopy suite, using nondisposable rigid instruments. Physicians skilled in bronchoscopy should find the semirigid pleuroscope easy to use because it has the same light source, video equipment, and manual controls as the fiberoptic bronchoscope [83, 84].Thus, it is considerably less invasive and less expensive than VATS. As an exception: VATS that allows huge biopsy samples can be taken, is preferred to medical thoracoscopy in patients with suspected mesothelioma. For diagnosis of mesothelioma and classification of its subtype, a large pleural biopsy specimen is often necessary. Immunohistochemical staining provides essential information in the diagnostic evaluation [6].

Medical thoracoscopy is primarily a diagnostic procedure [47, 87, 88]. In cases of undiagnosed exudative effusions with a high clinical suspicion for malignancy, some clinicians may proceed directly to thoracoscopy if the facilities for medical thoracoscopy are available. The procedure should be performed for diagnosis and possible talc poudrage [47].

The sensitivity of medical thoracoscopy was higher than that of cytology and closed pleural biopsy combined (96 versus 74%, pv0.001). Similar results have been reported by other investigators [89-92]. The reasons for false-negative thoracoscopy include insufficient and nonrepresentative biopsies that depend largely on the experience of the thoracoscopist [89, 92] and the presence of adhesions that prevent access to neoplastic tissue [87, 89].

The diagnostic yield of bronchoscopy is low in patients with undiagnosed pleural effusions and should not be undertaken routinely [93-95]. However, it is indicated when endobronchial lesions are suspected because of haemoptysis, atelectasis, or large effusions without contralateral mediastinal shift. Thoracotomy for diagnostic purposes is almost never indicated, because less invasive methods can provide diagnosis in up to 97% of cases [89, 96, 97].

7. Prognostic factors

Despite all the recent advances in cancer treatment management, MPE is suggestive of end stage disease with poor prognosis [51]. The mean survival is 3-6 months after diagnosis of malignant pleural effusion. Whereas, this period can take up to 4-12 months depending upon the histological subtype of the primary tumor such as in breast cancer, Hodgkin's disease, or lymphoma [98, 99]. The International Association for the Study of Lung Cancer reclassified MPE to the M1a descriptor, recognizing its prediction for poor long-term survival with an overall 5-year survival rate of 7% [100]. In addition, patients with malignant effusions, and a pH of less than 7:30 with wicked prognosis, shorter median survival, and poorer response to tetracycline pleurodesis and have a high rate of first finding of malignant cells in fluid cytology [61, 101]

On the other hand, malignant pleural effusion significantly affects the quality of life and reduced mobility of patients with malignant disease.The main goals of treatment for pleural effusion are to decrease symptoms and improve the quality of life [11].

8. Treatment

The aims of the treatment include drainage of pleural space, apposition of the visceral and pleural surfaces with complete expansion of the lung, and obliteration of the pleural surface with dispersion of a sclerosing agent throughout the pleural space [78]. Treatment options for malignant pleural effusion (MPE) are varied and often tailored to the clinician's specialty and expertise, the patient's physical performance status, hospitalization status, and individual desires [78].

Selection of optimal treatment for each individual patient requires a careful assessment of the benefits and the risks of the treatment. Primary treatment targets should involve palliation or elimination of dyspnea, improvement of a patient's overall quality of life in order to restore daily activities, and implementation of oncological therapies [102]. Treatment options include repeat thoracentesis, tube thoracostomy with drainage and sclerosis with chemical sclerosant agents, chronic indwelling pleural catheter, pleuroperitoneal shunt, intrapleural or systemic chemotherapy, thoracoscopy with drainage and talc insufflation, and pleurectomy [78].

8.1. Therapeutic thoracentesis

Therapeutic thoracentesis must be performed in all symptomatic patients with MPE. Up to 50% of patients may not have significant symptom relief due to comorbid conditions, generalized deconditioning from their malignancy, or incomplete re-expansion of the lung. Trapped lung may result from pleural-based malignancy or metastasis, pleural loculations, or bronchial obstruction with post-obstruction collapse [15]. A total of 98%–100% of patients will have reaccumulation of pleural fluid and recurrence of associated symptoms within 30 days of thoracentesis [103,104]. Therefore, recurrent thoracentesis may be a viable therapeutic approach for patients who have limited life expectancy or who are poor candidates for more definitive but invasive interventions [14].

Massive pleural effusions should be drained in a controlled fashion, avoiding evacuation of more than 1.5 l at one time or should be slowed down to about 500 ml/h. A massive evacuation of pleural fluid and rapid re-expansion of the lung can cause discomfort, bothersome cough, and hypotension. Reexpansion pulmonary oedema is a rare complication after rapid drainage of pleural effusion [105]. The mechanism of oedema progression is not fully clarified, but it is believed that it is mostly related to mechanical forces causing vascular stretching or injury, and increasing capillary permeability rather than the absolute level of negative pleural pressure [106].

8.2. Tube thoracostomy and pleurodesis

The aim of tube thoracostomy in MPE is primarily to drainage of the pleural cavity and demonstration of lung re-expansion before instillation of a chemical sclerosant. Typically a large bore chest tube is used though smaller bore tubes [10-14F) have been used for chemical pleurodesis [107-109]. Large bore chest tubes are associated with greater patient discomfort but have traditionally been used because of the concern of obstruction of smaller bore tubes by fibrin plugs. However, several randomized trials have compared small versus large bore chest tubes without significant difference in pleurodesis outcome [107, 110, 111].

Simple small bore drainage catheters have been used effectively. Gravity drainage of the pleural fluid can be accomplished and pleurodesis can be achieved with several agents. In one study, small-bore catheters yielded outcomes equivalent to patients receiving chest tube after diagnostic thoracoscopy, and in addition, they were more comfortable [107]. Additional small studies have been performed with early success using bleomycin or talc sclerotherapy [110, 112, 113].

An earlier randomized trial noted that pleurodesis following rapid drainage (median chest tube duration, 2 days) was equivalent to pleurodesis performed after drainage was less than 150 mL/day (median chest tube duration, 7 days). In summary, drainage of MPE using small bore catheter drainage and rapid pleurodesis achieves results similar to prolonged drainage prior to pleurodesis [78].

Lung re-expansion is necessary for a successful pleurodesis. A failure of the lung to expand completely after removal of fluid is suggestive of a trapped lung [114]. Radiographic appearance of lung re-expansion can determine an adequate timing for pleurodesis; the amount of pleural fluid drainage is not particularly significant in the timing and outcome of pleurodesis. After pleurodesis, the chest tube can be removed once the pleural fluid drainage is less than 150 ml/day [115, 116]. Failure of pleurodesis may be due to incomplete drainage of the effusion, unequal distribution of a sclerosing agent within the pleural cavity, or trapped lung syndrome [17].

Pleurodesis is performed by mixing the sclerosing agent of choice with 50–100 mL of sterile saline and then instilling it into the pleural cavity through the chest tube or small-bore catheter. The chest tube is clamped for 1–2 h and then reconnected to suction. No benefit in distribution of sclerosant or outcome or has been shown from rotating the patient [118, 119].

A number of antineoplastic and non-antineoplastic agents are used for pleurodesis. Sterilized asbestos-free talc consistently produces the highest success rates regardless of how it is implemented. Talc can be applied as poudrage or slurry. Poudrage is insufflation of talc powder after evacuation of fluid, while slurry is instillation of talc solution through the chest tube after tube thoracostomy and evacuation of an effusion [120]. Walker et al. reported success with the use of talc in 93% (153/165) of patients with MPE [120] Viallat et al. reported a 79% success rate in patients with malignant mesothelioma and an 89% success rate in patients with other malignancies underlying pleural metastasis [121]. Kılıc et al. reported that the success rates with talc insufflation by VATS were 81% in patients with pleural malignant mesothelioma and 91% in those with other malignancies, defined by a reacculumation ratio in 90 days of 19% (6/31) and 9% (2/24), respectively [122].

The video-assisted thoracoscopic talc poudrage with talc slurry via chest tube in patients with MPE has shown similar efficacy [30-day outcome: 78% for poudrage and 71% for slurry). Respiratory complications seem to be slightly higher after talc insufflations (i.e., insufflation 14% vs slurry 6%) [123]. Talc is usually well tolerated, and its most common side effects are pleuritic chest pain and fever. Acute respiratory distress syndrome has been reported with talc pleurodesis, which correlates with higher doses [124-126].

Tetracycline was commonly used in the past in association with tube thoracostomy. Instillation of the tetracycline solution provides a faster pleurodesis and pleural symphysis than chest tube drainage alone; however, it may cause significant pain. Doxycycline is an available alternative to tetracycline and is felt to have roughly equal effectiveness [127].

Bleomycin, an antineoplastic agent, is used in pleurodesis as a sclerosing agent. The precise mechanism of action of bleomycin and other antineoplastic agents is not fully understood, but the optimal dose is 1IU/kg (average 60 IU). In a study on 199 patients with malignant pleural effusion, bleomycin achieved a 54% (108 patients) complete response rate [120]. In the same study, 24% of patients had chest pain, 24% had fever, and 11% suffered from nausea. Hemoptysis, rashes, and diarrhea were also reported. Other rare side effects of bleomycin include alopecia and pulmonary fibrosis. Diacon et al. compared bleomycin with talc poudrage. The response to bleomycin was 59% whereas it was 87% for talc poudrage [128]. The disadvantages of bleomycin are its lower success rate and higher cost compared with tetracycline and talc.

Other agents tested for use for pleurodesis include cisplatin, cytarabine, doxorubicin, 5-FU, b-interferon, mitomycin C, and Corynebacterium parvum; however, these agents are not commonly used because of their high cost, adverse effects, and low efficacy [129].

8.3. Chronic indwelling pleural catheter

In patients not suitable for pleurodesis, or with recurrent MPE after pleurodesis, chronic intermittent drainage via a subcutaneous tunneled pleural catheter on an outpatient basis has been shown to relieve dyspnea effectively without serious complications [78,130]. A limited number of studies focused on the use of a chronic indwelling pleural catheter in patients with MPE. Putnam et al. summarized their experience with 100 consecutive patients with MPE treated with a chronic indwelling pleural catheter [78]. They concluded that placement of an indwelling pleural catheter was safe, effective and cost-effective. Hospitalization was only one day for patients treated with the pleural catheter, in contrast to 7 days with tube thoracostomy and sclerosis with doxycycline [12].

In a study by Pollak et al., the effectiveness of tunneled pleural catheter's in the treatment of malignant pleural effusions was assessed in 28 patients [130]. Dyspnea improved in 94% at 48th h and 91% on 30th day. Control of the MPE was achieved in 90% of patients. They concluded that the pleural catheter requires a shorter hospitalization and can be placed and managed on an outpatient basis. Other authors concluded that placement of an indwelling catheter was the right procedure in subjects with evidence of a trapped lung [131]. With respect to potential complications of pleural catheters, infections and dislocations of the catheter are seen most often. However, serious complications are uncommon.

8.4. Pleuroperitoneal shunt

The pleuroperitoneal shunt was introduced in 1982 for the management of pleural effusions. Pleuroperitoneal shunts transfer fluid from the pleural space to the peritoneal cavity actively when manually pumped (Denver shunt) or passively (LeVeen shunt). Several series have shown that effective palliation can be achieved in up to 90% of cases [132, 133]. It is used for patients who have failed pleurodesis or systemic chemotherapy, are not surgical candidates, or have trapped lung. The major disadvantage of the pleuroperitoneal shunt is the length of time required to drain the pleural space. The volume of pumping chamber is only 1.5 to 2mL, which translates into the necessity for frequent and protracted pumping sessions, a major inconvenience for patients. Infection and shunt occlusion are the most significant complications, occurring in up to 15% of cases [134].

8.5. Systemic or intrapleural chemotherapy

For the patients with chemosensitive tumors, including small cell lung cancer, lymphomas, and tumors of the breast, prostate, ovary, or thyroid, or those which have arisen from germ cells, systemic therapy can prove to be equally or more effective than local therapy for relieving malignant effusions. After the initial therapeutic thoracentesis, chemotherapy must be administered and pleurodesis, can be delayed until systemic treatment becomes ineffective [135].

Administration of chemotherapeutic agents directly into the pleural space has the potential to control the underlying malignancy and/or the MPE by producing high drug concentrations localized at the malignancy site while minimizing systemic toxicity [138]. Ideal agents would have a slow clearance rate from the intrapleural cavity, allowing greater exposure of cancer cells to the cytotoxic agent. Doxorubicin hydrochloride, cisplatin, cytarabine, mitomycin C, and 5-FU are some of the agents used.

Several studies have investigated the intrapleural use of several active cytokines. Interleukin-2 and interferon-β have been used. Their success varies but, in general, the results were poorer than that of talc [137, 138]. Staphylococcus aureus superantigen (SSAg) is one of the newer agents. Given current indwelling methods allowing chronic access to the pleural cavity, intrapleural chemotherapy remains a potential mechanism of drug administration, however, further studies are required.

8.6. Thoracoscopy

Tube thoracostomy and drainage with instillation of sclerosing agents is the most common treatment used for malignant pleural effusion. Chest tube drainage and pleurodesis does not allow lysis of adhesions to drain loculated effusions, which are often the reason for failure. The video-thoracoscopic approach allows for breaking of fibrin bridges and consequent loculations, insufflating talc uniformly on pleural surfaces, and full re-expansion of the lung [139].

The video-assisted thoracoscopy (VATS) should replace conventional instillation of talc slurry through tube thoracostomy as a procedure of choice to achieve pleurodesis. VATS pleurodesis offers reasonable palliation of MPE with low morbidity and rapid recovery. It is a safe and effective approach with an efficacy ranging from 88 to 97.5% [139, 140]. The VATS seems to be superior to simple chest tube drainage in management of MPE (92.3% vs 59.3%), with remission rates of 88.5 and 44.4% respectively [42,43]. In a series of 148 patients (VATS pleurodesis in 82 patients and tube thoracostomy with pleurodesis in 66 patients), VATS demonstrated longer recurrence-free survival and improved quality of life [142].

Thoracoscopic mechanical pleurodesis is a parietal pleura abrasion causing inflammation and adhesion of the parietal and visceral pleurae as a result of the healing process. Abrasion of the parietal pleura is initiated to yield uniform oozing. An injury to the visceral pleura should be avoided to reduce the risk of parenchymal injury, which would cause long-lasting postoperative air leak. Its efficacy was re-evaluated in a series of breast cancer patients (n=87) with MPE. Thoracoscopic mechanical pleurodesis and talc pleurodesis demonstrated similar success rates (92 and 91%, respectively) [143].

A VATS pleurectomy can provide excellent pleurodesis with less postoperative discomfort and pulmonary dysfunction compared to thoracotomy. Another benefit of VATS pleurectomy is a reduction of chest pain in patients with malignant tumors of the pleura and lung disease. In addition, it carries a lower risk of postoperative morbidity, less discomfort, and a better quality of life in terminally ill patients [144].

8.7. Pleurectomy

Pleurectomy, which is a palliative debulking procedure, is used to reduce the size of the tumor. However, it can also be done to relieve the lung and provide pleurodesis as a result of severe adhesions between the lung and the chest cavity. A posterolateral thoracotomy provides adequate access to the pleura. The pleura is stripped from the apex to the diaphragm. Dissection is continued in anterior, posterior, and apical aspects of the chest wall [144].

The procedure has a low mortality rate (1.5 to 5%), and it is well tolerated in patients with multiple morbidities [145]. Most authors concluded that thoracotomy was not indicated in patients with malignant effusion because of the high complication rate and prolonged hospitalization [146]. Most authors now agree that VATS is the only surgical approach that can be used in these patients [135, 147].

9. Conclusion

In conclusion, almost any cancer can produce an MPE which is a common clinical problem in thoracic surgery. MPE is prevalent disease and its therapy is essential. The presence of a malignant pleural effusion usually indicates advanced disease that is incurable with surgery alone. At all events, control of malignant pleural effusions is often difficult and inadequate. The risks of the therapy options should be considered meticulously. The survival time is short and expressed with months in patients with MPE. The goal of the treatment is to decrease the symptoms and the duration of hospitalization as well as to improve the quality of life of the patient. Also we aimed to return the patients and their families to daily life as earliest as possible. In order to achieve these targets, the therapy should be established for each patient according to the type, severity, localization and prognosis

Author details

Hidir Esme and Mustafa Calik

Konya Education and Research Hospital, Konya, Turkey

References

[1] Albertine KH, Wiener-Kronish JP, Bastacky J, et al: No evidence for mesothelial cell contact across the costal pleural space of sheep. J Appl Physiol 1999;170:123–134.

[2] Staub NC. Lung liquid and protein exchange: the four inhomogeneities. Ann Biomed Eng 1987;15(2):115–126.

[3] Miserocchi G. Physiology and pathophysiology of pleural fluid turnover. Eur Respir J 1997;10(1):219–225

[4] Cheng D, Rodriguez RM, Perkett EA, Rogers J, Bienvenu G, Lappalainen U, Light RW Vascular endothelial growth factor in pleural fluid. Chest 1999;116:760–765

[5] Bennett R, Maskell N Management of malignant pleural effusions. Curr Opin Pulm Med 2005;11:296–300.

[6] Robinson BWS, Lake RA: Advances in malignant mesothelioma. N Engl J Med 2005;353:1591–1603.

[7] Lombardi G, Zustovich F, Nicoletto MO, Donach M, Artioli G, Pastorelli D Diagnosis and treatment of malignant pleural effusion: a systematic literature review and new approaches. Am J Clin Oncol 2010;33:420–423.

[8] Johnston WW: The malignant pleural effusion. A review of cytopathologic diagnoses of 584 specimens from 472 consecutive patients. Cancer 1985;56:905–909

[9] Khaleeq G, Musani AI. Emerging paradigms in the management of malignant Respir Med. 2008 Jul;102(7):939-48.

[10] Putnam JB Jr, Light RW, Rodriguez RM, et al. A randomized comparison of indwelling pleural catheter and doxycycline pleurodesis in the management of malignant pleural effusions. Cancer 1999;86:1992–1999.

[11] Van den Toorn LM, Schaap E, Surmont VF, Pouw EM, van der Rijt KC, van Klaveren RJ. Management of recurrent malignant pleural effusions with a chronic indwelling pleural catheter. Lung Cancer. 2005 Oct;50(1):123-7.

[12] Chernow B, Sahn SA. Carcinomatous involvement of the pleura:an analysis of 96 patients. Am J Med. 1977;63:695–702.

[13] Musani AI, Haas AR, Seijo L, et al. Outpatient management of malignant pleural effusions with small-bore, tunneled pleural catheters. Respiration. 2004;71:559–66.

[14] Hsia David, Musani Ali I. Management of malignant pleural effusions Curr Respir Care Rep 2012;1:73–81

[15] Meyer PC. Metastatic carcinoma of the pleura.Thorax. 1966;21;437-443.

[16] Light RW, Hamm H. Malignant pleural effusion: would the real cause please stand up? Eur Respir J.1997;10:1701-1702.

[17] Antony VB, Loddenkemper R, Astoul P, Boutin C, Goldstraw P, Hott J, Rodriguez Panadero F, Sahn SA. Management of malignant pleural effusions. Eur Respir J. 2001 Aug;18(2):402-19.

[18] Martinez-Moragon E, Aparicio J, Sanchis J, Menendez R, Cruz Rogado M, Sanchis F. Malignant pleural effusion: prognostic factors for survival and response to chemical pleurodesis in a series of 120 cases. Respiration 1998;65:108—13

[19] Estenne M, Yernault JC, DeTroyer A. Mechanism of relief of dyspnoea after thoracentesis in patients with large pleural effusions. Am J Med 1983; 74: 813–819.

[20] Sahn SA. Malignancy metastatic to the pleura. Clin Chest Med 1998;19(2):351–361.

[21] Blackmore CC, Black WC, Dallas RV, Crow HC. Pleural fluid volume estimation: a chest radiograph prediction rule. Acad Radiol. 1996;3(2):103-109.

[22] Qureshi NR, Gleeson FV. Imaging of pleural disease. Clin Chest Med. 2006;27(2): 193-213.

[23] Shannon VR, Eapen GA, Jimenez CA, et al. Respiratory complications. In: Kufe DW, Blast Jr RC, Hait WN, et al., eds. Cancer Medicine 7. 7th edition. Philadelphia, PA, USA: BC Decker Inc;2006:2150-2173.

[24] Koh DM, Burke S, Davies N, Padley SP: Transthoracic US of the chest: clinical uses and applications. Radiographics 2002; Jan-Feb;22(1):e1.

[25] Heffner JE, Klein JS, Hampson C. Diagnostic utility and clinical application of imaging for pleural space infections. Chest. 2010;137:467-479.

[26] Mergo PJ, Helmberger T, Didovic J, et al: New formula for quantifi cation of pleural effusions from computed tomography. J Thorac Imaging 1999; 14:122–125.

[27] Mori K, Hirose T, Machida S, et al. Helical computed tomography diagnosis of pleural dissemination in lung cancer: comparison of thick-section and thin-section helical computed tomography. J Thorac Imaging 1998;13(3):211–218.

[28] Marom EM, Erasmus JJ, Pass HI, Patz EF Jr. The role of imaging in malignant pleural mesothelioma. Semin Oncol 2002;29(1): 26–35.

[29] Davis SD, Henschke CI, Yankelevitz DF, et al: MR imaging of pleural effusions. J Comput Assist Tomogr 1990;14:192–198.

[30] Gupta NC, Rogers JS, Graeber GM, et al. Clinical role of F-18 fluorodeoxyglucose positron emission tomography imaging in patients with lung cancer and suspected malignant pleural effusion. Chest 2002;122(6):1918–1924.

[31] Shamus R. Carr and Joseph S. Friedberg Malignant Effusions Oncology: An Evidence-Based Approach Editors Alfred E. Chang,Patricia A. Ganz,Daniel F. Hayes,Timothy Kinsella,Harvey I. Pass,Joan H. Schiller,Richard M. Stone,Victor Streche ;2006, Section seven, 1527-1534,

[32] Light RW. Pleural effusion. N Engl J Med 2002;346:1971–7.

[33] Light RW, MacGregor MI, Luchsinger PC, Ball WC Jr. Pleural effusions: the diagnostic separation of transudates and exudates. Ann Intern Med 1972;77(4):507–513.

[34] Burgess LJ, Maritz FJ, Taljaard JJ. Comparative analysis of the biochemical parameters used to distinguish between pleural transudates and exudates. Chest 1995;107(6): 1604–1609.

[35] Romero S, Candela A, Martin C, Hernandez L, Trigo C, Gil J. Evaluation of different criteria for the separation of pleural transudates from exudates. Chest 1993;104(2): 399–404.

[36] Heffner JE, Highland K, Brown LK. A meta-analysis derivation of continuous likelihood ratios for diagnosing pleural fluid exudates. Am J Respir Crit Care Med. 2003;167(12):1591-1599.

[37] Porcel JM, Alvarez M, Salud A, Vives M. Should a cytologic study be ordered in transudative pleural effusions? Chest. 1999;116:1836-1837.

[38] Ashchi M, Golish J, Eng P, O'Donovan P. Transudative malignant pleural effusions: prevalence and mechanisms. South Med J. 1998;91:23-26.

[39] Heffner JE, Klein JS.Recent advances in the diagnosis and management of malignant pleural effusions. Mayo Clin Proc. 2008 Feb;83(2):235-50

[40] Romero-Candeira S, Fernandez C, Martin C, et al. Influence of diuretics on the concentration of proteins and other components of pleural transudates in patients with heart failure. Am J Med 2001;110:681–6.

[41] Keller RR: Once more: Light's criteria revisited. Respiration 2000;67:11–12.

[42] Heffner JE, Brown LK, Barbieri CA: Diagnostic value of tests that discriminate between exudative and transudative pleural effusions. Chest 1997;111:970–980.

[43] Ferrer J, Roldan J, Teixidor J, et al. Predictors of pleural malignancy in patients with pleural effusion undergoing thoracoscopy. Chest 2005; 127:1017–22.

[44] Abouzgheib W, Bartter T, Dagher H, Pratter M, Klump W. A prospective study of the volume of pleural fluid required for accurate diagnosis of malignant pleural effusion. Chest. 2009;135:999-1001.

[45] Swiderek J, Morcos S, Donthireddy V, et al. Prospective study to determine the volume of pleural fluid required to diagnose malignancy. Chest. 2010;137:68-73.

[46] Ong KC, Indumathi V, Poh WT, Ong YY. The diagnostic yield of pleural fluid cytology in malignant pleural effusions. Singapore Med J. 2000; 41(1):19-23.

[47] Loddenkemper R. Thoracoscopy——state of the art. Eur Respir J 1998;11:213—21.

[48] Prakash UB, Reiman HM. Comparison of needle biopsy with cytologic analysis for the evaluation of pleural effusion: analysis of 414 cases. Mayo Clin Proc 1985;60:158 —64.

[49] Starr RL, Sherman ME: The value of multiple preparations in the diagnosis of malignant pleural effusions. A cost-benefi t analysis. Acta Cytol 1991;35:533–537.

[50] Ruckdeschel JC. Management of malignant pleural effusions. Semin Oncol 1995;22: 58—63.

[51] Light RW. Management of pleural effusions. J Formos Med Assoc 2000;99(7):523–531.

[52] Celikoglu F, Teirstein AS, Krellenstein DJ, Strauchen JA. Pleural effusion in non-Hodgkin's lymphoma. Chest 1992;101(5):1357–1360.

[53] Prakash UB, Reiman HM. Comparison of needle biopsy with cytologic analysis for the evaluation of pleural effusion: analysis of 414 cases. Mayo Clin Proc 1985;60(3): 158–164.

[54] Canto A, Rivas J, Saumench J, Morera R, Moya J. Points to consider when choosing a biopsy method in cases of pleurisy of unknown origin. Chest 1983;84(2):176–179.

[55] Chakrabarti B, Ryland I, Sheard J, Warburton CJ, Earis JE. The role of Abrams percutaneous pleural biopsy in the investigation of exudative pleural effusions. Chest. 2006;129(6):1549-1555.

[56] McLean AN, Bicknell SR, McAlpine LG, Peacock AJ. Investigation of pleural effusion: an evaluation of the new Olympus LTF semiflexible thoracofiberscope and comparison with Abram's needle biopsy. Chest. 1998;114(1):150-153.

[57] Maskell NA, Gleeson FV, Davies RJ. Standard pleural biopsy versus CT-guided cutting-needle biopsy for diagnosis of malignant disease in pleural effusions: a randomised controlled trial. Lancet. 2003;361(9366):1326-1330.

[58] Sahn SA. Thoracentesis and pleural biopsy. In: Shelhamer J, Pizzo PA, Parillo JE, Masur H, eds Respiratory disease in the immunosuppressed host. Philadelphia, J.B. Lippincott, 1991; p. 129.

[59] Villena V, Lopez Encuentra A, De Pablo A, et al. Ambulatory diagnosis of the patients requiring a pleural biopsy. Study of 100 consecutive cases Arch Bronconeumol 1997; 33: 395–8.

[60] Lesho EP, Roth BJ: Is pH paper an acceptable, low-cost alternative to the blood gas analyzer for determining pleural fl uid pH? Chest 1997;112:1291–1292.

[61] Sahn SA, Good JT Jr. Pleural fluid pH in malignant effusions: diagnostic, prognostic, and therapeutic implications. Ann Intern Med 1988; 108: 345–349.

[62] Sanchez-Armengol A, Rodriguez-Panadero F. Survival and talc pleurodesis in metastatic pleural carcinoma, revisited. Chest 1993; 104: 1482–1485.

[63] Rodriguez-Panadero F, Lopez-Mejias L. Low glucose and pH levels in malignant effusions; diagnostic significance and prognostic value in respect to pleurodesis. Am Rev Respir Dis 1989; 139: 663–667.

[64] Good JT, Taryle DA, Sahn SA. The pathogenesis of low glucose, low pH malignant effusions. Am Rev Respir Dis 1985; 131: 737–741.

[65] Rodriguez-Panadero F, Lopez-Majias L. Survival time of patients with pleural metastatic carcinoma predicted by glucose and pH studies. Chest 1989; 95:320–324.

[66] Sahn SA: State of the art. The pleura. Am RevRespir Dis 1988;138:184–234.

[67] Yam LT: Diagnostic signifi cance of lymphocytes in pleural effusions. Ann Intern Med 1967;66:972–982.

[68] Martinez-Garcia MA, Cases-Viedma E, Cordero-Rodriguez PJ, et al: Diagnostic utility of eosinophils in the pleural fluid. Eur Respir J 2000;15:166–169.

[69] Light RW, Erozan YS, Ball WC Jr: Cells in pleural fluid. Their value in differential diagnosis. Arch Intern Med 1973;132:854–860.

[70] Siyamek Neragi-Miandoab Malignant pleural effusion, current and evolving approaches for its diagnosis and management Lung Cancer 2006; 54, 1—9

[71] Terracciano D, Di Carlo A, Papa P, et al. New approaches in the diagnostic procedure of malignant pleural effusions. Oncol Rep 2004;12:79—83.

[72] Metintas M, Ozdemir N, Solak M, et al. Chromosome analysis in pleural effusions. Efficiency of this method in the differential diagnosis of pleural effusions. Respiration 1994;61:330—5.

[73] Grove CS, Lee YC: Vascular endothelial growth factor: the key mediator in pleural effusion formation. Curr Opin Pulm Med 2002;8:294–301.

[74] Cheng D, Lee YC, Rogers JT, et al: Vascular endothelial growth factor level correlates with transforming growth factor-beta isoform levels in pleural effusions. Chest 2000;118:1747–1753.

[75] Grogan DR, Irwin RS, Channick R, et al. Complications associated with thoracentesis. A prospective, randomized study comparing three different methods. Arch Intern Med 1990;150:873—7.

[76] Thomsen TW, DeLaPena J, Setnik GS. Videos in clinical medicine: thoracentesis. N Engl J Med. 2006;355(15):e16.

[77] McVay PA, Toy PTCY. Lack of increased bleeding after paracentesis and thoracentesis in patients with mild coagulation abnormalities. Transfusion 1991; 31:164–717.

[78] Putnam JB. Management of malignant pleural effusion: Sclerosis or chronic tube drainage. In: Ferguson MK. (ed.) Difficult Decisions in Thoracic Surgery. London: Springer; 2007. p 414-422

[79] Feller-Kopman D, Berkowitz D, Boiselle P, Ernst A. Large-volume thoracentesis and the risk of reexpansion pulmonary edema. Ann Thorac Surg.2007;84:1656-1661.

[80] Aaron M. Cheng, Douglas E. Wood Surgical and Endoscopic Palliation of Advanced Lung Cancer Surg Oncol Clin N Am 20 (2011) 779–790

[81] Tassi GF, Davies RJ, Noppen M. Advanced techniques in medical thoracoscopy. Eur Respir J. 2006;28(5):1051-1059.

[82] Mathur PN, Astoul P, Boutin C. Medical thoracoscopy: technical details. Clin Chest Med. 1995;16(3):479-486.

[83] Ernst A, Hersh CP, Herth F, et al. A novel instrument for the evaluation of the pleural space: an experience in 34 patients. Chest. 2002;122(5):1530-1534.

[84] Munavvar M, Khan MA, Edwards J, Waqaruddin Z, Mills J. The autoclavable semirigid thoracoscope: the way forward in pleural disease? Eur Respir J. 2007;29(3): 571-574

[85] Lewis RJ, Caccavale RJ, Sisler GE, MacKenzie JW. Video-assisted thoracic surgical resection of malignant lung tumors. J Thorac Cardiovasc Surg 1992;104(6):1679–1685; discussion 1685–1687.

[86] Cardillo G, Facciolo F, Carbone L, et al. Long-term follow-up ofvideo-assisted talc pleurodesis in malignant recurrent pleural effusions. Eur J Cardiothorac Surg 2002;21(2):302–305; discussion 305–306.).

[87] Loddenkemper R, Boutin C. Thoracoscopy: diagnostic and therapeutic indications. Eur Respir J 1993; 6:1544-1555

[88] Harris RJ, Kavuru MS, Rice TW, Kirby TJ. The diagnostic and therapeutic utility of thoracoscopy: a review. Chest 1995; 108: 828–841.

[89] Boutin C, Viallat JR, Cargnino P, Farisse P. Thoracoscopy in malignant pleural effusions. Am Rev Respir Dis 1981; 124: 588–592.

[90] Oldenburg FA Jr, Newhouse MT. Thoracoscopy: a safe accurate diagnostic procedure using the rigid thoracoscope and local anesthesia. Chest 1979; 75: 45–50.

[91] Menzies R, Charbonneau M. Thoracoscopy for thediagnosis of pleural disease. Ann Intern Med 1991;114: 271–276.

[92] Canto A, Blasco E, Casillas M, et al. Thoracoscopy in the diagnosis of pleural effusions. Thorax 1977; 32: 550–554.

[93] Kelly P, Fallouh M, O9Brien A, Clancy L. Fibreoptic bronchoscopy in the management of lone pleural effusion: a negative study. Eur Respir J 1990; 3: 397–398.

[94] Feinsilver SH, Barrows AA, Braman SS. Fiberoptic bronchoscopy and pleural effusion of unknown origin. Chest 1986; 90: 516–519.

[95] Poe RH, Levy PC, Israel RH, Ortiz CR, Kally MC. Use of fiberoptic bronchoscopy in the diagnosis of bronchogenic carcinoma: a study in patients with idiopathic pleural effusions. Chest 1994; 105: 1663–1667.

[96] Rusch VW, Mountain C. Thoracoscopy under regional anesthesia for the diagnosis and management of pleural disease. Am J Surg 1987;154(3):274–278.

[97] Hucker J, Bhatnagar NK, al-Jilaihawi AN, Forrester-Wood CP. Thoracoscopy in the diagnosis and management of recurrent pleural effusions. Ann Thorac Surg 1991;52(5):1145–1147.

[98] Bielsa S, Martin-Juan J, Porcel JM, Rodriguez-Panadero F. Diagnostic and prognostic implications of pleural adhesions in malignant effusions. J Thorac Oncol. 2008;3:1251-1256

[99] Fentiman IS, Millis R, Sexton S, Hayward JL. Pleural effusion in breast cancer: a review of 105 cases. Cancer 1981;47:2087—92.

[100] Detterbeck FC, Boffa DJ, Tanoue LT. The new lung cancer staging system. Chest 2009;136(1):260–71

[101] Heffner JE, Nietert PJ, Barbieri C. Pleural fluid pH as a predictor of survival for patients with malignant pleural effusions. Chest 2000;117:79–86.).

[102] Charpidou A., Harrington KJ, Syrigos KN. Management of Malignant Pleural Effusions. In: Syrigos KS., Nutting CM, Roussos C. (eds.) Tumors of the Chest Biology, Diagnosis and Management. Berlin: Springer; 2006. P563-573.

[103] Sorenson PG., Svendsen TL, Enk B. Treatment of malignant pleural effusion with drainage, with and without instillation of talc. Eur J Respir Dis. 1984;65:131–5.

[104] Groth G., Gatzemeier U, Haussingen K, et al. Intrapleural palliative treatment of malignant pleural effusions with mitoxantrone versus placebo (pleural tube alone). Ann Oncol. 1991; 2: 213–5.

[105] Tarver RD., Broderick LS, Conces DJ Jr. Reexpansion pulmonary edema. J Thorac Imaging 1996; 11: 198–209

[106] Sprung CL., Loewenherz JW, Baier H, Hauser JM. Evidence for increased permeability in re-expansion pulmonary edema. Am J Med 1981; 71: 497

[107] Clementsen P., Evald T, Grode G, et al. Treatment of malignant pleural effusion: pleurodesis using a small percutaneous catheter. A prospective randomized study. Respir Med. 1998; 92: 593–6.

[108] Goff BA., Mueller PR, Muntz HG, et al. Small chest-tube drainage followed by bleomycin sclerosis for malignant pleural effusions. Obstet Gynecol. 1993; 81: 993–6.

[109] Chen YM., Shih JF, Yang KY, et al. Usefulness of pig-tail catheter for palliative drainage of malignant pleural effusions in cancer patients. Support Care Canc. 2000; 8: 423–6.

[110] Parulekar W., Di Primio G, Matzinger F, et al. Use of small-bore vs. large-bore chest tubes for treatment of malignant pleural effusions. Chest. 2001; 120: 19–25.

[111] Caglayan B., Torun E, Turan D, et al. Efficacy of iodopovidone pleurodesis and comparison of small-bore catheter versus large bore chest tube. Ann Surg Oncol. 2008; 15: 2594–9.

[112] Marom EM., Patz EF Jr, Erasmus JJ, McAdams HP, Goodman PC, Herndon JE. Malignant pleural effusions: treatment with small-bore-catheter thoracostomy and talc pleurodesis. Radiology 1999; 210: 277–281.

[113] Bloom AI., Wilson MW, Kerlan RK Jr, Gordon RL, LaBerge JM. Talc pleurodesis through small-bore percutaneous tubes. Cardiovasc Intervent Radiol 1999; 22: 433–436.

[114] Perpina M., Benlloch E, Marco V, Abad F, Nauffal D. Effect of thoracentesis on pulmonary gas exchange. Thorax 1983; 38: 747–750.

[115] Sahn SA. Management of malignant pleural effusions. Monaldi Arch Chest Dis 2001; 56: 394–399.

[116] Yim AP., Chung SS, Lee TW, Lam CK, Ho JK. Thoracoscopic management of malignant pleural effusions. Chest 1996; 109: 1234–1238.

[117] Wong PS., Goldstraw P. Pleuroperitoneal shunts. Br J Hosp Med 1993; 50: 16–21.

[118] Dryzer SR., Allen ML, Strange C, et al. A comparison of rotation and nonrotation in tetracycline pleurodesis. Chest 1993;104:1763–9.

[119] Mager HJ., Maesen B, Verzijlbergen F, et al. Distribution of talc suspension during treatment of malignant pleural effusion with talc pleurodesis. Lung Cancer. 2002; 36: 77–81.

[120] Walker-Renard P., Vaughan LM, Sahn SA. Chemical pleurodesis for malignant pleural effusions. Ann Intern Med. 1994; 120: 56–64.

[121] Viallat J-R., Rey F, Astoul P, Boutin C. Thoracoscopic talc poudrage pleurodesis for malignant effusions. A review of 360 cases. Chest 1996; 110: 1387–93.

[122] Kilic D, Akay H, Kavukçu S, Kutlay H, Cangir AK, Enön S, Kadilar C. Management of Recurrent Malignant Pleural Effusion with Chemical Pleurodesis Surg Today. 2005; 35: 634-8

[123] Dresler CM., Olak J, Herndon JE II, Richards WG, Scalzetti E, Fleishman SB, Kernstine KH, Demmy T, Jablons DM, Kohman L, Daniel TM, Haasler GB, Sugarbaker DJ. Phase III intergroup study of talc poudrage vs talc slurry sclerosis for malignant pleural effusion. Chest 2005; 127: 909–915.

[124] de Campos JR., Vargas FS, de Campos Werebe E, Cardoso P, Teixeira LR, Jatene FB, Light RW Thoracoscopy talc poudrage: a 15-year experience. Chest 2001; 119: 801–806.

[125] Kennedy L., Rusch VW, Strange C, Ginsberg RJ, Sahn SA. Pleurodesis using talc slurry. Chest 1994; 106: 342–346

[126] Ferrer J., Villarino MA, Tura JM, Traveria A, Light RW. Talc preparations used for pleurodesis vary markedly from one preparation to another. Chest 2001; 119: 1901–1905

[127] Herrington JD., Gora-Harper ML, Salley RK. Chemical pleurodesis with doxycycline 1 g. Pharmacotherapy 1996; 16: 280–285.

[128] Diacon AH, Wyser C, Bolliger CT, Tamm M, Pless M, Perruchoud AP, et al. Prospective randomized comparison of thoracoscopic talc poudrage under local anesthesia versus bleomycin instillation for pleurodesis in malignant pleural effusions. Am J Respir Crit Care Med 2000; 162: 1445–9.

[129] Felletti R, Ravazonni C. Intrapleural Corynebacterium parvum for malignant pleural effusions. Thorax 1983; 38: 22–4.

[130] Pollak JS. Malignant pleural effusions: treatment with tunneled long-term drainage catheters. Curr Opin Pulm Med 2002; 83: 2—7.

[131] Pien GW., Gant MJ, Washam CL. Sterman DH. Use of an implantable pleural catheter for trapped lung syndrome in patients with malignant pleural effusion. Chest 2001; 119: 1641—6.

[132] Petrou M., Kaplan D, Goldstraw P. Management of recurrent malignant pleural effusions. The complementary role of talc pleurodesis and pleuroperitoneal shunting. Cancer (Phila) 1995; 75: 801–805.

[133] Lee KA, Harvey JC, Reich H, Beattie EJ. Management of malignant pleural effusions with pleuroperitoneal shunting. J Am Coll Surg 1994; 178: 568–586.

[134] Ponn RB., Blancaflor J, D'Agostino RS, Kiernan ME, Toole AL, Stern H. Pleuroperitoneal shunting for intractable pleural effusions. Ann Thorac Surg 1991; 51: 605–609

[135] Antony VB., Loddenkemper R, Astoul P, et al. Management of malignant pleural effusion. Am J Respir Crit Care Med 2000; 162: 1987.

[136] Perng RP, Chen YM, Wu MF, et al. Phase II trial of intrapleural paclitaxel injection for non-small-cell lung cancer patients with malignant pleural effusions. Respir Med. 1998; 92: 473–9.

[137] Kvale PA., Simoff M, Prakash UBS. Palliative care. Chest 2003; 123: 284

[138] Rosso R, Rimoldi R, Salvati F. İntrapleural natural beta interferon in the treatment of malignant pleural effusions. Oncology 1988; 45: 253.

[139] Marrazzo A., Noto A, Casà L, Taormina P, Lo Gerfo D, David M, Mercadante S. Video-Thoracoscopic Surgical Pleurodesis in the Management of Malignant Pleural Effu-

sion: The Importance of an Early Intervention J Pain Symptom Manage. 2005 ; 30: 75-9.

[140] Trotter D, Aly A, Siu L, Knight S. Video-assisted thoracoscopic (VATS) pleurodesis for malignant effusion: an Australian teaching hospital's experience. Heart Lung and Circulation 2005; 14: 93–97.

[141] Gu LJ, Wang WJ. Comparative study of video-assisted thoracoscopic surgery vs thoracic tube drainage in synthetic therapy for malignant pleural effusion secondary to non-small cell lung cancer. Nan Fang Yi Ke Da Xue Xue Bao 2006; 26: 1023–1026

[142] Luh SP, Chen CY, Tzao CY. Malignant pleural effusion treatment outcomes: pleurodesis via video-assisted thoracic surgery versus tube thoracostomy. Thorac Cardiovasc Surg 2006; 54: 332–336

[143] Crnjac A. The significance of thoracoscopic mechanical pleurodesis for the treatment of malignant pleural effusions. Wien Klin Wochenschr 2004; 116: 28–32

[144] Neragi-Miandoab S. Surgical and other invasive approaches to recurrent pleural effusion with malignant etiology. Support Care Cancer. 2008 Dec;16(12):1323-31.

[145] Rusch VW. Pleurectomy/decortication in the setting of multimodality treatment for diffuse malignant pleural mesothelioma. Semin Thorac Cardiovasc Surg 1997; 9: 367–372.

[146] Bernard A, de Dompsure R, Hagry O, Favre J. Early and late mortality after pleurodesis for malignant pleural effusion. Ann Thorac Surg 2002; 74: 213–217.

[147] Brega-Massone P, Conti B, Magnani B, Ferro F, Lequglie C. Minimally invasive thoracic surgery for diagnostic assessment and palliative treatment in recurrent neoplastic pleural effusion. Thorac Cardiovasc Surg 2004; 52: 191–195.

Chapter 5

Superior Sulcus Tumour with some Emphasis on the Anterior Approach

Haralabos Parissis, Alan Soo and Bassel Al-Alao

Additional information is available at the end of the chapter

http://dx.doi.org/10.5772/55724

1. Introduction

Superior sulcus tumours are rarely encountered in clinical practice, representing < 5% of all bronchogenic carcinomas [1, 2]. In 1932, Pancoast [3] published his classic article in which he reported four patients who had a similar presentation including pain in the shoulder and arm, weakness and wasting of the muscles of the hand, and ipsilateral Horner syndrome together with a lesion situated at the apex of the lung. Pancoast [3] rejected the pulmonary origin of the tumour that was recognised by Tobias [4], who described the same clinical syndrome in four other patients.

Pancoast syndrome is due to lesions extending to the superior thoracic inlet. Specific symptomatology mainly due to brachial plexus invasion accounts for the majority of those cases [5-7]. Pancoast tumour is a tumour of the apex of the lung with no intervening lung tissue between tumour and chest wall. Subsequently, there is an involvement of structures of the apical chest wall above the level of the second rib. Almost half of the treated cancers are squamous cell carcinomas (45-50%), while the rest are either adenocarcinomas (36-38%) or undifferentiated large-cell carcinomas (11-13%). The tumour rapidly involves the structures of the thoracic inlet & the root of neck. Due to its localisation in the apex of the lung, invasion of the lower part of the brachial plexus, first ribs, vertebrae, subclavian vessels or stellate ganglion, occurs [8-10]. The classical Pancoast presentation, with shoulder pain radiating to the ulnar side of the arm and the hand, is presented in 55 to 60% of the patients. Pain at the ulnar aspect of the forearm and hand is consistent with T1 involvement; furthermore symptomatology along the intrinsic hand muscles suggests the C8 root or lower trunk tumour deposits. Horner's syndrome is reported in up to 30% of the cases.

Superior sulcus tumours are not necessarily associated with the classic Pancoast syndrome. Though some controversy exists about their exact definition, it is generally accepted that they may be defined as primary lung cancers involving the apex of the chest wall and usually associated with pain in the shoulder and/or arm[9, 10].

Although those tumours represent a wide range of stage IIB to stage IV disease, (IIB (25-27%), stage IIIA (6-8%), stage IIIB (40-42%) and stage IV (21-23%) it is the T3, T4, N0-N1 subgroup of this spectrum that could be amenable to surgical intervention [11]. This subgroup of patients (less than 5% of Bronchogenic Carcinomas) however, is difficult to be treated surgically due to the location of the tumour and the complex anatomy of the area involved [12]. Historically, Pancoast tumours have been associated with high rates of incomplete resection, local recurrence, and death.

Pancoast tumours were thought to be located posteriorly and early attempts to resect those tumours were approached solely from the back. A percentage of these lesions might also be located at the front, with vascular rather than neuro-vertebral involvement. Various reports suggested spinal involvement in 15%, brachial plexus in 15% and subclavian vessels in 6% of the cases [13]. Therefore surgeons treating these cancers should be able to be familiar and adapt with the various approaches. An understanding of the posterior location of neural structures and somewhat anterior location of vascular structures is important for adequate operative planning.

This article alludes to the anatomy, initial assessment, and surgical approaches with an emphasis on the modified anterior approach for these cancers.

2. How does the treatment of pancoast tumours evolved the last decades

For more than 40 years the treatment of Pancoast tumours has centred on a bi-modality regimen consisting of preoperative external beam radiotherapy followed by surgery. Tri-modality treatment however with the addition of platinum based chemotherapy regimes has become currently the standard treatment, in order to achieve additive anti-tumour effects (chemotherapy as radiation sensitiser). According to Wright et al [14] induction chemo-radiotherapy (CT/RT) can be administered with low morbidity, a higher complete resection rate, a high pathologic response rate, a reduced loco-regional recurrence rate and improved survival. Further improvement in radiotherapy with the advent of 3-dimensional conformal radiotherapy, the total radiation dose that could be safely delivered was not anymore constrained by dose-limiting toxicities upon the nearby organs.

Careful patient selection for tri-modality treatment, on the basis of staging and comorbidity, is of vital importance in the treatment of Pancoast tumours. Nevertheless only 30% of M0 patients with Pancoast tumours were eligible for combined treatment according to Pourel et al [15]. Not only operability (patient fitness to surgery) but also ability to resect the tumour is of a major importance bearing in mind the difficulty of access, the crowded anatomy of this region and the tendency of the tumours in this area to involve important adjacent structures. As per the same group [15], following CT/RT, 67% of the patients were amenable to thoracotomy. The resection rate, which had remained unchanged at approximately 50% for almost 40 years with conventional preoperative radiotherapy, was improved to above 70% in SWOG [16] and JCOG [17] studies.

Preoperative radiotherapy was part of the standard treatment, but a recent prospective phase II study (Southwest Oncology Group 9416, INT 0160)[16], suggests that preoperative concurrent CT/RT (platinum-based chemotherapy and 45Gy of radiotherapy) improves the rate of complete resection, local recurrence, and intermediate-term survival. Like wise, the Japan Clinical Oncology Group JCOG trial 9806 [17]in a prospective report concluded along the same lines. Furthermore, Kwong et al [18] reported that high dose radiotherapy targeting up to 60 Gy (rather than 45 Gy) could be given in the neoadjuvant setting; it is successfully tolerated and associated with improved resection rate.

3. Applied surgical anatomy

The limited access and poor visualisation of the thoracic inlet is due to: 1) the unique course of the upper ribs downwards and outwards that render the neuro-vascular bundle inaccessible to posterior approaches, 2) the musculature of the area and also 3) the overlapping bulky pectoral-shoulder girdle with the clavicle and the manubrium to further restrict access from the neck. These anatomical idiosyncrasies create a hostile but challenging environment for the thoracic surgeon.

The main goal for cure is to achieve local control of the disease and aim for relapse-free, metastasis-free outcome. Local control is obtained by removing the upper lobe, chest wall and invaded structures (subclavian artery or vertebra), aiming for R0 resection margins. Radically resected cases yield better survival whereas R1 resections are associated with high incidence of local and distal recurrences. Involvement of the vertebral body or brachial plexus, once considered unresectable is nowadays amenable to advanced techniques of spinal reconstruction and should be planned jointly with a spine neurosurgeon. Finally, according to recent reports [16, 17], the rate of R0 resection could be above 85%, with the use of tri-modality protocols.

Contraindications for surgery would be due to metastasis, invasion of the brachial plexus above C7 & invasion of the spinal canal. Resection of the T1nerve root is usually well tolerated, but removal of the C8 root or lower trunk of the brachial plexus leads to loss of hand and arm function. N2 disease is a relative contraindication and some groups enrol those patients after extended hilar radiation. As per JCOG [17]rib involvement occurs in 77.2% of the patients (usually 3 ribs or more), vertebra involvement in 10.5% of the patients, and major vessels in 5.3%. T1 involvement is the commonest root involved in up to 85% of the cases.

4. Various treatment modalities and tumour down-staging

According to Wright et al [10], marked difference in pathologic response based on the induction therapy is favouring CT/RT. Surgical resection of Pancoast tumours after neoadjuvant high-dose CT/RT was carried out in 40.5% of patients according to Kwong et al [18].

Pathological downstaging although it does not correlate with the radiological appearance [16] is reported to be impressively above 30% in various series. As per Pourel et al [15], pathological complete response was observed in 39.5% of the patients, necrosis of tumoural tissues between 50% and 95% in 22.5% and less than 50% in 38% of the patients. Along the same lines JCOG reported [17] pathologic downstaging of the tumour in 40% of the patients; No residual viable tumour cells in the resected specimens, was achieved in 16% of the treated patients. Finally SWOG [16] summarised that pathologic no residual microscopic tumour was seen in one third of the resected specimens and minimal microscopic residual (few scattered tumour foci within a mostly necrotic or fibrotic mass), was observed in one third of the resected specimens.

5. What are the various surgical approaches

The approach of Paulson [19] is completely satisfactory in dealing with posteriorly located tumours; however, it is not fully adequate in the presence of invasion of anteriorly located structures (especially subclavian vessels or their branches). Therefore, different anterior approaches have been developed in the last 25 years, including the cervicosterno-thoracothomy[20] or the hemi-clamshell incision [21, 22], the transcervical-transthoracic approach with resection of the clavicle [23, 24], and the trans-manubrial approach [25]. Exact indications for these different approaches remain controversial, and few data are available about long-term outcome of patients treated by anterior approaches [22, 24, 26].

Posterior approach (Paulson)/ posterolateral-paravertebral thoracotomy: This is an extension of the conventional postero-lateral thoracotomy; the incision is extending around the tip of the scapula, then it continuous upwards and further midway between the posterior edge of the scapula and the spinous processes, up to the level of C7. By taking the scapula of the chest wall this incision allows good exposure of the posterior chest wall, including the transverse processes, the vertebrae and the roots of the thoracic nerves and the plexus [27]. Nevertheless the exposure of the neuro-vascular structures are limited. This is due to the fact that brachial plexus and vascular structures often lie above the tumour mass and access to such structures, is significantly limited using approaches from below.

According to Vanakesa et al [28], Posterior approach, does not provide adequate access to the many important structures which may be involved by apical chest tumours of bronchogenic origin. This restricted access may be one of the reasons for the high rate of incomplete resections [29] and high surgical morbidity and mortality using this approach [10]. The anterior-cervical entry [24] proved to be the answer to the problem of limited exposure. It appears to be the optimal approach to anterior lung apex or first rib lesions [30].

We would facilitate a case like the one presented in Figure 1 by using an anterior-manubrial-sternal approach for access.

Accurate and thorough staging & re-staging (Radiological response is defined according to the RECIST criteria [31]following neoadjuvant treatment is necessary prior to surgery (see Figure 2) and typically includes CT-PET and magnetic resonance imaging (Contrast-enhanced MRI of Chest and Brain). MRA is a noninvasive diagnostic method complementary to MR imaging for detecting vascular involvement in bronchogenic carcinoma with Pancoast syndrome [32].

http://dx.doi.org/10.5772/55724

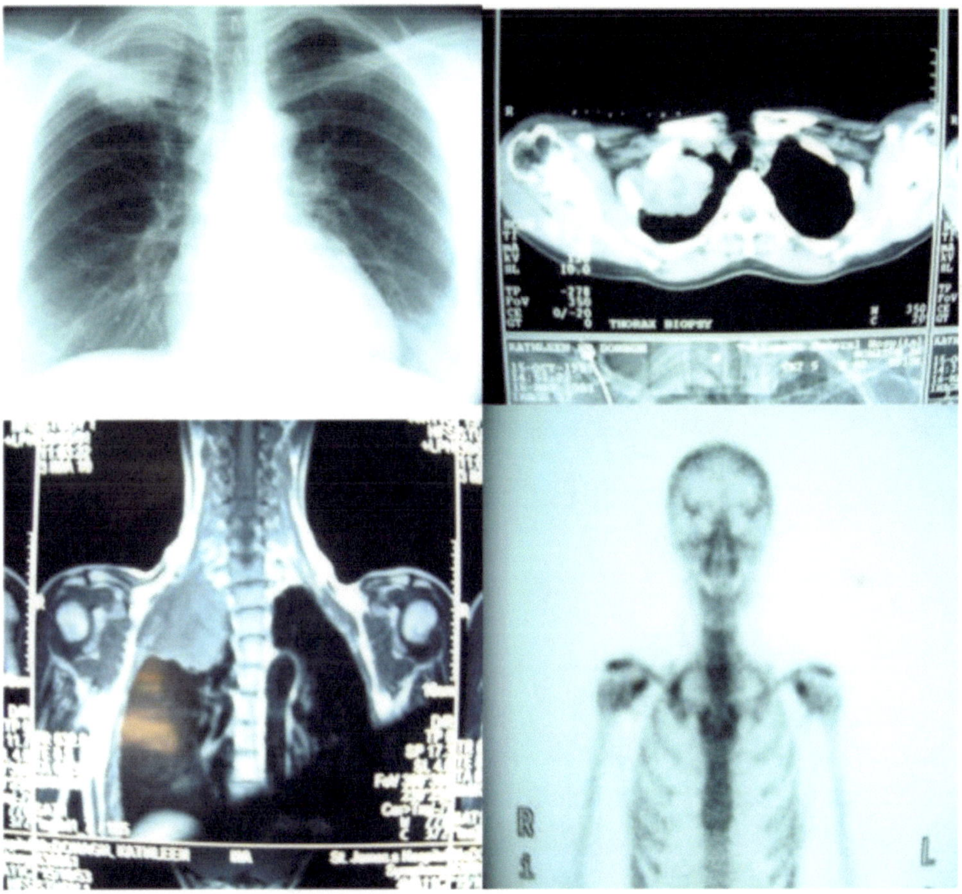

Figure 1. CXR, CT Chest imaging, MRI and bone scan of a Pancoast tumor of a 47 yrs old female, Ex smoker (25 cigs per day up to 13 years ago). Six weeks history of shoulder pain radiating to the median aspect of the right arm. CXR mass at apex of right chest. Percutanteous Biopsy NSCLC. PMH: Hysterectomy for Ca cervix 1996 - no evidence of recurrence. Clinical examination fullness in right supra-clavicular fossa.

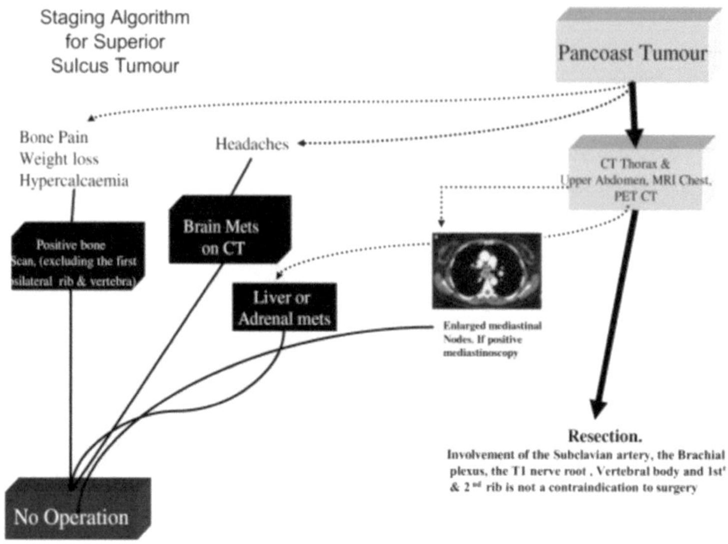

Figure 2. Staging algorithm for patients prior to resection of a Pancoast Tumor. MRI of the thoracic inlet may yield further information's on the status of vertebra involvement.

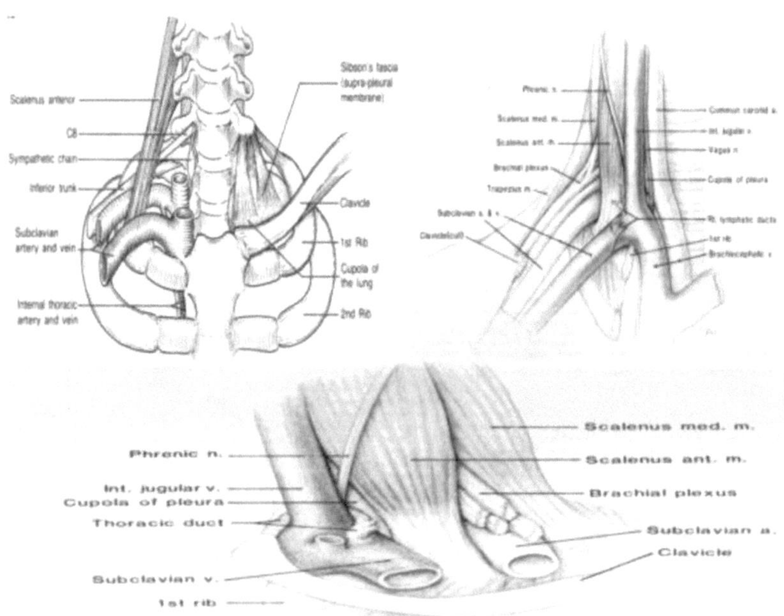

Figure 3. Root of neck anatomy, depicting carefully the relationship of the most important neurovascular structures to the scalene musculature and the first rib.

http://dx.doi.org/10.5772/55724

Root of neck anatomy as in Figure 3 is depicting carefully the relationship of the most important neuro-vascular structures to the scalene musculature and the first rib. The anterior and middle scalene muscles are attached to the first rib and can be used as landmarks: in front of the anterior scalene muscle situated the subclavian and internal jugular veins and the sternocleidomastoid and omo-hyoid muscles.

The subclavian artery, the trunks of the brachial plexus, and the phrenic nerve are emerging above the lateral part of the1st rib between the anterior and middle scalene muscles. The nerve roots of the brachial plexus, the stellate ganglion, and the vertebral column are situated behind the middle scalene muscle.

6. Exposure and surgical steps (Figure 4)

We favour a modified Dartevelle approach [24] an L shaped incision at the anterior edge of Sterno-cleido-mastoid (a). Division of the upper sternum extended into 2nd intercostal space (b). This is a modified access something between Grunenwald [25] and Klima et al [33] approach. Grunenwald has described a trans-manubrial approach, which avoids division of the clavicle. Klima and colleagues suggested extending the L-shaped section of the manubrium down to the first intercostal space. We prefer to divide the sternum down to the angle of Luis and then extend the incision horizontally along the 2nd intercostal space, thus allowing the surgeon to lift the clavicle, subclavian muscle, and transected part of the manubrium and superior body of the sternum without dividing the first costal cartilage and ligament. The internal mammary artery is encountered and divided during the horizontal intercostal incision.

Mobilisation & excision of the supra-clavicular fat pad (c), allows exposure of the structures at the thoracic inlet; further division of the subclavious, omohyoid with preservation of the accessory nerve is carried out.

The distal part of the jugular veins is divided to expose the subclavian and innominate veins. If the subclavian vein is affected then it is resected. Following this, the scalenus anterior muscle is divided by taking care to preserve the phrenic nerve (d) & (e). The subclavian artery is mobilised by, dividing most of its branches. Care is taken to preserve the vertebral artery and resection of the vessel is done only if it is involved with the tumour and no substantial extracranial occlusive disease can be detected on preoperative Doppler ultrasound.

If the subclavian artery is taken up by tumour, the affected portion is resected and reconstructed, usually with a 6-8 mm PTFE vascular graft. Small dose of heparin is usually administered during vascular clamping.

Following anterior traction of the subclavian artery, the scalenus medius muscle comes into good view. The muscle is divided above its insertion on the first rib, giving access to the branchial plexus. Familiarity with the anatomy of the plexus is important. At this stage, the anterior surface of the vertebral bodies of C7 and T1 are in view. The sympathetic chain and stellate ganglion are lying in front of the anterior surface of the vertebral bodies of C7 and T1.

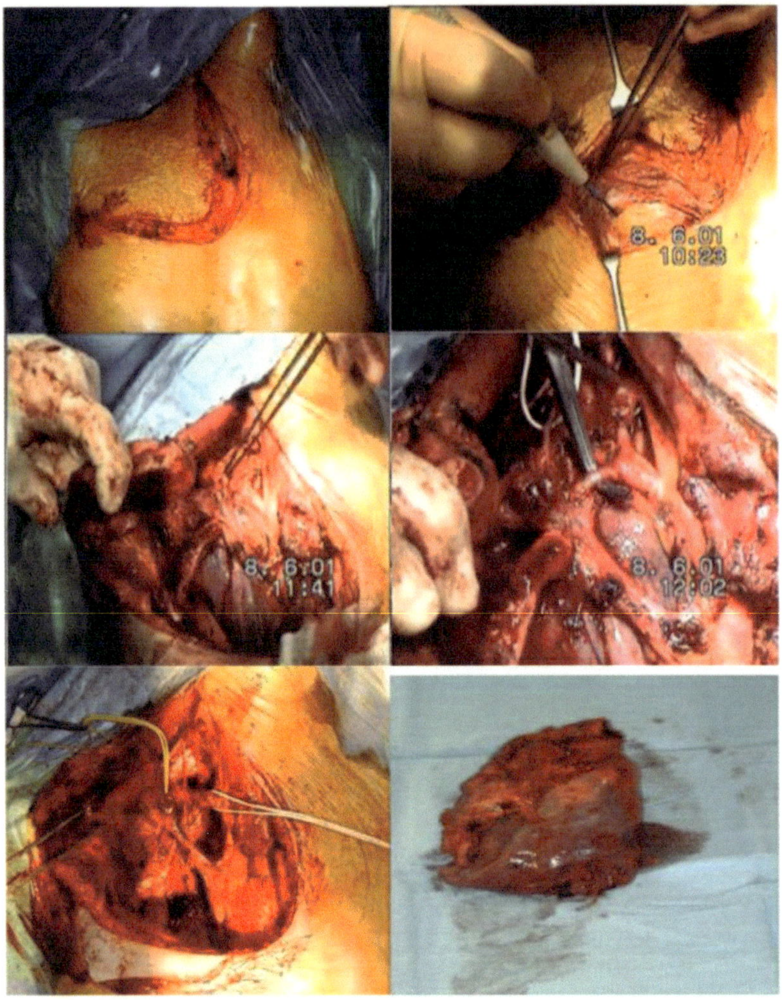

Figure 4. Step by step resection of a Pancoast tumor through an Antero-cervical approach. Incision at the anterior edge of Sterno-cleido-mastoid (a). Division of the upper sternum extended into 2nd intercostal space(b). Mobilisation-Excision of supraclavicular fat pad (c). Exposure of the structures at the thoracic inlet by dividing the subclavius, omohyoid with preservation of the accessory nerve. Division of the Scalenus anterior with preservation of the phrenic nerve (d) & (e). Right upper Lobectomy (f): can be performed through the neck incision or a posterolateral thoracotomy.

The C8 and T1 nerve roots are visualised and dissected medially up to the lower trunk of the brachial plexus. The C8 nerve component of the plexus is preserved if possible, for better functional outcome of the upper limp.

Care is taken then, to access tumour invasion and plan with the neurosurgeon the "spinal component" of the operation.

Chest wall resection is carried out by dividing the first 2-3 ribs at the sternal-costo-chondral junction following by disarticulation of the ribs from the transverse processes at the back. The last part of the resection consists of the upper Lobectomy (f). The access to perform a lobectomy and mediastinal lymph node clearance through the anterior incision is usually limited, therefore like others [34] we perform a traditional postero-lateral thoracotomy through the 5th inter-costal space. Routine coverage of the bronchial stump with an intercostal or serratus muscle flap is advocated by some groups [18] to counteract any potential damage on the stump from the neoadjuvant radiation. Chest wall reconstruction may be necessary in up to 40% of the cases [34].

For Pancoast carcinomas affecting the spine, a posterior midline approach can be added by a neurosurgeon, for multilevel unilateral laminectomy[35], nerve root division inside the spinal canal, and vertebral body division along the midline. The tumour then is removed en bloc with the lung, ribs, and vessels through the posterior incision. Fixation of the spine is mandatory.

7. Anterior approach: Advantages and dis-advantages

7.1. Advantages

According to Machiarini et al [36] one of the major advances in the treatment of Pancoast tumours has been the introduction of anterior approaches for resection. These approaches increase the likelihood of complete resection and permit resection of tumours that were previously considered technically unresectable [37].

Furthermore anterior approach facilitates: 1) Direct visualisation of major structures (eg. Subclavian artery, superior vena cava) thus allowing control and elective sacrifice of the artery if necessary and reconstruct directly to a safe outcome. 2) Excellent exposure of the brachial plexus, sympathetic chain, and stellate ganglion. 3) Carry out hemi-vertebrectomy if the anterior body of the vertebra are involved. 4) Resection of the lower parts of the Brachial plexus, especially of the C8, T1 roots; however T1 root resection results in diffuse weakness of the intrinsic muscles of the hand, whereas resection of the C8 nerve root of the lower trunk of the brachial plexus results in permanent paralysis of the hand muscles. 5) Optimal access, for resection of the chest wall. 6) Oncological clearance of the structures of the Thoracic inlet, because the tumour is the last to be encountered. 7) Lower morbidity than the posterior approach.

Moreover as per Vanakesa et al [28]the cervical-trans-sternal approach has several advantages, chiefly that of avoiding disfigurement and loss of function of the pectoral girdle, whilst providing excellent exposure of the brachial plexus, sympathetic chain, and stellate ganglion. Such an approach results in a short postoperative stay (3–6 days), and yet allows extension as per Grunenwald [25], or by a high, anterior thoracotomy if necessary.

7.2. Disadvantages

Removal of transverse processes and the head of the ribs in order to disarticulate them, could be difficult with the anterior access; furthermore more posterior seated tumours with vertebra involvement may require a complimentary posterior incision.

There are concerns about functional and aesthetic results with the trans-clavicular approach, which includes removal of the medial half of the clavicle.

8. Results from literature review

Unfavourable outcome is due to incomplete resection and life-threatening complications Current reports are quoting peri-operative mortality not higher than for any other lung resection [16, 17].

The prognosis of this tumour remained poor until 1961 when Shaw et al [38] reported their satisfactory experience with a bi-modality treatment based on preoperative radiotherapy followed by surgery through a posterior thoracotomy approach. Several other reports [2, 10, 19, 29, 38-41] confirmed that 5-year survivals of approximately 10 to 35% could be achieved with this combined approach, which became the standard treatment. Although radiotherapy was performed prior to surgery in most series, in the experience of others [24, 26]it was often carried out postoperatively.

Adverse prognostic factors are including the presence of mediastinal nodal metastases (N2 disease), spine or subclavian-vessel involvement (T4 disease), and limited resection (R1 or R2) [42-44]. Along the same lines Ginsberg et al [2] found Horner's syndrome, N2/N3 disease, T4 disease and incomplete resection, in general, to be adverse prognostic factors. Okubo and associates [29][16] found that incomplete resection particularly tumour invasion to the brachial plexus, influenced the prognosis.

9. Recurrence & survival

With bi-modality regimes the local recurrence rates were reported to be above 70% [10, 13]. Despite the advent in treatment regimes, local recurrence still occurs in about 40% of the patients [43]; it is expected that local recurrence rate is higher in patients with T4 disease because complete resection can be achieved in less than half of the patients with c-T4 disease [17]. More specifically [44] complete resection rate was achieved in only 64% of tumour stage T3 and nodal stage N 0 and 39% of T4N0 tumours. It is apparent however, that loco-regional relapse is predominant in R1-2 resections, whereas distant recurrence is frequent in R0 resections.

One would expect that a shift in the trend of clinical recurrences towards distant metastasis is to be currently expected because of the fact that tri-modality treatment facilitates better R0 resection. As per Pourel et al [15] the most frequent site of relapse was distant metastasis in 66% of the patients, (mainly brain) with the loco-regional recurrence rate of 18%. Likewise Kwong et al [18] reported brain metastasis in 25% and local recurrence rate in 19% of the cases. A small series that had bi-modality treatment however had an incidence of loco-regional recurrence of 17.2% [14].

Survival has been extensively reviewed by Attar et al [45]. Overall survival at 5 years after surgery was 46% for T3N0, 13% for T4N0, and 0% for lesions with N2 disease [44]. Particularly noteworthy [17]was the reproducibility of the favourable survival data, with a 5-year overall survival rate of 44% in the United States trial (SWOG) and 56% in JCOG trial, which were clearly superior to the historical value of 30%.

There is wide variability in overall 5-year survival rates reported in larger series,[19, 24, 26, 39, 41, 44, 46] with figures ranging 10 to 35% probably because of the heterogeneity in studied populations, operative techniques, and preoperative and postoperative treatments. Such heterogeneity is probably responsible for the difference in the percentage of T3 and T4 tumours as well as in the rates of complete resection. Comparison of long-term results of different studies is difficult also for the frequent lack of information about survival according to the pathologic stage.

10. Future thoughts

In the future new neoadjuvant regimes including aggressive protocols of accelerated radiotherapy would potentially increase the pool of surgical candidates from patients diagnosed with a Pancoast tumour (currently 23% of the patients as per Kappers et al [13]. However, several questions still remain unresolved:

1) The role of PET-CT in re-staging tumours (eg. The role of "late wash out" images in differentiating between inflammation and residual tumour) following neo-adjuvant treatment; Schmuecking et al [47] have shown that metabolic response after induction CT/RT evaluated within 1 week following its completion, is highly predictive of pathological response. 2) What is the significance and implications of ipsilateral supra-clavicular lymph node disease: The argument being that these nodes are in close vicinity of the tumour and therefore could have the characteristics of the biological behaviour of "N1 disease". 3) Recruiting patients with N2 disease: The argument being that inclusion of the hilar and mediastinal nodes in the irradiation field promotes downstaging. Kwong et al [18] did not exclude patients with positive mediastinal nodes from tri-modality treatment and found no difference in survival. In most papers, however, results of patients with persistent N2 disease turned out to be clearly inferior to those of patients with N0/1 only. On the other hand, no clinical trial has yet compared various tri-modality treatment regimes for patients with N2 disease. 4) The role of prophylactic cranial irradiation: Due to good loco-regional control with tri-modality treatment, distant metastases now represent the most common site of failure. Furthermore, the incidence of brain metastasis as a first site of recurrence in Pancoast tumour is between 15-30% [34, 48]. The negative impact of brain metastasis on survival has to be weighted against the risks benefits ration of the impact of prophylaxis with radiation to the brain. 5) The role of high dose of RT (up to 60Gy): Are there specific subgroups (eg. for patients with clinical T4 disease complete resection is feasible in less than 50% of the cases) that they would benefit. 6) The role of Adjuvant postoperative chemotherapy: distant metastases now represent the most common site of failure following treatment for Pancoast tumours therefore

preventing distant metastasis has now become the challenge in the treatment of these patients. Large randomised trials concluded a 5—15% survival benefit at 5 years of adjuvant chemotherapy in patients with radically resected stages I—IIIA NSCLC [49, 50]. However, many patients with Pancoast tumours may not tolerate more extensive treatment. Moreover Martinod et al [26] reported that preoperative radiotherapy significantly improved the 5-year survival for stage IIB—IIIA, while postoperative radiotherapy and chemotherapy did not significantly alter survival. 7) Is the Survival with the use of anterior approach better versus posterior approach for the same stage of Pancoast tumours?

11. Conclusion

Pancoast tumours represent a small percentage of Lung cancer population (1-5%). Due to poor performance status and/or advanced tumour stages, only 30-40 % [10, 13] of those patients are eligible to be enrolled in multi-modality protocols of treatment.

Careful patient selection and adherence to protocols enables Clinical groups to get an impression of the efficacy of an intervention and to compare results between studies.

Superior sulcus tumours remain an extremely severe condition, but cure may be achieved in a large percentage of cases. The surgical approach should be adapted to the different clinical and radiologic presentations in order to achieve a complete surgical resection, which represents the most important positive prognostic factor. Surgery carries a high operative risk, especially if a combined approach is needed, so every effort should be made to identify patients expected to derive a benefit that outweighs risks.

No single surgical approach however, provides the best access to all of the heterogeneous tumours of the thoracic inlet. The thoracic surgeon must be familiar with the potential advantages that the anterior approach offers under given circumstances. This knowledge enables the thoracic surgeon to explore new avenues and exciting challenges. Dartevilles approach and the various modifications are technically demanding, however once the anatomy has been appreciated, direct visualisation of the major structures of the Thoracic inlet aids to facilitate complete oncological clearance. Whether the anterior approach results in less loco-regional recurrences and possibly better 5 year survival, remains to be seen.

12. Summary

12.1. Introduction

Pancoast syndrome is due to lesions extending to the superior thoracic inlet. Pancoast tumour is a tumour of the apex of the lung with no intervening lung tissue between tumour and chest wall. The tumour rapidly involves the structures of the thoracic inlet & the root of neck.

Pain at the ulnar aspect of the forearm and hand is consistent with T1 involvement; furthermore symptomatology along the intrinsic hand muscles suggests the C8 root or lower trunk tumor deposits.

An understanding of the posterior location of neural structures and somewhat anterior location of vascular structures is important for adequate operative planning.

Pancoast tumours were thought to be located posteriorly and early attempts to resect those tumors were approached solely from the back. A percentage of these lesions might also be located at the front, with vascular rather than neuro- vertebral involvement. Therefore surgeons treating these cancers should be able to be familiar and adapt with the various approaches.

12.2. Surgical Approaches

1. Posterior approach (Paulson)/ posterolateral-paravertebral thoracotomy: This is an extension of the conventional postero-lateral thoracotomy; the incision is extending around the tip of the scapula, then it continuous upwards and further midway between the posterior edge of the scapula and the spinous processes, up to the level of C7. By taking the scapula of the chest wall this incision allows good exposure of the posterior chest wall, including the transverse processes, the vertebrae and the roots of the thoracic nerves and the plexus. Never the less the exposure of the neurovascular structures are limited.
2. The anterior-cervical approach proved to be the answer to the problem of limited exposure. It appears to be the optimal approach to anterior lung apex and first rib lesions.

We favour a modified Dartevelle approach We prefer to divide the sternum down to the angle of Luis and then extend the incision horizontally along the 2nd intercostal space, thus allowing the surgeon to lift the clavicle, subclavian muscle, and transected part of the manubrium and superior boby of the sternum without dividing the first costal cartilage and ligament.

Mobilisation & excision of the supraclavicular fat pad, allows exposure of the structures at the thoracic inlet; further division of the subclavius, omohyoid with preservation of the accessory nerve is carried out.

The distal part of the jugular veins is divided to expose the subclavian and innominate veins. If the subclavian vein is affected then it is resected. Following this, the scalenus anterior muscle is divided by taking care to preserve the phrenic nerve.

The subclavian artery is mobilized by, dividing most of its branches. Care is taken to preserve the vertebral artery and resection of the vessel is done only if it is involved with the tumor and no substantial extracranial occlusive disease can be detected on preoperative Doppler ultra-sound.

12.3. The advantages of the anterior- cervical approach

1. Direct visualization of major structures (eg. Subclavian artery), allowing control and elective sacrifice if necessary the artery and reconstruct directly to a safe outcome.

2. Carry out hemi-vertebrectomy if the anterior body of the vertebra are involved.
3. Provide complete oncological clearance of the structures of the Thoracic inlet. The structures which may be sacrificed if involved are the Subclavian artery, the Brachial plexus the T1 nerve root and Vertebral body

12.4. Down-staging

Pathological down-staging although it does not correlate with the radiological appearance is reported to be impressively above 30% in various series.

JCOG reported pathologic down-staging of the tumour in 40% of the patients; No residual viable tumour cells in the resected specimens, was achieved in 16% of the treated patients. Also SWOG summarised that pathologic no residual microscopic tumour was seen in one third of the resected specimens and minimal microscopic residual (few scattered tumour foci within a mostly necrotic or fibrotic mass), was observed in one third of the resected specimens.

12.5. Results

Unfavorable outcome is due to incomplete resection and life-threatening complications.

Current reports are quoting perioperative mortality not higher than for any other lung resection.

Adverse prognostic factors are including the presence of mediastinal nodal metastases (N2 disease), spine or subclavian-vessel involvement (T4 disease), and limited resection (R1 or R2.

Author (year)	No. of Cases	5 year survival (%)	Mortality (%)
Paulson DL (1985)	79	35	3
Maggi et al (1994)	60	17.4	5
Ginberg et al (1994)	100	26	4
Okubo et al (1995)	18	38.5	5.6
Hagan et al (1999)	34	33	0
Dartevelle P (1999)	70	34	0

Table 1. Survival with the use of the anterior versus posterior approach

12.6. Recurrence

With bimodality regimes the local recurrence rates were reported to be above 70%. Despite the advent in treatment regimes, local recurrence still occurs in about 40% of the patients; it is expected that local recurrence rate is higher in patients with T4 disease because complete resection can be achieved in less than half of the patients with c-T4 disease.

More specifically complete resection rate was achieved in only 64% of tumour stage T3 and nodal stage N 0 and 39% of T4N0 tumours.

It is apparent however, that locoregional relapse is predominant in R1-2 resections, whereas distant recurrence is frequent in R0 resections.

In the future new neoadjuvant regimes including aggressive protocols of accelerated radiotherapy would potentially increase the pool of surgical candidates from patients diagnosed with a Pancoast tumor (currently 23% of the patients as per Kappers et al). However, several questions still remain unresolved such as the role of PET, nodal involvement especially recruiting patients with N2 disease. Lastly the role of trimodality treatment and prophylactic cranial irradiation

12.7. Conclusion

Pancoast tumors represent a small percentage of Lung cancer population (1-5%). Due to poor performance status and/or advanced tumor stages, only 30-40 % of those patients are eligible to be enrolled in multimodality protocols of treatment.

No single surgical approach however, provides the best access to all heterogeneous tumors of the thoracic inlet. What probably provides the most favorable outcome would be a team approach, where the thoracic surgeon coordinates with an experience neuro-spinal surgeon, in a background of limited disease that is responding well to neoadjuvant chemoradiotherapy.

Author details

Haralabos Parissis*, Alan Soo and Bassel Al-Alao

*Address all correspondence to: hparissis@yahoo.co.uk

Cardiothoracic Surgery Department, Royal Victoria Hospital, Belfast, Northern Ireland

References

[1] Bridgewater B KR, Walton P. Sixth National Adult Cardiac Surgical Database Report. Society for Cardiothoracic Surgery in Great Britain and Ireland2008. Report No.: ISBN 1-903968-23-2. 2009.

[2] Ginsberg RJ, Martini N, Zaman M, Armstrong JG, Bains MS, Burt ME, McCormack PM, Rusch VW, Harrison LB. Influence of surgical resection and brachytherapy in the management of superior sulcus tumor. Ann Thorac Surg1994 Jun;57(6):1440-5.

[3] Pancoast H. Superior pulmonary sulcus tumor: tumor characterized by pain, Horner's syndrome, destruction of the bone and atrophy of hand muscles. JAMA1932;99:1391-6.

[4] Tobias J. Sindrome apico-costo-vertebral-doloroso por tu- mor apexiano: su valor diagnostico en le cancer primitivo pulmonar. Rev Med Lat-Amer1932;17:1522-56.

[5] Arcasoy SM, Jett JR. Superior pulmonary sulcus tumors and Pancoast's syndrome. N Engl J Med1997 Nov 6;337(19):1370-6.

[6] 6.Jett JR. Superior sulcus tumors and Pancoast's syndrome. Lung Cancer2003 Dec;42 Suppl 2:S17-21.

[7] Tsao JW, Garlin AB, Marder SR. Pancoast's syndrome. N Engl J Med1998 Mar 12;338(11):765-6.

[8] Pitz CC, de la Riviere AB, van Swieten HA, Duurkens VA, Lammers JW, van den Bosch JM. Surgical treatment of Pancoast tumours. Eur J Cardiothorac Surg2004 Jul; 26(1):202-8.

[9] Mansour K. Extended resection of bronchial carcinoma in the superior pulmonary sulcus. In: Shields T, editor. General thoracic surgery. Baltimore: Williams and Wilkins; 1994. p. 572-8.

[10] Wright CD, Moncure AC, Shepard JA, Wilkins EW, Jr., Mathisen DJ, Grillo HC. Superior sulcus lung tumors. Results of combined treatment (irradiation and radical resection). J Thorac Cardiovasc Surg1987 Jul;94(1):69-74.

[11] Komaki R, Putnam JB, Jr., Walsh G, Lee JS, Cox JD. The management of superior sulcus tumors. Semin Surg Oncol2000 Mar;18(2):152-64.

[12] Rusch VW. Management of Pancoast tumours. Lancet Oncol2006 Dec;7(12):997-1005.

[13] Kappers I, Belderbos JS, Burgers JA, van Zandwijk N, Groen HJ, Klomp HM. Non-small cell lung carcinoma of the superior sulcus: favourable outcomes of combined modality treatment in carefully selected patients. Lung Cancer2008 Mar;59(3):385-90.

[14] Wright CD, Menard MT, Wain JC, Donahue DM, Grillo HC, Lynch TJ, Choi NC, Mathisen DJ. Induction chemoradiation compared with induction radiation for lung cancer involving the superior sulcus. Ann Thorac Surg2002 May;73(5):1541-4.

[15] Pourel N, Santelmo N, Naafa N, Serre A, Hilgers W, Mineur L, Molinari N, Reboul F. Concurrent cisplatin/etoposide plus 3D-conformal radiotherapy followed by surgery for stage IIB (superior sulcus T3N0)/III non-small cell lung cancer yields a high rate of pathological complete response. Eur J Cardiothorac Surg2008 May;33(5):829-36.

[16] Rusch VW, Giroux DJ, Kraut MJ, Crowley J, Hazuka M, Johnson D, Goldberg M, Detterbeck F, Shepherd F, Burkes R, Winton T, Deschamps C, Livingston R, Gandara D. Induction chemoradiation and surgical resection for non-small cell lung carcinomas of the superior sulcus: Initial results of Southwest Oncology Group Trial 9416 (Intergroup Trial 0160). J Thorac Cardiovasc Surg2001 Mar;121(3):472-83.

[17] Kunitoh H, Kato H, Tsuboi M, Shibata T, Asamura H, Ichinose Y, Katakami N, Nagai K, Mitsudomi T, Matsumura A, Nakagawa K, Tada H, Saijo N. Phase II trial of pre-

operative chemoradiotherapy followed by surgical resection in patients with superior sulcus non-small-cell lung cancers: report of Japan Clinical Oncology Group trial 9806. J Clin Oncol2008 Feb 1;26(4):644-9.

[18] Kwong KF, Edelman MJ, Suntharalingam M, Cooper LB, Gamliel Z, Burrows W, Hausner P, Doyle LA, Krasna MJ. High-dose radiotherapy in trimodality treatment of Pancoast tumors results in high pathologic complete response rates and excellent long-term survival. J Thorac Cardiovasc Surg2005 Jun;129(6):1250-7.

[19] Paulson DL. Carcinomas in the superior pulmonary sulcus. J Thorac Cardiovasc Surg1975 Dec;70(6):1095-104.

[20] Masaoka A, Ito Y, Yasumitsu T. Anterior approach for tumor of the superior sulcus. J Thorac Cardiovasc Surg1979 Sep;78(3):413-5.

[21] Bains MS, Ginsberg RJ, Jones WG, 2nd, McCormack PM, Rusch VW, Burt ME, Martini N. The clamshell incision: an improved approach to bilateral pulmonary and mediastinal tumor. Ann Thorac Surg1994 Jul;58(1):30-2; discussion 3.

[22] Korst RJ, Burt ME. Cervicothoracic tumors: results of resection by the "hemi-clamshell" approach. J Thorac Cardiovasc Surg1998 Feb;115(2):286-94; discussion 94-5.

[23] Dartevelle P, Levasseur P, Rojas-Miranda A, Merlier M, Le Brigand H. [Combined cervical and thoracic approach to the removal of tumours responsible for the Pancoast and Tobias syndrome (author's transl)]. Nouv Presse Med1981 Mar 21;10(13): 1051-4.

[24] Dartevelle PG, Chapelier AR, Macchiarini P, Lenot B, Cerrina J, Ladurie FL, Parquin FJ, Lafont D. Anterior transcervical-thoracic approach for radical resection of lung tumors invading the thoracic inlet. J Thorac Cardiovasc Surg1993 Jun;105(6):1025-34.

[25] Grunenwald D, Spaggiari L. Transmanubrial osteomuscular sparing approach for apical chest tumors. Ann Thorac Surg1997 Feb;63(2):563-6.

[26] Martinod E, D'Audiffret A, Thomas P, Wurtz AJ, Dahan M, Riquet M, Dujon A, Jancovici R, Giudicelli R, Fuentes P, Azorin JF. Management of superior sulcus tumors: experience with 139 cases treated by surgical resection. Ann Thorac Surg2002 May; 73(5):1534-9; discussion 9-40.

[27] Kent MS, Bilsky MH, Rusch VW. Resection of superior sulcus tumors (posterior approach). Thorac Surg Clin2004 May;14(2):217-28.

[28] Vanakesa T, Goldstraw P. Antero-superior approaches in the practice of thoracic surgery. Eur J Cardiothorac Surg1999 Jun;15(6):774-80.

[29] Okubo K, Wada H, Fukuse T, Yokomise H, Inui K, Ike O, Mizuno H, Aoki M, Hitomi S. Treatment of Pancoast tumors. Combined irradiation and radical resection. Thorac Cardiovasc Surg1995 Oct;43(5):284-6.

[30] Ducic Y, Crepeau A, Ducic L, Lamothe A, Corsten M. A logical approach to the thoracic inlet: the Dartevelle approach revisited. Head Neck1999 Dec;21(8):767-71.

[31] Therasse P, Arbuck SG, Eisenhauer EA, Wanders J, Kaplan RS, Rubinstein L, Verweij J, Van Glabbeke M, van Oosterom AT, Christian MC, Gwyther SG. New guidelines to evaluate the response to treatment in solid tumors. European Organization for Research and Treatment of Cancer, National Cancer Institute of the United States, National Cancer Institute of Canada. J Natl Cancer Inst2000 Feb 2;92(3):205-16.

[32] Laissy JP, Soyer P, Sekkal SR, Tebboune D, Servois V, Sibert A, Menu Y. Assessment of vascular involvement with magnetic resonance angiography (MRA) in Pancoast syndrome. Magn Reson Imaging1995;13(4):523-30.

[33] Klima U LA, Haverich A. ransmanubrial approach reproposed: reply. Ann Thorac Surg1999;68:1888.

[34] Marra A, Eberhardt W, Pottgen C, Theegarten D, Korfee S, Gauler T, Stuschke M, Stamatis G. Induction chemotherapy, concurrent chemoradiation and surgery for Pancoast tumour. Eur Respir J2007 Jan;29(1):117-26.

[35] Fadel E, Missenard G, Chapelier A, Mussot S, Leroy-Ladurie F, Cerrina J, Dartevelle P. En bloc resection of non-small cell lung cancer invading the thoracic inlet and intervertebral foramina. J Thorac Cardiovasc Surg2002 Apr;123(4):676-85.

[36] Macchiarini P. Resection of superior sulcus carcinomas (anterior approach). Thorac Surg Clin2004 May;14(2):229-40.

[37] Tamura M, Hoda MA, Klepetko W. Current treatment paradigms of superior sulcus tumours. Eur J Cardiothorac Surg2009 Oct;36(4):747-53.

[38] Shaw RR, Paulson DL, Kee JL. Treatment of Superior Sulcus Tumor by Irradiation Followed by Resection. Ann Surg1961 Jul;154(1):29-40.

[39] Devine JW, Mendenhall WM, Million RR, Carmichael MJ. Carcinoma of the superior pulmonary sulcus treated with surgery and/or radiation therapy. Cancer1986 Mar 1;57(5):941-3.

[40] Hilaris BS, Martini N, Luomanen RK, Batata M, Beattie EJ, Jr. The value of preoperative radiation therapy in apical cancer of the lung. Surg Clin North Am1974 Aug; 54(4):831-40.

[41] Sartori F, Rea F, Calabro F, Mazzucco C, Bortolotti L, Tomio L. Carcinoma of the superior pulmonary sulcus. Results of irradiation and radical resection. J Thorac Cardiovasc Surg1992 Sep;104(3):679-83.

[42] Alifano M, D'Aiuto M, Magdeleinat P, Poupardin E, Chafik A, Strano S, Regnard JF. Surgical treatment of superior sulcus tumors: results and prognostic factors. Chest2003 Sep;124(3):996-1003.

[43] Pfannschmidt J, Kugler C, Muley T, Hoffmann H, Dienemann H. Non-small-cell superior sulcus tumor: results of en bloc resection in fifty-six patients - non-small-cell pancoast. Thorac Cardiovasc Surg2003 Dec;51(6):332-7.

[44] Rusch VW, Parekh KR, Leon L, Venkatraman E, Bains MS, Downey RJ, Boland P, Bilsky M, Ginsberg RJ. Factors determining outcome after surgical resection of T3 and T4 lung cancers of the superior sulcus. J Thorac Cardiovasc Surg2000 Jun;119(6): 1147-53.

[45] Attar S, Krasna MJ, Sonett JR, Hankins JR, Slawson RG, Suter CM, McLaughlin JS. Superior sulcus (Pancoast) tumor: experience with 105 patients. Ann Thorac Surg1998 Jul;66(1):193-8.

[46] Maggi G, Casadio C, Pischedda F, Giobbe R, Cianci R, Ruffini E, Molinatti M, Mancuso M. Combined radiosurgical treatment of Pancoast tumor. Ann Thorac Surg1994 Jan;57(1):198-202.

[47] M. Schmuecking CPS, N. Presselt, R. P. Baum, J. Leonhardi, K. Hoeffken, A. Niesen, K. M. Mueller, T. G. Wendt, R. Bonnet, LUCAS-MD Study Group, editor Are timing of chemoradiation and early therapy response as detected by PET prognostic factors of a multimodality treatment approach for NSCLC stage III? (LUCAS-MD). 2007 ASCO Annual Meeting; 2007.

[48] Komaki R, Derus SB, Perez-Tamayo C, Byhardt RW, Hartz A, Cox JD. Brain metastasis in patients with superior sulcus tumors. Cancer1987 May 1;59(9):1649-53.

[49] Arriagada R, Bergman B, Dunant A, Le Chevalier T, Pignon JP, Vansteenkiste J. Cisplatin-based adjuvant chemotherapy in patients with completely resected non-small-cell lung cancer. N Engl J Med2004 Jan 22;350(4):351-60.

[50] Erman M, Moretti L, Soria JC, Le Chevalier T, Van Houtte P. Adjuvant chemotherapy and radiotherapy in non-small cell lung cancer. Semin Radiat Oncol2004 Oct;14(4): 315-21.

Chapter 6

Malignant Pleural Mesothelioma and the Role of Non–Operative Therapies

Kelvin K.W. Lau and Calvin S.H. Ng

Additional information is available at the end of the chapter

http://dx.doi.org/10.5772/55722

1. Introduction

Malignant pleural mesothelioma (MPM) is a primary malignancy of the pleura. The main aetiological agent is asbestos. The latency period lasts several decades, and in countries where its use was banned in the 1950's and 1960's, the incidence is expected to peak within the coming decade. However, in the many other countries it continues to be mined and used. The incidence in these countries can be expected to continue to rise.

The prognosis for MPM is dismal and the median survival from the time of diagnosis is 12 to 18 months. Current therapies are blunt weapons that are very morbid but at the same time ineffective. They have barely made an impact on the poor outcomes of mesothelioma.

In this chapter, we will review the current knowledge on mesothelioma pathogenesis, epidemiology, biology and treatment. We will focus on nonoperative therapies and the role of surgery will be covered in another chapter.

2. Epidemiology and aetiological factors

2.1. The history of asbestos and mesothelioma

Following the earliest descriptions of mesothelioma, it remained an exceptionally rare malignancy until after industrialisation. For a long time, primary pleural malignancies were so rare that their very existence was disputed [1]. In the early 1950s, a number of reports noted small clusters of MPM but it was not until the late 1950s in South Africa when Kit Sleggs noted that patients with tuberculous pleurisy from the east of Kimberly were recovering with streptomycin and isoniazid, but a number of patients apparently with the same disease from the west of Kimberly continued to die. The pathologist Christopher Wagner observed that these patients had in fact a rare cancer of the pleura but yet without any other primary tumours, leading to the conclusion they had primary mesothelioma. In the same period, there were no mesotheliomas observed amongst 10,000 lungs examined from other areas of South Africa. This begged the question of why they were diagnosing so many of these rare tumours in west Kimberly. Wagner observed asbestos bodies in the lung beneath the tumour and surmised their association with mesothelioma, from that moment on the link was made [2]. His publication "Diffuse pleural mesothelioma and asbestos exposure in the North Western Cape Province" became the most cited paper in industrial medicine. This started a lifelong investigation into the association of MPM with asbestos [3].

Asbestos is a family of long, thin, fibrinous, hydrated magnesium-silicate crystals. The first record of its human use is from over 5,000 years ago, and Persians were known to make cloth with it that could be cleansed by throwing it into the fire [4]. They are classified according to their morphology into the straight and rod-like amphiboles, and the curly serpentines fibres. The amphiboles, which include crocidolite, amosite and tremolite, are strongly associated with the development of mesothelioma. The serpentine fibre chrysotile, believed to be less carcinogenic by some and non-carcinogenic by others, continues to be mined and sold in Canada to this day. The carcinogenicity of different asbestos preparations is also related to the fibre dimensions, with long, thin fibres being most strongly carcinogenic [5].

Asbestos is a versatile material valued for being weavable, resistant to heat, electricity and chemicals, being readily available and cheap. It is used in the building and construction, machinery, shipbuilding and transport industries, hence asbestos-related diseases including mesothelioma are mainly industrial work-related and therefore more common in males. The main cohorts with exposure are *occupational* - those working directly with the mining and preparation of asbestos (eg. mixing asbestos cement, cutting sheets, lagging) and end-users of asbestos such as builders, plumbers and shipyard workers, *paraoccupational* - in people living with people working with asbestos and *environmental* - from exposure to naturally occurring asbestos.

The background incidence of mesothelioma is approximately 1 per million, rising to 7 per million in Japan, 12 per million in the United States, 33 per million in the United Kingdom and 40 per million in Australia in a pattern consistent with the distribution of asbestos exposure. In Wittenoon, Western Australia where crocidolite was mined in the 1930s, follow-up records of 6,493 employees found MPM caused 3.4% deaths in exposed male workers [6]. The predicted peak incidence is expected to occur between 2005 and 2025 in countries which banned its use [7]. It is more common in males, and with a latency period between three and four decades [8], the median age at diagnosis is in the sixth and seventh decades, although there are instances when it can present in the second decade, often with a history of perinatal exposure.

There is an exposure dose-response relationship between asbestos and mesothelioma, both in terms of historic exposure (duration and episodes) and lung asbestos fibre content [9], [10] [11]. The risk is highest with crocidolite and amosite, and less with chrysotile. However, there is a background rate of mesothelioma, and virtually all mankind has been exposed to asbestos at some point – fibres have been found in the lungs of the general population. Because of this, it has not been possible to determine a threshold level below which exposure could be deemed safe [12] and this has important implications for legislation.

As of August 2012, 54 countries have banned the use of all types of asbestos [13]. For the rest of the countries, nearly all of the asbestos mined and consumed today is chrysotile asbestos. Developing countries are the highest consumers of asbestos, with China topping the list. With its rapid growth, China's production could not keep pace with its insatiable domestic appetite and needs to import a quarter of its asbestos. Russia, the world's largest producer with reserves that will last over a century, exports most of its asbestos [14]. Whilst the European Union and United States have complete bans on asbestos, Canada continues to mine chrysotile asbestos and is the fifth largest exporter of chrysotile to developing countries. This is in spite of severe restrictions on its domestic use. Although international agencies have long condemned the use of asbestos, it has been difficult to come to an agreement for an international ban. In June 2011, Canada for a third time objected to the inclusion of chrysotile asbestos under Annex III of the Rotterdam Convention.

2.2. The chrysotile controversy

The carcinogenicity of the amphiboles is now indisputable, but for chrysotile this has been fiercely debated. Most of the asbestos mined and utilised today is chrysotile, on the belief that this fibre is safe. This assumption is based on studies showing lesser biopersistence of the fibres, which is likely the result of the fibre's fragility, leading to fragmentation and quicker clearance from the lungs. Epidemiological studies which suggest chrysotile causes mesothelioma were dismissed by blaming contamination by amphiboles – the so-called 'Amphibole hypothesis' [15]. The experimental methodologies behind these studies have been questioned [16] [17] and it has become clear that even though chrysotile may be less potent at inducing mesothelioma, the heightened risks of asbestosis, lung cancer and death is still a glaring reality [18, 19].

2.3. Other implicated aetiological factors

2.3.1. Erionite and genetic susceptibility

An epidemic of malignant mesothelioma unfolded in 3 villages in Cappadocia, Turkey in the 1980's accounting for an unprecedented 50% of deaths in the region. In comparison to unaffected neighbouring villages, villages with mesothelioma also had high levels of airborne erionite, a fibrous zeolite with some similarities to asbestos [20]. Certainly, in animal models erionite is a very potent inducer of mesothelioma [21]. However, the incidence of mesothelioma in a nearby village with similar erionite levels was significantly lower, implicating other factors at play. Lineage studies have since incriminated an autosomal dominant transmission of susceptibility to fibre carcinogenesis to explain the disparity [22], but exposure to erionite itself remains the dominant driver of carcinogenesis [23].

Whilst erionite is also present in other parts of the world, mesothelioma directly attributable to erionite is still very rare [24]. Nevertheless, with a long latency period over three decades, the possibility of a future epidemic in erionite-rich areas, such as parts of America, is a concern [25].

2.3.2. SV40

SV40 is a polyoma virus which has long been studied as a carcinogen. The concerns over SV40 arose from the widespread administration of SV40-contaminated polio vaccines which were distributed worldwide in the 1960's. Certainly in the laboratory, SV40 virus has the ability to transform human cells and induce mesothelioma in experimental animals both directly, and as a co-carcinogen acting synergistically with asbestos [26] [27]. However, its relevance to clinical mesothelioma is less clear and the evidence is largely circumstantial. SV40 DNA fragments have been identified in 40 to 60% of mesothelioma samples [28] [29], but the copy numbers were exceedingly low (less than one per cell) [29]. Furthermore, there is no current treatment for SV40 infection.

2.3.3. Irradiation

Irradiation causes cancer and mesothelioma is no exception, Thorotrast is an alpha-emitting thorium dioxide radiocontrast used between 1930s and 1950s. It has a physical half-life of 10^{10} years and a biological half-life of several hundred years, and so it is retained lifelong, constantly exposing tissue including mesothelium to irradiation. Thorotrast is associated with many malignancies including mesothelioma [30]. Patients with lymphoma who underwent mantle radiotherapy represent another cohort with irradiation to the pleura. They also have a higher risk of mesothelioma compared to population with similar levels of asbestos exposure [31] [32].

3. Pathogenesis and biology

3.1. How asbestos causes cancer

Since most mesothelioma is associated with asbestos exposure, a lot of research has focused on how this inorganic fibre causes cancer. The physical properties of asbestos are more important for its carcinogenicity than its chemical composition. Many studies have confirmed that long (≥8 μm), thin (≤0.25 μm) fibres are most strongly associated with mesothelioma. Fibres of that size have aerodynamic features that are fine enough to allow them on the one hand to be deposited beyond the ciliated airways where they escape mechanical clearance, and on the other, large enough to frustrate phagocytosis by macrophages. Having been deposited, they migrate through still poorly understood pathways to the parietal pleura where they promote oncogenesis on the mesothelium. The chemical properties of the fibre are important insofar as they determine the biopersistence of the fibre. Chrysotile fibres, for example, are weak and fracture easily into shorter fibres which are easier to clear. Their apparent weak association with mesothelioma has been attributed to the fibre's lower biopersistence [33].

Asbestos is specifically cytotoxic to mesothelial cells in culture but not to fibroblasts [34], [35], therefore other processes must be involved *in vivo* to prevent cell death, promote cell survival and drive malignant transformation. The most widely accepted hypothesis invokes a chronic and genotoxic inflammatory response which over time drives tumourigenesis. As the long fibres become deposited and transported to the parietal pleura, they are progressively taken up by macrophages. However, because of their sheer size and biopersistence, they could not be cleared effectively, markedly lengthening their dwell time at the mesothelium compared to other particulates. Furthermore, macrophages are unable to engulf the entirety of these large fibres. Such frustrated phagocytosis is a potent stimulation of the macrophage's inflammatory response which results in respiratory bursts and secretion of toxic metabolites such as reactive oxygen species, growth factors and cytokines. The asbestos fibres have also themselves been implicated in carcinogenesis through direct interference with the mitotic apparatus, and direct generation of free radicals through its interaction with mobilisable iron on the fibre surface [36]. Over a long period of time, it could be envisaged the unrelenting exposure to these mutagens and growth signals could drive neoplastic transformation.

3.2. Molecular pathogenesis

A central player which promotes mesothelial transformation is believed to be tumour necrosis factor-alpha (TNF-α). Asbestos stimulates both macrophages and human mesothelial cells to express TNF-α. TNF-α has been shown to promote mesothelial cell survival in the face of asbestos exposure *in vitro*, and the effect appears to be mediated through Nuclear Factor Kappa-light-chain-enhancer of Activated B Cells (NF-κB) [35]. NF-κB activation results in release of a p16 subunit which translocates to the nucleus to induce expression of antiapoptotic genes. Meanwhile, activated macrophages also secrete a host of other cytokines and growth factors including interleukins, vascular endothelial growth factor (VEGF) and hepatocyte growth factor (HGF), as well as reactive oxygen and nitrogen species which directly causes DNA and chromosomal damage. Together, this sustained insult of mutagens and growth stimulators causes the first genetic alterations behind malignant mesothelioma.

Whilst most cancers have inactivation of the p53 and pRb tumour suppressor genes, mutation of these genes in mesothelioma is surprisingly rare [37] [38]. In contrast, over 70% of mesotheliomas have deletions of 9p21 and about 40% mesothelioma have loss of heterozygosity at the 22q12 locus [39] [40] [41] [42] [43]. 9p21 contains the INKa/ARF locus which encodes two proteins p16INK4a and p14ARF alternatively spliced from the same mRNA. Functionally, p14ARF stabilises p53 whilst p16INK4a inhibits the inactivation of pRb, thereby restricting progression through the cell cycle G1 checkpoint. Thus, mutations in the INKa/ARF locus effectively lead to loss of both tumour suppressor pathways. Positional cloning also identified the neurofibromatosis NF2 gene within the 22q12 locus, which encodes for the protein merlin. Merlin integrates signals from various adhesion molecules and cytoskeletal components and promotes cell adhesion, establishes apical polarity and mediates contact inhibition. It also has the capacity to migrate to the nucleus to modulate gene expression.

The precise mechanism of NF2 tumour suppression remains unclear [44] but it is likely to have a salient role. Whilst only 40% mesothelioma have truncations of NF2 or merlin, in the remaining cases, merlin is functionally inactivated through increased phosphorylation at Ser518 [45] and changes in microRNA expression [46]. Simultaneous loss of both INKa/ARF and NF2 appears to be important in the pathogenesis of mesothelioma. In experimental models of asbestos-induced mesothelioma, loss of the remaining NF2 allele is accompanied by the concomitant loss of INKa/ARF [47]. Indeed functionally, loss of INKa/ARF appears to be permissive for NF2 tumourigenesis [48]. Thus, the evidence points to mutations in INKa/ARF and NF2/merlin as driver mutations central to the pathogenesis of mesothelioma. As a result of the genetic instability conferred by these tumour suppressor gene mutations, a large number of genetic lesions appear causing dysregulation of growth factor expression and signalling, angiogenesis and apoptosis, conferring on the cell the phenotype of malignancy.

4. Diagnosis

Pleural diseases are common and the causes are diverse, but there is also considerable overlap in the clinical manifestatations of these conditions. Because of this, MPM is notoriously difficult to diagnose, both radiologically and pathologically.

4.1. Radiology

Radiologically, pleural malignancy is often suspected on clinical history and an abnormal chest radiograph showing pleural effusion or thickening. Computed tomography can be helpful in distinguishing malignant from benign pleural processes [49]. Whilst direct invasion of surrounding structures is diagnostic of malignancy, mediastinal pleural thickening, nodules in the pleura and thickness >1cm predict malignancy with a sensitivity of 40-70% and specificity of 64-96%. In differentiating mesothelioma from secondary pleural malignancies, mediastinal pleural involvement and rind-like encasement of the lung shows a sensitivity/specificity of 85%/67% and 70%/85% respectively. Magnetic resonance imaging (MRI) has a similar performance to CT at distinguishing benign from malignant processes on the basis of morphology, but signal intensity is a useful additional feature which improves the ability to differentiate between the two [50] [51]. PET-CT is less helpful for the differentiation of benign from malignant pleural diseases and is more valuable in staging than in diagnosis [52]. Interpretation is confounded by inflammatory and infective pleural conditions and recent talc pleurodesis [53] [54]. Nevertheless, none of these modalities are absolutely specific so, irrespective of radiological findings, diagnosis of mesothelioma requires pathological confirmation.

4.2. Obtaining tissue for diagnosis

The mesothelium is a flattened layer of pluripotent mesodermal-derived epithelial cells on the surface of the pleura and mesothelioma can be morphologically diverse. Two main issues face the pathologist trying to establish a diagnosis of mesothelioma. Firstly, mesothelial proliferation is common in benign conditions, and differentiating benign from malignant mesothelial proliferation can be very difficult with many benign processes showing atypical features and mimicking invasion. Secondly, of the malignant pathologies affecting the mesothelium, secondary malignancies are by far the most common and mesothelioma is rare. Determining that a pleural malignancy is primary can also be very difficult.

The quality of tissue available to the pathologist greatly influences the ability to make a diagnosis. Fluid from a pleural effusion is helpful at narrowing the differential diagnosis but it has poor sensitivity (about 50-60%) for the diagnosis of malignancy, and in most studies the negative predictive value is around 70% [55]. However, a diagnosis may be more forthcoming when aspiration cytology is repeated [56]. For the specific diagnosis of mesothelioma, cytology has an overall sensitivity of about 30-50%, and is almost useless at diagnosing sarcomatoid mesothelioma (20% sensitivity) [57].

Tissue for histopathology can be obtained by percutaneous or thoracoscopic means. Of the percutaneous methods, the Abram's needle has the highest yield, but is only similar to cytological diagnosis [58] [59]. Although pneumothorax can be expected in 15% of patients, few require intervention and the overall complication rate is low in safe hands [60] [61]. The addition of image guidance to target areas with >5mm pleural thickening significantly improves the diagnostic yield to >80% and reduces the rate of complications [61].

Thoracoscopy allows direct visual inspection and target selection, at the same time enabling greater amounts of tissue to be obtained, thereby improving the diagnostic yield for malignancy to about 95%. Video-assisted thoracoscopy requires a general anaesthetic and single lung ventilation and may be less suited to frail patients, however, it offers the opportunity to proceed to other procedures such as opening up loculations, pleurodesis or insertion of an indwelling drain in case of trapped lung.

Thoracotomy and pleural excision remains the gold-standard for diagnosis of mesothelioma. Whilst pleural biopsy, both open and close, have a high sensitivity for the diagnosis of mesothelioma, the sensitivity for the determination of tissue subtype is approximately 80-86% and is less accurate for non-epithelioid subtypes [62] [63].

4.3. Differentiating benign from malignant mesothelial proliferation

The separation of benign from malignant mesothelial proliferation can be extremely difficult. Most processes that affect the pleural space, from pneumothorax to thoracic surgery, pulmonary diseases to systemic diseases cause a degree of pleuritis with a degree of reactive mesothelial hyperplasia. This hyperplasia can be accompanied by quite florid cytological atypia, sometimes more florid than seen in some mesothelioma. Therefore, cytological features of a specimen are not helpful in the diagnosis of malignant mesothelioma [64].

Whilst invasion necessarily implies malignancy, benign processes in the pleura can also produce features that mimic invasion. To demonstrate invasion requires surrounding fat and stroma within the biopsy specimen, that is a reason why the diagnostic yield is higher with larger surgical specimens which contain the full thickness of the pleura and the deeper surrounding tissue. To illustrate the difficulty in clinching a diagnosis, even expert members of the US-Canadian Mesothelioma Reference Panel disagree 22% of the time on selected cases referred to them [65] [66].

Some benign histological features can appear ominous, one such is entrapment, where organising pleuritis within the pleural space overlying a pleural surface gives the deceptive appearance of mesothelial invasion. This can be complicated by the concomitant appearance of fat-like spaces within the organising pleuritis further giving the appearance of fat invasion [67]. Reactive proliferation of the surrounding stroma fibroblasts and spindled mesothelial cells can resemble sarcomatoid mesothelioma, whilst dense, fibrous pleuritis with low cellular content can resemble desmoplastic sarcomatoid mesothelioma.

Because of the difficulties differentiating benign from malignant mesothelial cells on morphological grounds, other techniques have been developed to this end. Unfortunately, immunohistochemistry is of limited value, with poor sensitivity and specificity [68], but the identification of mutated genes may be more fruitful. The discovery that the majority of mesothelioma has loss of 9q21 led to the recent development of fluorescence in-situ hybridisation techniques looking for homozygous deletions of the p16INK4a gene. Loss of p16 in this assay appears to be 100% specific for mesothelioma [40] [69]. Another avenue which has found commercial application is diagnosis through the pattern of downregulation of specific microRNAs [70].

4.4. Differentiating MPM from other pleural malignancies

Immunohistochemistry is indispensable for the differentiation between primary pleural mesothelioma and secondary malignancies. A number of markers for each of mesothelioma and the carcinoma should be used to improve the diagnostic specificity. The International Mesothelioma Interest Group (IMIG) recommends the use of at least 2 mesothelial markers and 2 markers of the tumour under consideration, and if no diagnosis could be arrived at, an expanded panel could be used [64]. Epithelioid mesothelioma markers include Wilms Tumour 1 (WT-1), calretinin. cytokeratin 5 or 5/6. Thyroid transcription factor-1 (TTF-1) is useful for the differentiation of lung adenocarcinoma, whilst CYFRA 21-1, SCCA and p63 are useful squamous cell carcinoma markers. Markers can also be selected for secondary malignancies of other tissue origin.

4.5. Histological subtypes

Many subtypes of mesothelioma have been described, but a single tumour can harbour several subtypes, so they are best broadly grouped into three types: epithelioid, sarcomatoid and mixed or biphasic. The epithelioid type is the most common (60%) whilst the other two types comprise 20% each [71]. The histological type not only determines the main differential diagnoses, but is also a predictor of response to treatment and one of the most powerful prognostic predictor [72] [73] [74].

5. Clinical features

The symptoms of MPM typically present insidiously with vague symptoms [75]. The characteristic symptoms are pain in half the patients, breathlessness in a third, and constitutional symptoms in less than 10%. At the beginning, symptoms are usually ill-defined and mild, but as the disease progresses, the initial heaviness becomes an ache and pain that interferes with

http://dx.doi.org/10.5772/55722

sleep, and the breathlessness would often force the patient to stop working. Medical attention is usually only sought after a median of 3.5 months of progressing symptoms [76].

Physical examination is helpful insofar as suggesting a pleural effusion or pleural thickening, but is nonspecific for the diagnosis of MPM. Peripheral stigmata of pulmonary diseases such as clubbing and hypertrophic pulmonary osteoarthropathy are not features of MPM, and palpable lymphadenopathy is rare.

In those with large effusion, drainage may lead to rapid improvement of symptoms but a trapped lung is also common. As the disease progresses, less fluid is produced and there is progressively more pleural thickening, eventually the fluid disappears and the chest becomes contracted and filled with tumour. Local invasion of the chest wall can result in intractable pain and paresthesia, whilst invasion of the contralateral pleural space, pericardial space or through the diaphragm usually herald a rapid deterioration. Distant spread is common but is usually less symptomatic than the primary site.

The outlook for patients with mesothelioma is bad. For patients who present asymptomatically on a chest radiograph, the median survival is 20 months with best supportive care [76], and it is with this baseline in mind that we should evaluate noncomparative studies on new therapies.

6. Staging of mesothelioma

The purpose of staging is threefold: it allows stratification of patients by the anatomical extent of disease into groups with similar prognosis, enables comparison of results between studies and facilitates treatment decision-making by determining the role of specific therapies in these subgroups. However, the staging of mesothelioma is hampered by two difficulties, firstly it has a non-spherical and non-concentric plate-like growth pattern and secondly, there is a lack of understanding of the natural history of mesothelioma. This is reflected in the fact there has been six different staging systems over the last 30 years [77] [78] [79] [80] [81] [82] [83]. Only the later systems adopted the TNM model, and most have not been independently validated.

The lack of an organ within which mesothelioma grows and the way it encroaches insidiously onto contiguous structures make clinical staging by imaging challenging. This is particularly the case with T-staging. The latest International Mesothelioma Interest Group (IMIG) staging system recognises that mesothelioma starts on the parietal pleura (T1a), and the spreads onto the visceral pleura as isolated and scattered foci (T1b), which becomes confluent (T2). These features are not easily resolvable on imaging and require direct visualisation with thoracoscopy or open surgery. Nevertheless, most tumours present at the T3 and T4 stages. Here, the preoperative determination of invasion into the chest wall, mediastinum, diaphragm or pericardium is crucial to the separation of potentially resectable (T3) from unresectable (T4) tumour, but in practice this is not an exact science. The visual distinction between a contiguous structure and an invaded structure can be a difficult call. When compared to the pathological stage, both CT and MRI have an accuracy of only 50-60% in most categories, but MRI may be marginally more superior in the diagnosis of diaphragmatic and chest wall invasion on account of the signal changes in these structures [84].

Nodal metastases portends a grave prognosis in patients with mesothelioma who underwent resection [80] [85] and so accurate staging of nodal involvement is crucial for the selection of patients for radical treatment and prognostication. However, several factors complicate the assessment of nodal disease. Firstly, our knowledge of nodal staging is hampered by the fact that bronchopulmonary nodes are not routinely sampled in radical pleurectomy-decortication, or routinely reported in extrapleural pneumonectomy specimens. Secondly, the current IMIG staging system adopted the lung cancer nodal classification for mesothelioma. However, early anatomical studies has already showed that lymphatic drainage of the pleura occurs first to the chest wall (internal mammary) and paravertebral lymph nodes, whilst there is little flow upstream through the lung parenchyma to the N1 stations [86]. Indeed, the survival of patients with N1 disease does not appear to be any better than those with N2 disease [87] [88] [89] whilst the extramediastinal nodes (internal mammary, pericardial, diaphragmatic) are associated with better prognosis [90]. Finally, within the mediastinal nodes there are differences in outcomes: involvement of upper mediastinal nodes is associated with worse prognosis [90]. This is compatible with the hypothesis that mesothelioma starts basally and progresses apically.

Radiologically, the nodes are frequently obscured by the pleural thickening, and there is little correlation between nodal size and disease involvement in mesothelioma [85], so that imaging modalities based on structural criteria perform poorly at discriminating between involved and uninvolved nodes. CT and MRI has an accuracy of about 50% for nodal staging and so cannot be relied on [84]. For this reason, functional imaging such as PET and PET-CT have been investigated for their role in staging. PET alone has poor spatial resolution, but when combined with CT, increases the specificity of the PET and the sensitivity of the CT. PET-CT is more accurate for staging resectable disease than CT, MRI or PET, through its ability to diagnose distant metastases [91]. For nodal staging, the accuracy for mediastinal nodal involvement in PET-CT is about 60-66% [92] [93], therefore invasive techniques such as mediastinoscopy are still required for accurate nodal staging given its potent impact on prognosis [90]. In practice, in a population with a 'resectable tumour on CT' and mandatory mediastinoscopy, PET-CT was able to prevent futile surgery in an additional 29% patients [92].

The current staging system has several deficiencies. Firstly, it was developed with surgical patients in mind and requires intraoperative and pathological assessment. As a result, clinical staging is highly inaccurate and correlates with pathological staging less than 50% of the time [89]. Secondly, it successfully stratifies survival in only some [94] and not other surgical series [83]. Thirdly, most patients end up belonging to stage III with little differentiation within. Fourthly, it does not predict survival in nonsurgical patients such as those following chemotherapy alone [95]. There are other prognostic factors which are more powerful at stratifying prognosis of mesothelioma patients. Cell type is an important prognostic determinant, the hazard ratio for death following trimodality therapy is several fold higher than nodal status and overall stage [83] [95].

Numerous other prognostic factors have been found to be associated with survival in mesothelioma. They include *clinical factors* such as age, performance status and asbestos burden, *laboratory indices* such as haemoglobin, platelet count, white cell count and serum lactate dehydrogenase, and *biomarkers* such as mesothelin and megakaryocyte potentiating factor [96] [95] [97]. These have been variously combined into different prognostic scores. Amongst the various scores, different factors take on different prognostic significance in different series and ultimately, the few consistent predictive factors are age, performance status, histology and stage. A gene ratio based test for molecular staging using the relative expression of four genes, namely *TM4SF1, PKM2, ARHGDIA*, and *COBLL1*, has been described and internally validated in a prospective patient set from the same institution [98]. This test was more powerful at predicting overall survival than either histology or lymph node involvement, and when combined with these, was able to differentiate three subgroups with very different outcomes [99]. Nevertheless, the test suffers the same limitation as the current staging system in its requirement for pathological data following resection.

7. Assessment of treatment response

Many tumours grow as spherical masses and linear measurements which correlate well to tumour volume can usually be taken on cross-section imaging for the assessment of response to treatment. The sheet like growth pattern of MPM over many different topologically complex surfaces meant objective measure of mesothelioma responses is difficult and subject to significant interobserver variation, the standard criteria for response assessment may therefore be unsuited to it.

The WHO criteria was introduced in 1979 to determine whether there was a complete response, partial response, stable disease or disease progression [100] and was based in part on evaluation of breast cancer response by palpation. Without stipulating the assessment protocol or measurement process, it proposed taking bidimensional measurements and obtaining the product of the longest tumour diameter with the greatest perpendicular measurement. This led to significant variation in the assessment method, and made comparison of reporting from different trials difficult. The Response Evaluation Criteria In Solid Tumour (RECIST) guideline was proposed in 2000 to try to address some of these problems [101]. It moved onto unidimensional assessment and measured changes in the longest tumour diameter on standardised imaging protocols. However, for tumours like mesothelioma, the choices of longest tumour diameter are many and subject to interpretation and bias. To improve on this, a modification of the RECIST criteria for mesothelioma was proposed to assess response by summating the perpendicular thickness of the tumour rind in two positions at three levels into a unidimensional measurement, and repeating the measurements at the same position [102]. Where appropriate for a lesion, bidimensional assessment can still be used. Within this system, a complete response is defined as complete disappearance of all tumour, a partial response by at least 30% reduction in the measurement on two occasions 4 weeks apart, progressive disease as increase in the measurement by 20% or appearance of new lesions, and stable disease as those who fulfilled neither the partial response nor progressive disease criteria.

This system was validated and showed correlation to lung function and survival outcomes [102]. Nevertheless, there is still significant overlap in survival between those with stable disease and those with partial response, even following optimisation of the cut-off criteria for each group [103]. This has significant implications for the clinical relevance of studies which use response as their primary outcome measure instead of survival.

8. Treatment

8.1. From single to multi-modality treatment

The results of mesothelioma treatment in the 1970s and 1980s were disappointing. Radical surgery alone was associated with high morbidity and mortality, whilst its impact on long term outcomes was questionable [77]. The response rate to chemotherapy was poor amongst most agents and responses were not durable with 80% of patients developing recurrent disease within 2 years. Mesothelioma cells are radiosensitive in the laboratory [104], but the use of radiotherapy to treat mesothelioma was associated with significant toxicity resulting from the extensive volume that needs to be treated and the proximity of vital organs. The disease burden is great from both local progression and distant metastases, but none of the modalities when used alone were effective. In 1980, Karen Antman at the then Sidney Farber Cancer Institute in Boston, proposed the combination of resection with radiotherapy and systemic chemotherapy in limited disease to maximise local control and minimise distant relapse.

Studies of surgery alone have reported that following extrapleural pneumonectomy, local recurrence occurs in a third of patients and distant recurrence in half the patients [105] [106]. Therefore, there was room to improve local control, but systemic control should also be part of the treatment for all patients. Early work focused on adding adjuvant chemotherapy and postoperative radiotherapy after EPP, but compliance with early chemotherapy following lung resection was often poor due to a prolonged postoperative recovery [107]. With this in mind, and the discovery of significant responses from platinum doublets, the Swiss investigators adopted a strategy of neoadjuvant chemotherapy followed by surgery and hemithoracic radiotherapy to ensure all patients received systemic treatment [108]. They showed that surgery after neoadjuvant chemotherapy was safe and outcomes were at least comparable if not improved. With this strategy, compliance with chemotherapy was near 100% and overall compliance with all three treatment modalities was 60-70% [109].

Since then, each of the therapeutic modalities have undergone refinement and a number of groups reported improved outcomes in selected patients undergoing multimodality treatment when compared to historical results. This has led to a number of randomised trials designed to tease out the role of various components of multimodality treatment.

In this section we will review the current state of knowledge on the treatment of mesothelioma. The role and nuances of surgery will be covered in another chapter, and here we will focus on radiation therapy and systemic treatment. We will review the roles of these treatments in palliation and as part of multimodality therapy with radical intent.

8.2. Symptom palliation

The symptoms of mesothelioma are severe and debilitating, leaving many patients miserable for their remaining time. In particular, the severity of pain and breathlessness exceeds that in non-small cell lung cancer patients [110].

Early on in the disease, breathlessness is due to pleural effusion compressing the lung and can be managed effectively by drainage. If the lung reexpands following drainage, pleurodesis can prevent reaccumulation. Most studies concern the management of malignant pleural effusions in general which include some cases of mesothelioma. Randomised trials for the use of sclerosant (drainage alone vs drainage with sclerosant), between different sclerosants and between techniques (bedside vs thoracoscopic) for malignant pleural effusions in general favoured the use of talc pleurodesis and thoracoscopy [111] [112]. One subsequent large randomised trial did suggest equivalence between bedside talc slurry and thoracoscopic talc pleurodesis [113], but the frequent need to obtain tissue for diagnosis usually favours the thoracoscopic approach. The recurrence rate following thoracoscopic pleurodesis remains however at 20-30%.

As the disease progresses, a trapped lung develops where the visceral tumour forms a constricting cortex over the lung preventing pleural apposition. Talc pleurodesis in such situations risks infection from long term drainage and contamination of a fixed space. VATS pleurectomy and decortication has been advocated as a palliative procedure which does not aim for complete macroscopic clearance, but tries to achieve lung reexpansion. There seems to be some short-term improvement in pain and dyspnoea [114] without detriment to survival [115] [116]. Recruitment to the randomised trial for VATS decortication (MesoVATS) has now closed, and the results should be available in the near future [117].

Recently, the use of long term tunnelled pleural catheters for effusions with underlying trapped lung has shown promise with very short hospital stay, low morbidity and better patient tolerability. It compared favourably with bedside talc slurry [118]. Even in patients with trapped lung, long term drainage could ultimately result in pleural symphysis, and the drain could eventually be removed in a fifth of patients [119]. Furthermore, chemotherapy can safely continue in the presence of such drains.

As the disease progresses, the effusion disappears and is replaced by a constricting tumour and a contracted hemithorax. Management of breathlessness at this stage is difficult. A palliative pleurectomy could be performed to relieve the restriction on ventilation and chest wall pain but there is significant morbidity associated with such an extensive operation. On the other hand, self-help breathlessness management techniques and opioids can help to relieve the sensation of dyspnoea.

Pain is also a significant symptom that could be difficult to manage. In addition to the WHO pain ladder, radiotherapy can improve chest wall pain in 50-60% patients [120] although unfortunately in most cases the relief is not sustained [121]. There is some suggestion that hyperthermia may increase the response rate to radiotherapy for pain control [122]. In addition, there is a significant neuropathic component to the pain, so early referral to a specialist pain management team may help to improve the quality of life in the final months.

The question of whether palliative chemotherapy has additional benefit on top of best supportive treatment was addressed by a three-armed randomised trial [123]. This was an important landmark - whilst there were numerous phase II trials addressing different chemotherapy agents, prior to this trial there were no randomised evidence to show that chemotherapy was beneficial over best supportive care, and most retrospective comparisons suffered from significant selection bias. Unfortunately, the trial experienced slow accrual and was revised to amalgamate two chemotherapy arms, which then also closed early from falling recruitment following the results of other randomised trials. This rendered it underpowered to show a survival difference. The trial was also criticised for employing non-standard chemotherapy regimens which may have led to nonsignificant results [124]. Within these limitations, it concluded the addition of chemotherapy did not improve symptoms or quality of life to any significant degree, in part because the few symptoms which improved were outweighed by the significant morbidity associated with chemotherapy.

The role of chemotherapy was indirectly addressed by other studies. The MED trial randomised 43 malignant mesothelioma (M) patients with stable symptoms to early (E) chemotherapy or to delayed (D) chemotherapy when there was symptom progression. It found patients who received early chemotherapy had a longer freedom from symptom progression and a better quality of life; furthermore, despite the small number of patients, there was a trend towards prolonged survival in the early chemotherapy group [125]. In addition to this study, a number of comparative randomised phase III studies found benefit for one regimen over another. Unless the control arms led to worse outcome than best supportive care, which is unlikely, these studies indirectly showed that a benefit for chemotherapy exists. Together, they showed that chemotherapy not only has a role in palliation as well as improving survival, but that it should be given early rather than late, and before symptoms worsen.

8.3. Chemotherapy

MPM is a particularly aggressive condition which responds poorly to treatment and chemotherapy is no exception. In the rush to make an impact, numerous studies have been carried out and almost all agents have been tried. Yet amongst these, most are small, noncomparative phase II studies, so attempts to draw conclusions about the efficacy of each treatment were frustrated by heterogeneity of the populations and variations in treatment schedules, assessment of response and reporting of outcomes, not to mention selection and publication biases. Frequently, promising outcomes in smaller trials were not replicated in larger and better conducted trials.

8.3.1. Towards cisplatin-based chemotherapy

In general, the single agent studies have been hard pressed to obtain response rates of over 20% and complete responses were rare. Of the single agent chemotherapy trials, many agents such as the vinca alkaloids (with the exception of vinorelbine) had no efficacy, and responders were few for the alkylating agents [126] [127] [128] [129]. The three classes of agents which showed some degree of response, albeit with response rates that rarely exceeded 20%, were the anthracyclines, platinum compounds and the antimetabolites/antifolates [130]. On the basis of this, Berghmans and colleagues carried out a metaanalysis, grouping studies into four subgroups: those which contained cisplatin without doxorubicin, doxorubicin without cisplatin, both doxorubicin and cisplatin and those that contained neither agents [131]. The composite response rate was highest for the two groups that contained cisplatin, with a higher response rate in the group that contained also doxorubicin (28.5%). On the other hand, doxorubicin alone (11.3%) was not better than trials which contained neither cisplatin nor doxorubicin (11.6%), suggesting cisplatin was the active agent.

A more recent metaanalysis [132] found the combined intention-to-treat (ITT) response rate for phase II single agent trials was indeed highest for cisplatin (20.0%) whilst almost all other classes of drugs including the anthracyclines had a rate of <10%. When used in combination, the non-platinum combination regimens had a slight improvement over single agents (overall response rate of 10.4%), but still remained some way behind single-agent cisplatin. On the other hand, certain combination therapies containing cisplatin appeared to show an improvement on single-agent cisplatin such as with anthracyclines (32.4%) and gemcitabine/irinotecan (26.1%).

These trials seemed to suggest that cisplatin is the more potent agent, and that combination therapy could improve on the results of single-agent cisplatin. Nevertheless, these phase II trials were hampered by their non-comparative nature, and the use of response rate as a surrogate outcome whilst often without reporting of survival outcomes. In fact, these responses were rarely sustained, and the link between radiological response and improved survival is tenuous.

8.3.2. The antimetabolites

Gemcitabine is a false nucleotide antimetabolite that gets misincorporated into DNA and hence interferes with DNA synthesis and repair. It showed broad activity against many solid and haematological malignancies, and has been evaluated in mesothelioma. The single agent trials were however inconsistent, with three trials showing widely differing response rates of 0%, 7% and 31% [133] [134] [135]. The overall ITT response rate was a disappointing 6.9%. There was significant heterogeneity in patient selection, chemotherapy dose and schedule, and response evaluation to explain some of the differences seen.

Cisplatin and gemcitabine are synergistic in the killing of neoplastic cells *in vitro* [136]. It is efficacious for several malignancies including non small cell lung cancer for which it became a standard of care prior to 2008 [137]. In a single institution phase II study from Australia, Byrne and colleagues administered a 6-cycle regimen of cisplatin and gemcitabine to 21 patients with confirmed mesothelioma. Tumour response was assessed by what was to become the modified RECIST criteria. There was an impressive 47.6% response rate that exceeded the results of both drugs as single agents, and a number of patients, including non-responders, found symptom relief [138]. This led to a multicentre phase II study of 53 patients using the same regimen [139]. However, the overall response rate this time was only 33% with a median duration of response of 5.4 months; the overall survival from diagnosis was a median of 17.3 months. In Europe, a phase II trial using a different dosing and scheduling regimen, obtained a response rate of 16% for the 25 patients using the WHO criteria for assessment [140].

In the absence of better phase III results, cisplatin and gemcitabine became widely adopted at the turn of the millenium and was also appropriated into multimodality regimens. In a single institution Swiss trimodality study, neoadjuvant chemotherapy with cisplatin and gemcitabine gave a response rate of 32% without increasing perioperative morbidity or mortality, and the ITT overall survival was 23 months [108]. A similar study from Memorial Sloan-Kettering Cancer Centre with 21 patients with advanced MPM reported a response rate of 26% to neoadjuvant cisplatin and gemcitabine. There were no postoperative mortality despite neoadjuvant treatment. The median survival was 33.5 months for those who completed all three modalities [141].

8.3.3. *The antifolates*

The other class of drugs which showed promise was the antifolate family of antimetabolites. Antifolates interfere with DNA synthesis through disrupting nucleotide synthesis, a process which requires folate. A trial of 63 patients with unresectable mesothelioma in the 1980s treated with high dose methotrexate found a 37% response rate (albeit with a looser definition of 'response') [142]. Another phase II trial of edatrexate, a drug very similar to methotrexate but for a single carbon to nitrogen substitution and greater potency, showed a response rate of 25% but with significant toxicity (20% early deaths) [143]. This required a protocol amendment with the use of leucovorin rescue. Unfortunately, this alteration also reduced the response rate.

Pemetrexed is a new generation antifolate which inhibits multiple folate-dependent processes including thymidylate synthase, dihydrofolate reductase and glycinamide ribonucleotide formyltransferase (GARFT), all of which are involved in thymidine and purine nucleotide synthesis. However, folate competes with pemetrexed for cellular uptake. Low folate levels result in higher intracellular accumulation of pemetrexed and thus higher cytotoxicity. Homocysteine levels has been found to be a marker of overall folate status and correlates clinically with pemetrexed toxicity [144]. However, a threshold level below which homocysteine levels could be considered safe could not be established. From 1999, it became a requirement to supplement folic acid and vitamin B12 in studies with pemetrexed, but trials straddling that period would include both non-supplemented and then supplemented patients.

Pemetrexed on its own showed efficacy similar to other single agents. In a multicentre phase II trial, 64 patients with confirmed MPM received pemetrexed [145], the response rate was 14.6%. Therapy was better tolerated by the supplemented patients, who also fared better with a response rate of 16.3% and median survival of 13.0 months. This was in contrast to 9.5% and 8.0 months in the nonsupplemented patients.

A large, international, multicentre, single-blinded phase III study comparing cisplatin and pemetrexed with cisplatin alone was carried out between 1999 and 2001[146]. In this pivotal study, 456 chemonaïve patients with unresectable disease or who were not surgical candidates were randomised to receive cisplatin and pemetrexed or cisplatin alone. Of these, 8 patients were randomised but were not able to receive treatment. At mid-trial, the protocol was modified to include folate and vitamin B12 supplementation to all enrolled patients. Supplementation greatly reduced toxicity: comparing patients who were never supplemented with those who were fully supplemented, the instance of neutropenic sepsis fell from 6.3% to 0.6%, vomiting from 34.4% to 10.7% and diarrhoea from 9.4 to 3.6%.

The trial found a significantly better response rates, time to progressive disease and survival in the combination therapy arm. The headline response rate was a remarkable 41.3% in the combination arm and 16.7% in the cisplation-only arm ($p<0.0001$), all responses were partial responses. However, true to the difficulty of assessing response, an independent review of imaging by the FDA confirmed only 47 of the 94 reported responses in the combination arm, but there were nevertheless still more responses in the combination arm [147].

In the final analysis, the median survival was 12.8 months in the combination arm versus 9.0 months in the cisplatin-only arm, with a hazard ratio of 0.74 [148]. Importantly, the use of vitamin supplementation did not appear to impact on the response rate or survival outcomes. On the basis of an advantage on survival, and in spite of the discrepant response rate data, pemetrexed became the first agent to be approved by the FDA for the treatment of MPM in patients whose disease is not resectable or who are otherwise not candidates for curative surgery [149].

A validated quality of life instrument (Lung Cancer Symptom Scale – mesothelioma) was also administered to all patients on the trial, and the overall symptom score was significantly in favour of the combination arm. Pain scores had worsened on the cisplatin arm but improved on the combination arm; dyspnoea scores had also worsened on the cisplatin arm but remain unchanged on the combination arm. The authors concluded that combination cisplatin and pemetrexed offered both symptomatic and survival benefit [150].

The trial was notable for its scale, rigorous execution and striking findings. However, it has also attracted a number of criticisms [151] [152]. The study was single blinded and this may have contributed to the discrepancy in observed response rates between the investigators and the FDA reviewers. There was concern that the control group was not the standard of care, ie. cisplatin doublet, but was instead single agent cisplatin which was not widely used. Furthermore, the outcome of the cisplatin-alone arm was unusually poor and this may have resulted in the combination arm appearing more efficacious. In fact, the survival benefit only reached borderline significance (p=0.051) suggesting the conclusion would have been very sensitive to small differences in outcome. The low toxicity seen in the vitamin supplemented patients may suggest that the optimal dosage of pemetrexed has not been reached, as the trial dosage was derived from the maximum tolerated dose from phase I studies carried out without supplementation.

Whilst the evidence and the FDA approval was for nonsurgical disease, on the basis of the survival benefits of the Vogelzang trial, several phase II studies of trimodality treatment adopted cisplatin and pemetrexed as their neoadjuvant chemotherapy from 2003. Krug and colleagues reported a multicentre phase II trial of 77 patients with cT1-3,N0-2,M0 histologically confirmed MPM undergoing trimodality therapy with this combination [153]. 64 patients (81.3%) were able to complete 4 cycles of chemotherapy. The radiological response rate with this regimen was 32.4%, of which 3 had pathological complete response at extrapleural pneumonectomy. The ITT median survival was 16.8 months, and for the 52% who completed all three modalities, the median survival was 29.1 months. In a similar vein, a multicentre European Organisation for Research and Treatment of Cancer (EORTC) trial in 2005-2007 recruited 58 patients with earlier stage (cT1-3,N0-1,M0) histologically-confirmed MPM for 3 cycles of cisplatin and pemetrexed followed by EPP and radical radiotherapy [154]. The radiological response after chemotherapy was a remarkable 43.9% (24.6% complete response and 19.3% partial response). The ITT median survival was 18.4 months. 37 patients completed all 3 modalities and their median survival was about estimated at 33 months, although the median was barely reached within the follow-up period and so does not allow a confident estimate.

Another new generation antifolate which has been tested in a randomised phase III setting in MPM is raltitrexed. Unlike pemetrexed, raltitrexed is a selective inhibitor of only one folic enzyme - thymidylate synthase. In a phase II study, single agent raltitrexed gave a response rate of 20.8% with only mild toxicity, without requiring vitamin supplementation [155]. This led to a multicentre randomised phase III study of cisplatin/ raltitrexed against cisplatin alone in patients with MPM not amenable to surgical resection [156]. 250 patients were randomised between the two groups. The radiological response rates were 14% for the cisplatin-only group and 24% for combination cisplatin-raltitrexed. There was a borderline significant increase in median survival for the combination chemotherapy arm (8.8 months vs 11.4 months, p=0.048). The study also assessed quality-of-life but did not find difference in the measures between the two arms.

Aside from the scale of the trials, the magnitude of benefits seen in the pemetrexed and raltitrexed randomised trials were very similar. An economic analysis recently found raltitrexed/cisplatin to be much more cost effective than pemetrexed/cisplatin combination chemotherapy [157]. Raltitrexed however, is not available in the US, and so the standard of care there remains cisplatin with pemetrexed or gemcitabine [124].

8.3.4. Second-line chemotherapy

The response rate for existing chemotherapy is poor and many patients have disease progression during first line therapy. Even for those who respond, the improvement is not durable. This relentless progression inevitably leads to a question of second line chemotherapy. The evidence for second-line therapy is however, limited, and many studies are confounded by rampant immortal time bias – that only patients who can survive to and are fit enough to receive second-line chemotherapy will receive it, so that treatment benefits will be arbitrarily overestimated.

For pemetrexed-naïve patients, both pemetrexed and non-pemetrexed-containing regimens have been used. There is little difference between the two and the outcomes were generally poor with a median time to progression of several months. Janne et al. reported on the outcomes of the extended access program for pemetrexed on 153 pemetrexed-naïve patients [158]. Some patients received single-agent pemetrexed, and others combination cisplatin and pemetrexed. The response rate and median survival was 32.5% and 7.6 months for combination therapy and 5.5% and 4.1 months for single agent therapy. There is an element of selection bias as patients who were older, have poorer performance status were more likely to receive only single agent therapy. They were also more likely to receive fewer chemotherapy cycles.

A multicentre phase III randomised trial also addressed the benefits of pemetrexed alone as second line chemotherapy versus best supportive care in pemetrexed-naïve patients. 243 patients were randomised, but 60% patients died or progressed on the trial treatment. The response rate was 18.7% with pemetrexed and 1.7% without, and progression free survival and time to progression were all in favour of pemetrexed. However, there was no difference in overall survival observed which may relate the large number of patients on the best supportive care arm who went onto receive early post-discontinuation therapy including pemetrexed. Quality of life was difficult to assess because of the rapid rate of attrition of these patients.

For pemetrexed-pretreated patients, both pemetrexed-containing and non-pemetrexed-containing regimens have been reported in noncomparative studies. For non-pemetrexed containing regimens, the response rates were reported as <10% and the time to progression was 2-3 months [159] [160]. Pemetrexed retreatment have also been investigated in pretreated patients. In one Italian institutional series, 31 pretreated patients were retreated at disease progression. There was a 19% response rate and a progression free survival of 3.8 months. They also noted that patients who had a longer progression free survival after first line chemotherapy also derived a longer progression free survival after second line retreatment [161], so that the ability to respond to the drug is not lost after first line treatment. In a larger multicentre retrospective observational study, the same authors reviewed 120 pemetrexed pretreated patients of which 42 were retreated with a pemetrexed regimen and 78 with a non-pemetrexed regimen. Those who received the pemetrexed regimen had a higher disease-control rate, and those rechallenged with platinum/pemetrexed combination therapy had a significantly longer progression free and overall survival than those receiving monotherapy (HR 0.11) [162].

However, the results of second line therapy remain poor and there is no standard therapy, this has made it a platform to test new agents. Many of the new targeted therapy drugs have been investigated as part of second line therapy, but this stage of the disease also places extraordinary demands on a new agent to prove a therapeutic value, and a negative trial on this platform risks writing off an effective agent.

8.4. Targeted therapy

In addition to the classical and largely indiscriminant cytotoxic chemotherapy, the landscape of oncology has recently been transformed with the arrival of targeted agents which target the many molecular alterations identified on the malignant cells. The successes of these agents in other malignancies have also led to them being tested in mesothelioma. There are many such agents, some of which have been or are investigated for mesothelioma. In this section we will outline the main targets, but the list is by no means exhaustive. The prevailing theme, nevertheless, is that the agents tested to date have not been successful.

8.4.1. Vascular Endothelial Growth Factor (VEGF)

Angiogenesis is crucial for tumour growth and mesothelioma is no exception. Indeed, angiogenesis is itself a poor prognostic factor for mesothelioma [163]. VEGF is not only a paracrine growth factor for blood vessels but also an autocrine signal for mesothelioma cells which expresses the VEGF receptors (VEGFR) -1, -2 and -3 [164]. A number of angiogenesis inhibitors are now available, and some has demonstrated effectiveness against malignancies such as colorectal cancer, non-small cell lung cancer (NSCLC) and multiple myeloma.

A number of anti-VEGF agents have been tested in mesothelioma but the results have been disappointing. Bevacizumab (Avastin) is a humanised anti-VEGF-A antibody which has showed effectiveness in metastatic colorectal cancer and NSCLC. In a phase II trial of patients with mesothelioma not amenable to curative intent surgery, they were randomised to cisplatin/gemcitabine with either bevazicumab or placebo. There was no difference in progression free or overall survival [165]. In a similar vein, the addition of bevazicumab to cisplatin and pemetrexed in a noncomparative trial did not result in improvements in response rates or survival compared to historical results [166]. A randomised trial of pemetrexed-cisplatin with or without bevacizumab is currently ongoing in Europe (MAPS trial).

Thalidomide has been resurrected in the 1990s when it was shown to be a powerful antiangiogenic agent. Clinically, it has showed effectiveness in multiple myeloma. In a dose escalation study, it was given to 40 patients with MPM irrespective of previous treatment [167]. Response was not formally reported, but only 27.5% patients were free from progression at 6 months.

Many other agents targeting the angiogenesis pathways such as sunitinib, vatalanib, sorafenib and NGR-hTNF have been tested in MPM alone or in addition to a cisplatin doublet, however, they mostly showed no or only very modest activity against MPM [168] [169] [170] [171].

8.4.2. Epidermal Growth Factor Signalling

EGF receptors (EGFR) is overexpressed in MPM. The tyrosine kinase inhibitors targeting EGFR, such as erlotinib and gefitinib, have been so successful in various types of cancer they too have been tested in MPM. Unfortunately, in phase II trials, these two agents did not show any significant activity against MPM: in both erlotonib trials, no objective response was observed [172] [173] whilst the gefitinib trial only showed a 4% response rate [174].

8.4.3. Histone deactylase inhibitors

Acetylation of histones is an important mechanism of epigenetic regulation of gene expression: acetylation frees the DNA from histones and increases gene expression, at the same time promoting cell cycle arrest or apoptosis. Histone deacetylase (HDAC) inhibitors have been developed and investigated in MPM. In the largest randomised trial in MPM to date, 660 patients pretreated were randomised to vorinostat, (a HDAC inhibitor) or placebo. The results were reported at the European Multidisciplinary Cancer Congress in September 2011. The triallists reported that vorinostat did not improve the response rate or overall survival compared to placebo [175].

8.4.4. NF-κB pathway

The NF-κB pathway is important in the pathogenesis of mesothelioma. Two agents that target the pathway have been investigated in mesothelioma. Bortezomib, a proteasome inhibitor which induces apoptosis in mesothelioma cells is currently studied in several trials [176]. In a phase II trial of monotherapy bortezomib, the response rate was 4.8%, and the majority of patients had disease progression on treatment within the first two cycles [177]. Ranpirnase is a ribonuclease found in the Northern Leopard Frog oocyte. It is a tRNase that also prevents NF-κB nuclear translocation. In a large phase II study of single-agent ranpirnase which included patients who previously did not respond to chemotherapy, the response rate was 5% and the ITT median survival was 6 months [178]. In a phase III randomised trial of doxorubicin with or without ranpirnase for both chemonaïve and pretreated patients, there was no difference in ITT overall survival. However, a survival benefit could be seen in the preplanned subgroup analysis of the pretreated subgroup [179].

9. Radiotherapy

Radiotherapy has been studied in three roles for the management of mesothelioma: the palliation of symptoms, prevention of tract site metastases and with radical intent to improve survival alone or as part of multimodality treatment. The first of these was covered earlier and we will focus our discussion here on the other two roles.

9.1. Prophylactic irradiation

Mesothelioma has been known to seed along interventional tracts to form painful subcutaneous nodules and radiotherapy is commonly used in the prevention of such metastases. In general, the more invasive the procedure, the higher the likelihood is of getting tract metastases [180]. The carte blanche to give prophylactic irradiation came from a randomised trial in 1995 [181]. Boutin et al. randomised 40 patients following thoracoscopy to local irradiation with 21Gy of 12.5-15 MeV electrons in 3 fractions within 15 days of the procedure. They found an incidence of subcutaneous nodules of 40% in the untreated patients and 0% in the irradiated patients. Since then, prophylactic irradiation of intervention sites has become entrenched in guidelines [182] [183] and clinical practice [184] [185].

Two subsequent randomised trials found an incidence of subcutaneous nodules of only about 10% of patients, and that prophylactic irradiation offered no protection against the development of these nodules [186] [187]. The interpretation of these results was confounded by different radiotherapy techniques in these trials [188]. Bydder et al. employed a single fraction of 10Gy of 9MeV electrons delivered up to 15 days following intervention, and O'Rourke employed 21Gy in 3 fractions of 9-12 MeV electrons up to 21 days following intervention. Furthermore, all three trials were underpowered, and in none of them was histological confirmation of subcutaneous nodules obtained.

Further questions which confuse the issue for prophylactic irradiation included the degree to which these nodules are symptomatic - reports varied between 25% and 75% [187] [189], and to what degree these nodules impact on the quality of life of patients. To illustrate the confusion and debate surrounding the use of prophylactic irradiation, we need look no further than the evidence-based guidelines. The latest British Thoracic Society guideline continue to recommend prophylactic irradiation [190], whilst the European Society of Medical Oncology and the European Respiratory Society were not able to recommend it [191, 192]. In the penumbra of all this equipoise, a new randomised trial is being conducted to assess the role of prophylactic irradiation in the modern era of chemotherapy, in an adequately powered multicentre study [193].

9.2. Radical radiotherapy

Radiotherapy has been used both alone and as part of trimodality therapy in the radical treatment of MPM. A number of trials in the 1980's examined the use of radiotherapy alone with radical intent and found no survival benefit [194]. The use of radiotherapy for mesothelioma is complicated by the extensive field which it is required to covered, but at the same time juxtaposition of vital structures such as lung, oesophagus, spine, heart, liver and kidneys which limits the dose that can be delivered. Following irradiation of the hemithorax for mesothelioma, the loss of lung function is complete and equivalent to a pneumonectomy [195]. There is a real risk of treatment-related deaths, reaching 2 out of 12 in one retrospective series [196]. Because of this, it is felt radical radiotherapy should be delivered only after extrapleural pneumonectomy, to avoid the morbidity and mortality associated with life-threatening toxicity to the in-field ipsilateral lung.

The local relapse rate following surgery alone is 70-80% [105], and the focus of radiotherapy has shifted over the years to improving local control within the model of multimodality treatment. However, the rate of local recurrence from single modality radical treatment 53% [197], 35% [198] and 11% [199]. There is a suggestion of a dose-response relationship between radiation dosage and local recurrence but this has not yet been established [199] [200]. Beyond these observational series there is no randomised evidence yet to support or refute the use of postoperative radiotherapy. A multicentre randomised trial for radiotherapy within trimodality therapy is currently recruiting, but the trial will reach completion only in late 2017 [201]. At present, it is common to include postoperative hemithoracic irradiation to 54Gy within trimodality therapy.

With the tumour abutting a number of radiosensitive vital structures, there has been great interest in the use of intensity-modulated radiotherapy (IMRT) to deliver radiation in a field which conforms much more tightly to the target volume, in an effort to improve delivery to the tumour whilst reducing bystander irradiation. It is much more complex to deliver and requires significantly longer planning and treatment times. Whilst there is a growing body of evidence in support of the benefits of IMRT in various cancers, its use in mesothelioma appears to be harmful. In a series from Boston, fatal pneumonitis in the remaining lung occurred in 6 of 13 patients [202], whilst in MD Anderson, 23 of 63 patients died within 6 months of IMRT, of which 6 were from pulmonary causes [203]. The factor which predicted pulmonary complications appeared to be V20 (volume of lung receiving over 20Gy irradiation) [204]. At the same time, however, the locoregional failure rate remained at 13% [203]. Several subsequent series together corroborated the findings of a relationship between pulmonary complications and V20 [205] [206] [207]. As it stands, there is no evidence for additional benefit from IMRT, whilst there are significant concerns about harm. IMRT has not replaced conventional radiotherapy and its use should be confined to carefully monitored clinical trials.

Historically, EPP has been reserved for patients who are fit to undergo pneumonectomy, whilst patients who are less fit and/or have unresectable disease are often offered radical pleurectomy/decortication (P/D). However, despite this strategy, patients who underwent EPP not only have a survival advantage over those who underwent P/D, but actually had more morbidity, mortality and worse survival [208]. In recent years, the enthusiasm for EPP has waned and many surgeons has shifted to offering the less morbid P/D, to the extent that the proposed MARS2 trial intends to abandon EPP and instead randomise patients between radical P/D and no surgery [209].

The implication this has on delivering radiotherapy within multimodality therapy is significant. Whilst local control becomes even more pertinent, the risk of radiotherapy is also higher because of toxicity to the unresected lung. With the poor results of single modality radical radiotherapy, there is little experience of radiotherapy after pleurectomy-decortication. Some groups have delivered prophylactic radiotherapy to the surgical wounds with occasional boost radiation to at-risk areas, and therefore although described as trimodality therapy, these studies did not reflect the radical doses resembling that after EPP [210].

When higher dose external-beam radiation was used after pleurectomy-decortication, there was significant treatment-related mortality and morbidity. Likewise, the addition of intraoperative brachytherapy to the pleural space was associated with worse, not better survival. Nevertheless, there was some suggestion that delivery of >40 Gys was associated with better outcome although there is inevitably selection and immortal time bias [211]. There has been interest therefore in the use of IMRT after pleurectomy-decortication to improve delivery of therapeutic doses to disease area whilst keeping normal tissue irradiation to a minimum. Planning is challenging, and for MPM requires over 20 planning cycles. A phase I study found IMRT up to 50Gy was feasible but severe pneumonitis occurred in 20% patients. The median survival of 26 months after receiving all three modalities was comparable to the results after trimodality treatment with EPP [212].

10. Conclusion

In conclusion, MPM is an aggressive malignancy which presents insidiously, is difficult to diagnose and is resistant to most standard treatments. There have been a lot of developments over the years but the prognosis remains bleak. A number of ongoing current trials are looking to refine the treatment of this cancer, but it will probably take a quantum leap in thinking to really make a dent in the outcomes.

Author details

Kelvin K.W. Lau and Calvin S.H. Ng

Department of Cardiothoracic Surgery, Chinese University of Hong Kong, Prince of Wales Hospital, Shatin, New Territories, Hong Kong, China

References

[1] Smart, J, & Hinson, K. F. Pleural neoplasms. Br J Tuberc Dis Chest, (1957). , 319-330.

[2] Wagner, J. C, Sleggs, C. A, & Marchand, P. Diffuse pleural mesothelioma and asbestos exposure in the North Western Cape Province. Br J Ind Med, (1960). , 260-271.

[3] Wagner, J. C. The discovery of the association between blue asbestos and mesotheliomas and the aftermath. Br J Ind Med, (1991). , 399-403.

[4] Ross, M, & Nolan, R. P. History of asbestos discovery and use and asbestos-related disease in context with the occurrence of asbestos within the ophiolite complexes, in Ophiolite Concept and the Evolution of Geological Thought, Y. Dilek and S. Newcomb, Editors. (2003). The Geological Society of America, Inc.: Boulder, Colorado. , 447.

[5] Loomis, D, et al. Increased lung cancer mortality among chrysotile asbestos textile workers is more strongly associated with exposure to long thin fibres. Occupational and Environmental Medicine, (2012). , 564-568.

[6] Berry, G, et al. Malignant pleural and peritoneal mesotheliomas in former miners and millers of crocidolite at Wittenoom, Western Australia. Occup Environ Med, (2004). , e14.

[7] Robinson, B. W, & Lake, R. A. Advances in malignant mesothelioma. N Engl J Med, (2005). , 1591-1603.

[8] Lanphear, B. P, & Buncher, C. R. Latent period for malignant mesothelioma of occupational origin. J Occup Med, (1992). , 718-721.

[9] Iwatsubo, Y, et al. Pleural mesothelioma: dose-response relation at low levels of asbestos exposure in a French population-based case-control study. Am J Epidemiol, (1998). , 133-142.

[10] Hansen, J, et al. Environmental exposure to crocidolite and mesothelioma: exposure-response relationships. Am J Respir Crit Care Med, (1998). , 69-75.

[11] Rogers, A. J, et al. Dose-Response Relationship Between Airborne and Lung Asbestos Fibre Type, Length and Concentration, and the Relative Risk of Mesothelioma. Annals of Occupational Hygiene, (1994). inhaled particles VII): , 631-638.

[12] Hillerdal, G. Mesothelioma: cases associated with non-occupational and low dose exposures. Occup Environ Med, (1999). , 505-513.

[13] Kazan-allen, L. Current asbestos bans and restrictions. (2012). Available from: http://ibasecretariat.org/alpha_ban_list.php.

[14] LaDouJ., et al., The case for a global ban on asbestos. Environ Health Perspect, (2010). , 897-901.

[15] Mossman, B. T, et al. Asbestos: scientific developments and implications for public policy. Science, (1990). , 294-301.

[16] Pezerat, H. Chrysotile biopersistence: the misuse of biased studies. Int J Occup Environ Health, (2009). , 102-106.

[17] Mirabelli, D, et al. Excess of mesotheliomas after exposure to chrysotile in Balangero, Italy. Occup Environ Med, (2008). , 815-819.

[18] Wang, X, et al. A 37-year observation of mortality in Chinese chrysotile asbestos workers. Thorax, (2012). , 106-110.

[19] Deng, Q, et al. Exposure-response relationship between chrysotile exposure and mortality from lung cancer and asbestosis. Occup Environ Med, (2012). , 81-86.

[20] Baris, Y. I, et al. Malignant mesothelioma and radiological chest abnormalities in two villages in Central Turkey. An epidemiological and environmental investigation. Lancet, (1981). , 984-987.

[21] Carthew, P, et al. Intrapleural administration of fibres induces mesothelioma in rats in the same relative order of hazard as occurs in man after exposure. Hum Exp Toxicol, (1992). , 530-534.

[22] Dogan, A. U, et al. Genetic predisposition to fiber carcinogenesis causes a mesothelioma epidemic in Turkey. Cancer Res, (2006). , 5063-5068.

[23] Metintas, M, et al. Endemic malignant mesothelioma: exposure to erionite is more important than genetic factors. Arch Environ Occup Health, (2010). , 86-93.

[24] Kliment, C. R, Clemens, K, & Oury, T. D. North american erionite-associated mesothelioma with pleural plaques and pulmonary fibrosis: a case report. Int J Clin Exp Pathol, (2009). , 407-410.

[25] Carbone, M, et al. Erionite exposure in North Dakota and Turkish villages with mesothelioma. Proc Natl Acad Sci U S A, (2011). , 13618-13623.

[26] Robinson, C, et al. A novel SV40 TAg transgenic model of asbestos-induced mesothelioma: malignant transformation is dose dependent. Cancer Res, (2006). , 10786-10794.

[27] Kroczynska, B, et al. Crocidolite asbestos and SV40 are cocarcinogens in human mesothelial cells and in causing mesothelioma in hamsters. Proc Natl Acad Sci U S A, (2006). , 14128-14133.

[28] Carbone, M, et al. Simian virus 40-like DNA sequences in human pleural mesothelioma. Oncogene, (1994). , 1781-1790.

[29] Strickler, H. D. A multicenter evaluation of assays for detection of SV40 DNA and results in masked mesothelioma specimens. Cancer Epidemiol Biomarkers Prev, (2001). , 523-532.

[30] Van Kaick, G, et al. The German Thorotrast study: Recent results and assessment risks. Radiation Research, (1999). , S64-S71.

[31] Hodgson, D. C, et al. Long-Term Solid Cancer Risk Among 5-Year Survivors of Hodgkin's Lymphoma. Journal of Clinical Oncology, (2007). , 1489-1497.

[32] De Bruin, M. L, et al. Malignant mesothelioma after radiation treatment for Hodgkin lymphoma. Blood, (2009). , 3679-3681.

[33] Bernstein, D. M, Rogers, R, & Smith, P. The biopersistence of brazilian chrysotile asbestos following inhalation. Inhal Toxicol, (2004). , 745-761.

[34] Bocchetta, M, et al. Human mesothelial cells are unusually susceptible to simian virus 40-mediated transformation and asbestos cocarcinogenicity. Proc Natl Acad Sci U S A, (2000). , 10214-10219.

[35] Yang, H, et al. TNF-alpha inhibits asbestos-induced cytotoxicity via a NF-kappaB-dependent pathway, a possible mechanism for asbestos-induced oncogenesis. Proc Natl Acad Sci U S A, (2006). , 10397-10402.

[36] Srivastava, R. K, et al. Cyto-genotoxicity of amphibole asbestos fibers in cultured human lung epithelial cell line: role of surface iron. Toxicol Ind Health, (2010). , 575-582.

[37] Papp, T, et al. Mutational analysis of N-ras, p53 p16INK4a, p14ARF and CDK4 genes in primary human malignant mesotheliomas. Int J Oncol, (2001). p. 425-33.

[38] Kratzke, R. A, et al. Immunohistochemical analysis of the p16INK4cyclin-dependent kinase inhibitor in malignant mesothelioma. J Natl Cancer Inst, (1995). p. 1870-5.

[39] Xio, S, et al. Codeletion of p15 and p16 in primary malignant mesothelioma. Oncogene, (1995). p. 511-5.

[40] Takeda, M, et al. deletion in the diagnosis of malignant mesothelioma, using fluorescence in situ hybridization analysis. Pathol Int, (2010). p. 395-9., 21.

[41] Bianchi, A. B, et al. High frequency of inactivating mutations in the neurofibromatosis type 2 gene (NF2) in primary malignant mesotheliomas. Proc Natl Acad Sci U S A, (1995). , 10854-10858.

[42] Sekido, Y, et al. Neurofibromatosis type 2 (NF2) gene is somatically mutated in mesothelioma but not in lung cancer. Cancer Res, (1995). , 1227-1231.

[43] Cheng, J. Q, et al. Frequent mutations of NF2 and allelic loss from chromosome band 22q12 in malignant mesothelioma: evidence for a two-hit mechanism of NF2 inactivation. Genes Chromosomes Cancer, (1999). , 238-242.

[44] Li, W, et al. Merlin: a tumour suppressor with functions at the cell cortex and in the nucleus. EMBO Rep, (2012). , 204-215.

[45] Thurneysen, C, et al. Functional inactivation of NF2/merlin in human mesothelioma. Lung Cancer, (2009). , 140-147.

[46] Guled, M, et al. CDKN2A, NF2, and JUN are dysregulated among other genes by miRNAs in malignant mesothelioma-A miRNA microarray analysis. Genes Chromosomes Cancer, (2009). , 615-623.

[47] Lecomte, C, et al. Similar tumor suppressor gene alteration profiles in asbestos-induced murine and human mesothelioma. Cell Cycle, (2005). , 1862-1869.

[48] Jongsma, J, et al. A conditional mouse model for malignant mesothelioma. Cancer Cell, (2008). , 261-271.

[49] Metintas, M, et al. Computed tomography features in malignant pleural mesothelioma and other commonly seen pleural diseases. Eur J Radiol, (2002). , 1-9.

[50] Falaschi, F, et al. Usefulness of MR signal intensity in distinguishing benign from malignant pleural disease. AJR Am J Roentgenol, (1996). , 963-968.

[51] Hierholzer, J, et al. MRI and CT in the differential diagnosis of pleural disease. Chest, (2000). , 604-609.

[52] Orki, A, et al. The role of positron emission tomography/computed tomography in the diagnosis of pleural diseases. Thorac Cardiovasc Surg, (2009). , 217-221.

[53] Elboga, U, et al. The role of FDG PET-CT in differential diagnosis of pleural pathologies. Rev Esp Med Nucl, (2011).

[54] Genestreti, G, et al. FDG PET/CT Response Evaluation in Malignant Pleural Mesothelioma Patients Treated with Talc Pleurodesis and Chemotherapy. J Cancer, (2012). , 241-245.

[55] Motherby, H, et al. Diagnostic accuracy of effusion cytology. Diagn Cytopathol, (1999). , 350-357.

[56] Garcia, L. W, Ducatman, B. S, & Wang, H. H. The value of multiple fluid specimens in the cytological diagnosis of malignancy. Mod Pathol, (1994). , 665-668.

[57] Rakha, E. A, et al. The sensitivity of cytologic evaluation of pleural fluid in the diagnosis of malignant mesothelioma. Diagn Cytopathol, (2010). , 874-879.

[58] Adams, R. F, et al. Percutaneous image-guided cutting needle biopsy of the pleura in the diagnosis of malignant mesothelioma. Chest, (2001). , 1798-1802.

[59] Tomlinson, J. R, & Sahn, S. A. Invasive Procedures in the Diagnosis of Pleural Disease. Seminars in Respiratory Medicine, (1987). , 30-36.

[60] Hooper, C, Lee, Y. C, & Maskell, N. Investigation of a unilateral pleural effusion in adults: British Thoracic Society Pleural Disease Guideline (2010). Thorax, 2010. 65 Suppl 2: , ii4-i17.

[61] Maskell, N. A, Gleeson, F. V, & Davies, R. J. Standard pleural biopsy versus CT-guided cutting-needle biopsy for diagnosis of malignant disease in pleural effusions: a randomised controlled trial. Lancet, (2003). , 1326-1330.

[62] Bueno, R, et al. Pleural biopsy: a reliable method for determining the diagnosis but not subtype in mesothelioma. Ann Thorac Surg, (2004). , 1774-1776.

[63] Greillier, L, et al. Accuracy of pleural biopsy using thoracoscopy for the diagnosis of histologic subtype in patients with malignant pleural mesothelioma. Cancer, (2007). , 2248-2252.

[64] Husain, A. N, et al. Guidelines for Pathologic Diagnosis of Malignant Mesothelioma: (2012). Update of the Consensus Statement from the International Mesothelioma Interest Group. Arch Pathol Lab Med, 2012.

[65] Mccaughey, W. T, et al. Diagnosis of diffuse malignant mesothelioma: experience of a US/Canadian Mesothelioma Panel. Mod Pathol, (1991). , 342-353.

[66] Churg, A, et al. The separation of benign and malignant mesothelial proliferations. Am J Surg Pathol, (2000). , 1183-1200.

[67] Churg, A, et al. The fake fat phenomenon in organizing pleuritis: a source of confusion with desmoplastic malignant mesotheliomas. Am J Surg Pathol, (2011). , 1823-1829.

[68] King, J, et al. Sensitivity and specificity of immunohistochemical antibodies used to distinguish between benign and malignant pleural disease: a systematic review of published reports. Histopathology, (2006). , 561-568.

[69] Monaco, S. E, et al. The diagnostic utility of p16 FISH and GLUT-1 immunohistochemical analysis in mesothelial proliferations. Am J Clin Pathol, (2011). p. 619-27.

[70] Gee, G. V, et al. Downregulated microRNAs in the differential diagnosis of malignant pleural mesothelioma. International Journal of Cancer, (2010). , 2859-2869.

[71] Attanoos, R. L, & Gibbs, A. R. Pathology of malignant mesothelioma. Histopathology, (1997). , 403-418.

[72] Montanaro, F, et al. Survival of pleural malignant mesothelioma in Italy: a population-based study. Int J Cancer, (2009). , 201-207.

[73] Milano, M. T, & Zhang, H. Malignant pleural mesothelioma: a population-based study of survival. J Thorac Oncol, (2010). , 1841-1848.

[74] Musk, A. W, et al. Predicting survival in malignant mesothelioma. Eur Respir J, (2011). , 1420-1424.

[75] Elmes, P. C, & Simpson, J. C. The clinical aspects of mesothelioma. Q J Med, (1976). , 427-449.

[76] Brien, O. M.E.R., Malignant mesothelioma-the UK experience. Lung cancer, (2004)., S133-S135.

[77] Butchart, E. G, et al. Pleuropneumonectomy in the management of diffuse malignant mesothelioma of the pleura. Experience with 29 patients. Thorax, (1976)., 15-24.

[78] Mattson, K. Natural history and clinical staging of malignant mesothelioma. Eur J Respir Dis, (1982). suppl 124):, 87.

[79] Chahinian, A. P. Therapeutic modalities in malignant pleural mesothelioma, in Diseases of the pleura, J. Chretien and A. Hirsch, Editors. (1983). Masson: New York., 224-236.

[80] Sugarbaker, D. J, et al. Node status has prognostic significance in the multimodality therapy of diffuse, malignant mesothelioma. J Clin Oncol, (1993)., 1172-1178.

[81] Pleural Mesotheliomain American Joint Committee on Cancer Manual for Staging of Cancer, O.H. Beahrs, et al., Editors. (1992). JB Lippincott Co.: Philadelphia., 123-125.

[82] A Proposed New International TNM Staging System for Malignant Pleural Mesothelioma. CHEST Journal, 1995. 108(4): p. 1122-1128.

[83] Sugarbaker, D. J, et al. Resection margins, extrapleural nodal status, and cell type determine postoperative long-term survival in trimodality therapy of malignant pleural mesothelioma: results in 183 patients. J Thorac Cardiovasc Surg, (1999). discussion 63-5., 54-63.

[84] Heelan, R. T, et al. Staging of malignant pleural mesothelioma: comparison of CT and MR imaging. AJR Am J Roentgenol, (1999)., 1039-1047.

[85] Pilling, J. E, et al. The case for routine cervical mediastinoscopy prior to radical surgery for malignant pleural mesothelioma. Eur J Cardiothorac Surg, (2004)., 497-501.

[86] Singer, J. J. The Lymphatic Drainage of the Pleura as Demonstrated by Thorotrast. Cal West Med, (1942)., 28-29.

[87] Edwards, J. G, et al. The pattern of lymph node involvement influences outcome after extrapleural pneumonectomy for malignant mesothelioma. J Thorac Cardiovasc Surg, (2006)., 981-987.

[88] Flores, R. M, et al. The impact of lymph node station on survival in 348 patients with surgically resected malignant pleural mesothelioma: implications for revision of the American Joint Committee on Cancer staging system. J Thorac Cardiovasc Surg, (2008)., 605-610.

[89] Rusch, V. W, et al. Initial analysis of the international association for the study of lung cancer mesothelioma database. J Thorac Oncol, (2012)., 1631-1639.

[90] Nakas, A, et al. The new case for cervical mediastinoscopy in selection for radical surgery for malignant pleural mesothelioma. European Journal of Cardio-Thoracic Surgery, (2012)., 72-76.

[91] Plathow, C, et al. Computed tomography, positron emission tomography, positron emission tomography/computed tomography, and magnetic resonance imaging for staging of limited pleural mesothelioma: initial results. Invest Radiol, (2008). , 737-744.

[92] Sorensen, J. B, et al. Preoperative staging of mesothelioma by 18F-fluoro-2-deoxy-D-glucose positron emission tomography/computed tomography fused imaging and mediastinoscopy compared to pathological findings after extrapleural pneumonectomy. Eur J Cardiothorac Surg, (2008). , 1090-1096.

[93] Pilling, J, Dartnell, J. A, & Lang-lazdunski, L. Integrated positron emission tomography-computed tomography does not accurately stage intrathoracic disease of patients undergoing trimodality therapy for malignant pleural mesothelioma. Thorac Cardiovasc Surg, (2010). , 215-219.

[94] Rusch, V. W, & Venkatraman, E. The importance of surgical staging in the treatment of malignant pleural mesothelioma. J Thorac Cardiovasc Surg, (1996). discussion 825-6., 815-825.

[95] Ak, G, et al. Prognostic factors according to the treatment schedule in malignant pleural mesothelioma. J Thorac Oncol, (2009). , 1425-1430.

[96] Edwards, J. G, et al. Prognostic factors for malignant mesothelioma in 142 patients: validation of CALGB and EORTC prognostic scoring systems. Thorax, (2000). , 731-735.

[97] Hollevoet, K, et al. The effect of clinical covariates on the diagnostic and prognostic value of soluble mesothelin and megakaryocyte potentiating factor. Chest, (2012). , 477-484.

[98] Bueno, R. Making the case for molecular staging of malignant pleural mesothelioma. Semin Thorac Cardiovasc Surg, (2009). , 188-193.

[99] Gordon, G. J, et al. Four-gene expression ratio test for survival in patients undergoing surgery for mesothelioma. J Natl Cancer Inst, (2009). , 678-686.

[100] WHO Handbook for reporting results for cancer treatment(1979). Available from: http://whqlibdoc.who.int/publications/9241700483.pdf.

[101] Therasse, P, et al. New guidelines to evaluate the response to treatment in solid tumors. European Organization for Research and Treatment of Cancer, National Cancer Institute of the United States, National Cancer Institute of Canada. J Natl Cancer Inst, (2000). , 205-216.

[102] Byrne, M. J, & Nowak, A. K. Modified RECIST criteria for assessment of response in malignant pleural mesothelioma. Ann Oncol, (2004). , 257-260.

[103] Labby, Z. E, et al. Optimization of response classification criteria for patients with malignant pleural mesothelioma. J Thorac Oncol, (2012). , 1728-1734.

[104] Carmichael, J, et al. Radiation sensitivity of human lung cancer cell lines. Eur J Cancer Clin Oncol, (1989). , 527-534.

[105] Pass, H. I, et al. Surgically debulked malignant pleural mesothelioma: results and prognostic factors. Ann Surg Oncol, (1997). , 215-222.

[106] Rusch, V. W, Piantadosi, S, & Holmes, E. C. The role of extrapleural pneumonectomy in malignant pleural mesothelioma. A Lung Cancer Study Group trial. J Thorac Cardiovasc Surg, (1991). , 1-9.

[107] Pisters, K. M, et al. Induction chemotherapy before surgery for early-stage lung cancer: A novel approach. Bimodality Lung Oncology Team. J Thorac Cardiovasc Surg, (2000). , 429-439.

[108] Weder, W, et al. Neoadjuvant chemotherapy followed by extrapleural pneumonectomy in malignant pleural mesothelioma. J Clin Oncol, (2004). , 3451-3457.

[109] Weder, W, et al. The MARS feasibility trial: conclusions not supported by data. Lancet Oncol, (2011). author reply 1094-5., 1093-1094.

[110] Nowak, A. K, Stockler, M. R, & Byrne, M. J. Assessing quality of life during chemotherapy for pleural mesothelioma: feasibility, validity, and results of using the European Organization for Research and Treatment of Cancer Core Quality of Life Questionnaire and Lung Cancer Module. J Clin Oncol, (2004). , 3172-3180.

[111] Shaw, P, & Agarwal, R. Pleurodesis for malignant pleural effusions. Cochrane Database Syst Rev, (2004). , CD002916.

[112] Tan, C, et al. The evidence on the effectiveness of management for malignant pleural effusion: a systematic review. European Journal of Cardio-Thoracic Surgery, (2006). , 829-838.

[113] Dresler, C. M, et al. Phase III intergroup study of talc poudrage vs talc slurry sclerosis for malignant pleural effusion. Chest, (2005). , 909-915.

[114] Martin-ucar, A. E, et al. Palliative surgical debulking in malignant mesothelioma: Predictors of survival and symptom control. European Journal of Cardio-Thoracic Surgery, (2001). , 1117-1121.

[115] Nakas, A, et al. The role of video assisted thoracoscopic pleurectomy/decortication in the therapeutic management of malignant pleural mesothelioma. European Journal of Cardio-Thoracic Surgery, (2008). , 83-88.

[116] Halstead, J. C, et al. Improved survival with VATS pleurectomy-decortication in advanced malignant mesothelioma. Eur J Surg Oncol, (2005). , 314-320.

[117] MESOVATS Available from: http://public.ukcrn.org.uk/search/StudyDetail.aspx?StudyID=1352.

[118] Demmy, T. L, et al. Optimal management of malignant pleural effusions (results of CALGB 30102). J Natl Compr Canc Netw, (2012). , 975-982.

[119] Sioris, T, et al. Long-term indwelling pleural catheter (PleurX) for malignant pleural effusion unsuitable for talc pleurodesis. Eur J Surg Oncol, (2009). , 546-551.

[120] Jenkins, P, Milliner, R, & Salmon, C. Re-evaluating the role of palliative radiotherapy in malignant pleural mesothelioma. European Journal of Cancer, (2011)., 2143-2149.

[121] De Graaf-strukowska, L, et al. Factors influencing the outcome of radiotherapy in malignant mesothelioma of the pleura--a single-institution experience with 189 patients. Int J Radiat Oncol Biol Phys, (1999)., 511-516.

[122] Van Der Zee, J, & Van De, M. Pol, and J.O. Praag, Survey on the prophylactic as well as symptomatic treatment of intervention sites of malignant pleural mesothelioma in the Netherlands and Belgium. Radiotherapy and oncology : journal of the European Society for Therapeutic Radiology and Oncology, (2004)., 99.

[123] Muers, M. F, et al. Active symptom control with or without chemotherapy in the treatment of patients with malignant pleural mesothelioma (MS01): a multicentre randomised trial. Lancet, (2008)., 1685-1694.

[124] Vogelzang, N. J. Chemotherapy for malignant pleural mesothelioma. The Lancet, (2008)., 1640-1642.

[125] Brien, O, et al. A randomised trial in malignant mesothelioma (M) of early (E) versus delayed (D) chemotherapy in symptomatically stable patients: the MED trial. Ann Oncol, (2006)., 270-275.

[126] Sorensen, P. G, et al. Randomized trial of doxorubicin versus cyclophosphamide in diffuse malignant pleural mesothelioma. Cancer Treat Rep, (1985)., 1431-1432.

[127] Zidar, B. L, et al. A phase II evaluation of ifosfamide and mesna in unresectable diffuse malignant mesothelioma: A southwest oncology group study. Cancer, (1992)., 2547-2551.

[128] Martensson, G, Sorenson, S, & Phase, A. II study of vincristine in malignant mesothelioma--a negative report. Cancer Chemother Pharmacol, (1989)., 133-134.

[129] Cowan, J. D, et al. Phase II trial of five day intravenous infusion vinblastine sulfate in patients with diffuse malignant mesothelioma: a Southwest Oncology Group study. Invest New Drugs, (1988)., 247-248.

[130] Ryan, C. W, Herndon, J, & Vogelzang, N. J. A review of chemotherapy trials for malignant mesothelioma. Chest, (1998). Suppl):, 66S-73S.

[131] Berghmans, T, et al. Activity of chemotherapy and immunotherapy on malignant mesothelioma: a systematic review of the literature with meta-analysis. Lung Cancer, (2002)., 111-121.

[132] Ellis, P, et al. The use of chemotherapy in patients with advanced malignant pleural mesothelioma: a systematic review and practice guideline. J Thorac Oncol, (2006)., 591-601.

[133] Van Meerbeeck, J. P, et al. A Phase II study of gemcitabine in patients with malignant pleural mesothelioma. European Organization for Research and Treatment of Cancer Lung Cancer Cooperative Group. Cancer, (1999)., 2577-2582.

[134] Kindler, H. L, et al. Gemcitabine for malignant mesothelioma: A phase II trial by the Cancer and Leukemia Group B. Lung Cancer, (2001). , 311-317.

[135] Bischoff, H. E, et al. Gemcitabine (Gemzar) may reduce tumor load and tumor associated symptoms in malignant pleural mesothelioma. Proc Am Soc Clin Oncol, (1998). , 464a.

[136] Peters, G. J, et al. Preclinical combination therapy with gemcitabine and mechanisms of resistance. Semin Oncol, (1996). Suppl 10): , 16-24.

[137] Peters, S, et al. Metastatic non-small-cell lung cancer (NSCLC): ESMO Clinical Practice Guidelines for diagnosis, treatment and follow-up. Annals of Oncology, (2012). suppl 7): , vii56-vii64.

[138] Byrne, M. J, et al. Cisplatin and gemcitabine treatment for malignant mesothelioma: a phase II study. J Clin Oncol, (1999). , 25-30.

[139] Nowak, A. K, et al. A multicentre phase II study of cisplatin and gemcitabine for malignant mesothelioma. Br J Cancer, (2002). , 491-496.

[140] Van Haarst, J. W, et al. Multicenter phase II study of gemcitabine and cisplatin in malignant pleural mesothelioma (MPM). Lung Cancer, (2000). , 18.

[141] Flores, R. M, et al. Induction chemotherapy, extrapleural pneumonectomy, and postoperative high-dose radiotherapy for locally advanced malignant pleural mesothelioma: a phase II trial. J Thorac Oncol, (2006). , 289-295.

[142] Solheim, O. P, et al. High-dose methotrexate in the treatment of malignant mesothelioma of the pleura. A phase II study. Br J Cancer, (1992). , 956-960.

[143] Kindler, H. L, et al. Edatrexate (10-ethyl-deaza-aminopterin) (NSC #626715) with or without leucovorin rescue for malignant mesothelioma. Sequential phase II trials by the cancer and leukemia group B. Cancer, (1999). , 1985-1991.

[144] Niyikiza, C, et al. Homocysteine and methylmalonic acid: markers to predict and avoid toxicity from pemetrexed therapy. Mol Cancer Ther, (2002). , 545-552.

[145] Scagliotti, G. V, et al. Phase II study of pemetrexed with and without folic acid and vitamin B12 as front-line therapy in malignant pleural mesothelioma. J Clin Oncol, (2003). , 1556-1561.

[146] Vogelzang, N. J, et al. Phase III study of pemetrexed in combination with cisplatin versus cisplatin alone in patients with malignant pleural mesothelioma. J Clin Oncol, (2003). , 2636-2644.

[147] Hazarika, M, et al. Pemetrexed in malignant pleural mesothelioma. Clin Cancer Res, (2005). , 982-992.

[148] Vogelzang, N, et al. Long-term survival update from the randomized phase III study of pemetrexed plus cisplatin vs cisplatin in patients with malignant pleural mesothelioma (MPM). Lung Cancer, (2005). Supplement 2(0): , S230-S231.

[149] Hazarika, M, et al. FDA Drug Approval Summaries: Pemetrexed (Alimta®). The Oncologist, (2004). , 482-488.

[150] Boyer, M. J, et al. Symptom and quality of life advantages for pemetrexed + cisplatin versus cisplatin in treatment of malignant pleural mesothelioma. Lung Cancer, (2003). Supplement 2(0): , S19.

[151] Steele, J. P. The new front line treatment for malignant pleural mesothelioma? Thorax, (2003). , 96-97.

[152] Goudar, R. K. Review of pemetrexed in combination with cisplatin for the treatment of malignant pleural mesothelioma. Ther Clin Risk Manag, (2008). , 205-211.

[153] Krug, L. M, et al. Multicenter phase II trial of neoadjuvant pemetrexed plus cisplatin followed by extrapleural pneumonectomy and radiation for malignant pleural mesothelioma. J Clin Oncol, (2009). , 3007-3013.

[154] Van Schil, P. E, et al. Trimodality therapy for malignant pleural mesothelioma: results from an EORTC phase II multicentre trial. Eur Respir J, (2010). , 1362-1369.

[155] Baas, P, et al. The activity of raltitrexed (Tomudex) in malignant pleural mesothelioma: an EORTC phase II study (08992). Eur J Cancer, (2003). , 353-357.

[156] Van Meerbeeck, J. P, et al. Randomized phase III study of cisplatin with or without raltitrexed in patients with malignant pleural mesothelioma: an intergroup study of the European Organisation for Research and Treatment of Cancer Lung Cancer Group and the National Cancer Institute of Canada. J Clin Oncol, (2005). , 6881-6889.

[157] Woods, B, et al. Raltitrexed plus cisplatin is cost-effective compared with pemetrexed plus cisplatin in patients with malignant pleural mesothelioma. Lung Cancer, (2012). , 261-267.

[158] Janne, P. A, et al. Pemetrexed alone or in combination with cisplatin in previously treated malignant pleural mesothelioma: outcomes from a phase IIIB expanded access program. J Thorac Oncol, (2006). , 506-512.

[159] Xanthopoulos, A, et al. Gemcitabine combined with oxaliplatin in pretreated patients with malignant pleural mesothelioma: an observational study. J Occup Med Toxicol, (2008). , 34.

[160] Zucali, P. A, et al. Gemcitabine and vinorelbine in pemetrexed-pretreated patients with malignant pleural mesothelioma. Cancer, (2008). , 1555-1561.

[161] Ceresoli, G. L, et al. Retreatment with pemetrexed-based chemotherapy in patients with malignant pleural mesothelioma. Lung Cancer, (2011). , 73-77.

[162] Zucali, P. A, et al. Second-line chemotherapy in malignant pleural mesothelioma: results of a retrospective multicenter survey. Lung Cancer, (2012). , 360-367.

[163] Edwards, J. G, et al. Angiogenesis is an independent prognostic factor in malignant mesothelioma. Br J Cancer, (2001). , 863-868.

[164] Masood, R, et al. Malignant mesothelioma growth inhibition by agents that target the VEGF and VEGF-C autocrine loops. Int J Cancer, (2003). , 603-610.

[165] Kindler, H. L, et al. Multicenter, double-blind, placebo-controlled, randomized phase II trial of gemcitabine/cisplatin plus bevacizumab or placebo in patients with malignant mesothelioma. J Clin Oncol, (2012). , 2509-2515.

[166] Dowell, J. E, et al. A multicenter phase II study of cisplatin, pemetrexed, and bevacizumab in patients with advanced malignant mesothelioma. Lung Cancer, (2012). , 567-571.

[167] Baas, P, et al. Thalidomide in patients with malignant pleural mesothelioma. Lung Cancer, (2005). , 291-296.

[168] Nowak, A. K, et al. A phase II study of intermittent sunitinib malate as second-line therapy in progressive malignant pleural mesothelioma. J Thorac Oncol, (2012). , 1449-1456.

[169] Jahan, T, et al. Vatalanib in malignant mesothelioma: a phase II trial by the Cancer and Leukemia Group B (CALGB 30107). Lung Cancer, (2012). , 393-396.

[170] Dubey, S, et al. A phase II study of sorafenib in malignant mesothelioma: results of Cancer and Leukemia Group B 30307. J Thorac Oncol, (2010). , 1655-1661.

[171] Gregorc, V, et al. Phase II study of asparagine-glycine-arginine-human tumor necrosis factor alpha, a selective vascular targeting agent, in previously treated patients with malignant pleural mesothelioma. J Clin Oncol, (2010). , 2604-2611.

[172] Garland, L. L, et al. Phase II study of erlotinib in patients with malignant pleural mesothelioma: a Southwest Oncology Group Study. J Clin Oncol, (2007). , 2406-2413.

[173] Jackman, D. M, et al. Erlotinib plus bevacizumab in previously treated patients with malignant pleural mesothelioma. Cancer, (2008). , 808-814.

[174] Govindan, R, et al. Gefitinib in patients with malignant mesothelioma: a phase II study by the Cancer and Leukemia Group B. Clin Cancer Res, (2005). , 2300-2304.

[175] Krug, L. M, et al. VANTAGE 014: Vorinostat in patients with advanced malignant pleural mesothelioma (MPM) previously treated with pemetrexed and either cisplatin or carboplatin therapy: a phase III, randomized, double-blinded, placebo-controlled trial. 2011 European Multidisciplinary Cancer Conference, (2011). p. Abstract 3BA.

[176] Wang, Y, et al. Targeted proteasome inhibition by Velcade induces apoptosis in human mesothelioma and breast cancer cell lines. Cancer Chemother Pharmacol, (2010). , 455-466.

[177] Fennell, D. A, et al. Phase II clinical trial of first or second-line treatment with bortezomib in patients with malignant pleural mesothelioma. J Thorac Oncol, (2012). , 1466-1470.

[178] Mikulski, S. M, et al. Phase II trial of a single weekly intravenous dose of ranpirnase in patients with unresectable malignant mesothelioma. J Clin Oncol, (2002). , 274-281.

[179] Reck, M, et al. Randomized, multicenter phase III study of ranpirnase plus doxorubicin (DOX) versus DOX in patients with unresectable malignant mesothelioma (MM). ASCO Meeting Abstracts, (2009). S): , 7507.

[180] Agarwal, P. P, et al. Pleural mesothelioma: sensitivity and incidence of needle track seeding after image-guided biopsy versus surgical biopsy. Radiology, (2006). , 589-594.

[181] Boutin, C, Rey, F, & Viallat, J. R. Prevention of malignant seeding after invasive diagnostic procedures in patients with pleural mesothelioma. A randomized trial of local radiotherapy. Chest, (1995). , 754-758.

[182] BTS statement on malignant mesothelioma in the UK(2007). Thorax, 2007. 62 Suppl 2: , ii1-ii19.

[183] Scherpereel, A. Guidelines of the French Speaking Society for Chest Medicine for management of malignant pleural mesothelioma. Respir Med, (2007). , 1265-1276.

[184] De Ruysscher, D, & Slotman, B. Treatment of intervention sites of malignant pleural mesothelioma with radiotherapy: a Dutch-Belgian survey. Radiother Oncol, (2003). , 299-302.

[185] Lee, C, et al. Prophylactic radiotherapy to intervention sites in mesothelioma: a systematic review and survey of UK practice. Lung Cancer, (2009). , 150-156.

[186] Bydder, S, et al. A randomised trial of single-dose radiotherapy to prevent procedure tract metastasis by malignant mesothelioma. Br J Cancer, (2004). , 9-10.

[187] Rourke, O, et al. A randomised controlled trial of intervention site radiotherapy in malignant pleural mesothelioma. Radiother Oncol, (2007). , 18-22.

[188] Davies, H. E, Musk, A. W, & Lee, Y. C. Prophylactic radiotherapy for pleural puncture sites in mesothelioma: the controversy continues. Curr Opin Pulm Med, (2008). , 326-330.

[189] Froment, M. A, Frechette, E, & Dagnault, A. Prophylactic irradiation of intervention sites in malignant pleural mesothelioma. Radiother Oncol, (2011). , 307-310.

[190] Roberts, M. E, et al. Management of a malignant pleural effusion: British Thoracic Society Pleural Disease Guideline 2010. Thorax, (2010). Suppl 2: , ii32-ii40.

[191] Stahel, R. A, Weder, W, & Felip, E. Malignant pleural mesothelioma: ESMO clinical recommendations for diagnosis, treatment and follow-up. Ann Oncol, (2008). Suppl 2: , ii43-ii44.

[192] Scherpereel, A, et al. Guidelines of the European Respiratory Society and the European Society of Thoracic Surgeons for the management of malignant pleural mesothelioma. Eur Respir J, (2010). , 479-495.

[193] The SMART trial Available from: http://public.ukcrn.org.uk/search/StudyDetail.aspx?StudyID=11023.

[194] Ung, Y. C, et al. The role of radiation therapy in malignant pleural mesothelioma: a systematic review. Radiother Oncol, (2006)., 13-18.

[195] Maasilta, P. Deterioration in lung function following hemithorax irradiation for pleural mesothelioma. Int J Radiat Oncol Biol Phys, (1991)., 433-438.

[196] Ball, D. L, & Cruickshank, D. G. The treatment of malignant mesothelioma of the pleura: review of a 5-year experience, with special reference to radiotherapy. Am J Clin Oncol, (1990)., 4-9.

[197] De Perrot, M, et al. Risk factors for major complications after extrapleural pneumonectomy for malignant pleural mesothelioma. Ann Thorac Surg, (2008)., 1206-1210.

[198] Baldini, E. H, et al. Patterns of failure after trimodality therapy for malignant pleural mesothelioma. Ann Thorac Surg, (1997)., 334-338.

[199] Rusch, V. W, et al. A phase II trial of surgical resection and adjuvant high-dose hemithoracic radiation for malignant pleural mesothelioma. J Thorac Cardiovasc Surg, (2001)., 788-795.

[200] Allen, A. M, et al. Influence of radiotherapy technique and dose on patterns of failure for mesothelioma patients after extrapleural pneumonectomy. Int J Radiat Oncol Biol Phys, (2007)., 1366-1374.

[201] Pemetrexed Disodium and Cisplatin Followed by Surgery With or Without Radiation Therapy in Treating Patients With Malignant Pleural Mesothelioma Available from: http://clinicaltrials.gov/show/NCT00334594.

[202] Allen, A. M, et al. Fatal pneumonitis associated with intensity-modulated radiation therapy for mesothelioma. Int J Radiat Oncol Biol Phys, (2006)., 640-645.

[203] Rice, D. C, et al. Outcomes After Extrapleural Pneumonectomy and Intensity-Modulated Radiation Therapy for Malignant Pleural Mesothelioma. Ann Thorac Surg, (2007)., 1685-1693.

[204] Rice, D. C, et al. Dose-dependent pulmonary toxicity after postoperative intensity-modulated radiotherapy for malignant pleural mesothelioma. Int J Radiat Oncol Biol Phys, (2007)., 350-357.

[205] Kristensen, C. A, et al. Pulmonary toxicity following IMRT after extrapleural pneumonectomy for malignant pleural mesothelioma. Radiother Oncol, (2009)., 96-99.

[206] Miles, E. F, et al. Intensity-modulated radiotherapy for resected mesothelioma: the Duke experience. Int J Radiat Oncol Biol Phys, (2008)., 1143-1150.

[207] Buduhan, G, et al. Trimodality therapy for malignant pleural mesothelioma. Ann Thorac Surg, (2009). discussion 876., 870-875.

[208] Flores, R. M, et al. Extrapleural pneumonectomy versus pleurectomy/decortication in the surgical management of malignant pleural mesothelioma: results in 663 patients. J Thorac Cardiovasc Surg, (2008). e1-3., 620-626.

[209] MARS2 Proposal Form Available from: http://www.btog.org/editorimages/MARS2%20Proposal%20form%20120213.doc.

[210] Bolukbas, S, et al. Survival after trimodality therapy for malignant pleural mesothelioma: Radical Pleurectomy, chemotherapy with Cisplatin/Pemetrexed and radiotherapy. Lung Cancer, (2011). , 75-81.

[211] Gupta, V, et al. Hemithoracic radiation therapy after pleurectomy/decortication for malignant pleural mesothelioma. Int J Radiat Oncol Biol Phys, (2005). , 1045-1052.

[212] Rosenzweig, K. E, et al. Pleural intensity-modulated radiotherapy for malignant pleural mesothelioma. Int J Radiat Oncol Biol Phys, (2012). , 1278-1283.

Chapter 7

Recent Advances in Surgical Techniques for Multimodality Treatment of Malignant Pleural Mesothelioma

Christos Asteriou, Athanassios Kleontas and Nikolaos Barbetakis

Additional information is available at the end of the chapter

http://dx.doi.org/10.5772/53397

1. Introduction

Malignant mesothelioma is a tumour which arises from mesothelial or possibly more primitive sub-mesothelial cells. It occurs most commonly in the pleura, but also in the peritoneum and rarely in the pericardium or tunica vaginalis testis [1]. The vast majority of cases (almost 80%) arise from the pleural mesothelium, and of these, most (60-70%) are associated with asbestos exposure [2]. The first clear evidence of a causal link between asbestos exposure and primary malignant tumours of the mesothelium was the observation by Wagner et al. (1960) of 33 cases of pleural mesothelioma in the Northwest Cape Province of South Africa, 28 in individuals who had lived close to the crocidolite mines, mostly as children [3]. Subsequent studies, especially work by Selikoff and associates (1965) and Whitwell and Rawcliffe (1971) in the United States, confirmed that asbestos exposure was the major risk factor for malignant pleural mesothelioma [4–6]. The epidemiology of malignant pleural mesothelioma is now well understood, but its biological behavior remains an enigma and the treatment of this cancer is still controversial.

2. Incidence

The incidence of malignant pleural mesothelioma was increasing and reached a peak in the years 2000-2005 in the United States, because of the large number of individuals who were exposed to asbestos during the 1930s to 1960s in asbestos mines and asbestos-related industries, before the causal relationship between asbestos and malignant pleural mesothelioma was recognized [7]. The recent decline in incidence is attributable to declining asbestos exposure, and this trend is expected to continue [2]. On the other hand, asbestos use in Western Europe remained high until 1980, and substantial quantities are still used in several European countries. Peto et al. suggested that for the period 1995–2029 the number of men dying from mesothelioma in Western Europe each year will almost double over the next 20 years, from 5,000 in 1998 to about 9,000 around 2018, and then decline, with a total of about a quarter of a million deaths over the next 35 years [8]. The highest risk will be suffered by men born around 1945–50, of whom about 1 in 150 will die of mesothelioma. These projections are based on the fit of a simple age and birth cohort model to male pleural cancer mortality from 1970 to 1989 for six countries (Britain, France, Germany, Italy, The Netherlands and Switzerland) which together account for three-quarters of the population of Western Europe [8]. According to Surveillance, Epidemiology and End Results (SEER) Program data, the incidence of malignant mesothelioma in the United States is estimated to be between 1-2/million in states with minimal exposure to mineral fibers and 10-15/million in states where large amounts of asbestos were used [9]. The latest data available show that malignant mesothelioma is responsible for approximately 3,000 deaths per year in the United States and an additional 5,000 deaths in Western Europe [10], [11]. The latency period, which is the interval between first exposure and the development of malignant mesothelioma, ranges from about 25 to 71 years and appears to be influenced by the amount of exposure, because workers in trades with higher amounts of exposure may experience shorter latencies compared to those exposed to lower amount of asbestos [11], [12]. It is of crucial importance for the Thoracic Surgeons to be fully informed about malignant pleural mesothelioma in order to reach the correct diagnosis and recommend the appropriate treatment when dealing with it.

3. Epidemiology

The main risk factor in developing malignant mesothelioma is asbestos exposure [13]. Asbestos refers collectively to a group of naturally occurring hydrated mineral silicate fibers that include two major forms: serpentine, represented by chrysotile (white asbestos); and the amphiboles, including crocidolite (blue asbestos), amosite (brown asbestos), anthophyllite, actinolite and tremolite [13], [14]. Crocidolite fibers are regarded as the most oncogenic type of asbestos because they are long and thin, and are believed to persist longer in the pleura, but the exact way in which asbestos induces the development of malignant mesothelioma is still not well understood [13], [14]. Inflammation appears to play a critical role as following asbestos exposure in vivo, recruitment of mononuclear phagocytes (which differentiate into macrophages that in turn phagocytize asbestos) was observed, resulting in the release of tumour necrosis factor-alpha (TNF-a) by the phagocytes and mesothelial cells [14]. Exposure to asbestos can also lead to the accumulation of DNA damage in mesothelial cells through interaction with reactive nitrogen and oxygen species, which coupled to the activation of the NF-kB pathway by TNF-a perpetuates the survival of the DNA-damaged mesothelial cells [14–16].

Crocidolite asbestos is found only in South Africa and Western Australia but has been exported all over the world for various industrial uses [17]. Chrysotile accounts for 97% of worldwide asbestos production and has been mined principally in Russia, Canada (Quebec Province), South Africa, Italy, and Cyprus [17]. Chrysotile itself is not thought to cause malignant pleural mesothelioma but is often contaminated with amphibole fibers, such as tremolite or amosite [18], [19]. However, the issue of chrysotile as a cause of malignant mesothelioma remains still controversial [17–19].

Individuals can be exposed to asbestos in many situations because of its widespread use [17], [20]. However, the areas of the world that have a high incidence of malignant pleural mesothelioma are those with asbestos mines and countries that have shipyards, insulation, construction, and automobile industries that use large amounts of asbestos [17], [21–23].Regarding tobacco use, there is no evidence that smoking increases the risk of development of malignant mesothelioma [1], [24]. On the other hand, past radiotherapy is considered as a risk factor from case series [1], [25].

4. Biological behavior

The right pleural cavity is more commonly involved than the left. In the early stages of the disease, the tumour often appears as multiple nodules on the surface of the visceral and parietal pleurae [1]. Occasionally, a localized pleural mass may develop but more often the nodules coalesce to form a sheet of tumour which surrounds the lung, extends along the fissures and may invade the underlying parenchyma [1]. Pericardial and diaphragmatic invasion are common. Bronchial invasion, usually by spread from the pleura near the hilum, is uncommon and may lead to diagnostic confusion if tumour is visible at bronchoscopy [26]. At post-mortem examination, distant metastases are common, occurring in about two-thirds of the cases with sarcomatoid type and one-third of the patients with the epithelioid and mixed types [26].

Diffuse malignant mesothelioma is divided into three main histological types: epithelioid which is most common, sarcomatoid and mixed or biphasic. The epithelial variety displays several patterns including tubulopapillary and glandular [1]. Histochemical and immunohistochemical stains assist in differentiating epithelioid mesothelioma from adenocarcinoma, the most common and difficult differential diagnosis [27].

A small number of localized serosal/subserosal neoplasms with histopathologic, histochemical, immunohistochemical, and ultrastructural features identical to those of diffuse malignant mesothelioma have been described and given the designation "localized malignant mesothelioma" [28]. Crotty et al first described a series of 6 localized malignant mesotheliomas in 1994 [28]. Localized malignant mesotheliomas are extremely rare solitary circumscribed nodular tumors, attached either in a sessile or pedunculated manner to the surface of the pleura [29]. Most localized malignant mesotheliomas present as incidental findings or with nonspecific symptoms. Epithelial-type localized malignant mesotheliomas predominate, and very few tumors are purely sarcomatous [29]. However, as opposed to ordinary diffuse malignant mesotheliomas where epithelial forms have a better prognosis than sarcomatous forms and biphasic forms are intermediate, histologic subtype does not correlate with survival [29]. Tumor size also does not appear to affect the clinical course [28]. Because of the vastly different treatment and prognosis, it is crucial to separate localized malignant mesotheliomas from diffuse malignant mesotheliomas. Diffuse malignant mesotheliomas always show gross and/ or microscopic evidence of widespread tumor on the serosal surface, as individual tumor nodules, or as a rind around viscera or as tumor caking [29]. Recurrent spread of localized malignant mesothelioma in the manner of diffuse malignant mesothelioma has been reported [30]. The crucial feature of localized malignant mesothelioma is that many cases can apparently be cured by surgical excision [29]. Localized malignant mesotheliomas should be separated from diffuse malignant mesotheliomas because of their localized presentation, quite different biologic behavior, and far better prognosis.

5. Clinical presentation

The majority of cases occur in men, reflecting their greater frequency of occupational asbestos exposure. A careful occupational history should be taken when mesothelioma is suspected or confirmed [1]. Median age at presentation is in the seventh decade but the disease may occur at any age [31]. During the early stages of disease, dyspnea is the predominant symptom and is related to the presence of an effusion. When the effusion is drained, patients are asymptomatic [17], [32]. As the tumor grows, patients develop ill-defined, mild, but continuous chest discomfort. Dyspnea may actually improve during this phase of the disease because, with tumor growth, the pleural surfaces fuse and the effusion resolves [17], [33]. Only when the disease becomes locally advanced does the patient develop severe chest pain, which is related to tumor infiltration of the chest wall and intercostal nerves [17], [33]. This is accompanied by a sense of chest tightness and dyspnea caused by entrapment of the lung by tumor [17]. There may be anorexia, weight loss and general malaise. Profuse sweats, particularly at night, often occur [1]. In the final stages of disease, dyspnea and chest pain become severe and unremitting [17]. These symptoms are related to encasement of the chest wall, lung, and mediastinum, and are occasionally associated with mediastinal shift and compression of the contralateral lung [17], [32]. Subcutaneous nodules may develop, particularly at sites of previous pleural aspiration or biopsy [1]. Other late features may include superior vena caval obstruction, pericardial tamponade due to malignant effusion or pericardial constriction due to tumour invasion of the pericardium [1], [32]. The tumour may spread to the abdominal cavity causing ascites. Mesothelioma may metastasize widely to all areas including the contralateral pleura and lung, intra- and extra-thoracic lymph nodes, liver, bone and brain [1], [26].

6. The role of biomarkers in early detection of malignant pleural mesothelioma and in predicting patients' response after therapy and outcome

Because of mesothelioma's nonspecific presenting symptoms, patients often suffer a substantial diagnostic delay, resulting in a more advanced disease at diagnosis [34]. At present, the only instruments for screening and diagnosis are based on radiological tests, posing evident economic and radio-protectionist problems [35]. An adequate screening program and subsequent earlier detection might improve patient outcome [36]. Current guidelines on mesothelioma management do, however, not advocate the use of screening and recommend that the efficacy of any screening tool should be further evaluated in high-risk populations [37]. Soluble mesothelin (SM) and megakaryocyte potentiating factor (MPF) are serum biomarkers of mesothelioma [38], [39]. Mesothelin is a 40 kDa cell surface glycophosphatidylinositol- anchored protein expressed at a low level by normal mesothelial cells in the pleura, peritoneum, and pericardium. It is highly expressed in pancreatic cancer, ovarian cancer, mesotheliomas, and some other cancers [40]. Hollevoet et al. showed that the longitudinal behavior of SM and MPF in controls indicates that a biomarker-based screening approach can benefit from the incorporation of serial measurements and individual-specific screening rules, adjusted for age and glomerular filtration rate (GFR) in their prospective longitudinal cohort study in asbestos-exposed individuals [34]. Large-scale validation remains nevertheless mandatory to elucidate whether such an approach can improve the early detection of mesothelioma [34].

Other authors are evaluating different combination of biological indicators as screening and early diagnosis markers, such as plasma osteopontin (pOPN) and serum soluble mesothelin-related peptides (SMRP) [35]. OPN is a glycoprotein overexpressed in several human neoplasms such as lung, breast, and colon cancer [41]. OPN modulates cell-matrix interactions; high levels correlate with tumor invasion, progression, and metastasis [35]. Serum OPN (sOPN) levels in patients with malignant pleural mesothelioma have been reported to be higher than in healthy subjects [42], [43]. Cristaudo et al. showed for the first time that combined SMRP and pOPN measurements can increase both sensitivity and specificity, in diagnosis of epithelioid malignant pleural mesothelioma, in terms of combined risk index [35].

Biomarkers are also urgently needed for the selection of patients likely to benefit from multimodality therapy regimens while preventing aggressive but futile treatment interventions in ineligibles [37], [44]. Serum C-reactive protein (CRP) is known as a widely available routine marker for diagnosis and follow-up of patients affected by various inflammatory diseases [45]. Recently, a negative prognostic value has been assigned to elevated serum CRP levels in several malignant diseases including breast, ovarian, renal, and lung cancer [45–49]. The results of Ghanim et al. suggest that multimodality regimens including radical resection increase survival selectively in malignant pleural mesothelioma patients with normal pre-treatment serum CRP levels, in their retrospective multicenter analysis [50].

The last few years there is an increased focus on markers of resistance, which can be used to predict treatment efficacy and thereby guide treatment decisions. Cisplatin and carboplatin work by binding to the DNA forming adducts that lead to intra- or interstrand cross-links. The formation of these DNA cross-links inhibits the cell from replicating and drives it toward apoptosis. This proapoptotic signal can be counteracted by the cells' intrinsic ability to recognize and repair the DNA damage. Nucleotide excision repair is a highly conserved pathway that maintains DNA integrity by removing helix-distorting cross-links. This pathway seems to be a key element in mediating resistance toward platinum compounds. There are three important steps in this pathway. First, the DNA damage is recognized then excised, and finally, the excised area is resynthesized. Excision repair cross-complementation group 1 enzyme (ERCC1) plays a rate-limiting step in this process by forming a complex with xeroderma pigmentosum complementation group F that excises the damaged DNA [51–54]. Two studies have recently addressed the possible predictive and prognostic role of ERCC1 in malignant pleural mesothelioma [51]. In an observational study by Righi et al., immunohistochemistry was used to detect ERCC1 in a cohort of 45 malignant pleural mesotheliomas treated with different platinum-based therapies (cisplatin-pemetrexed or carboplatin-pemetrexed in different regimens) [55]. In this series, there was no association between ERCC1 status and treatment response, but the authors did find high ERCC1 levels to be associated with a better prognosis regardless of the chemotherapy regimen used [51], [55]. Zucali et al. also used immunohistochemistry to detect ERCC1 in a retrospective cohort of 67 malignant pleural mesotheliomas treated with a combination of pemetrexed and carboplatin [56]. These authors found no association between ERCC1 protein status and clinical outcome in terms of disease control, progression-free survival and overall survival [51], [56]. The retrospective study of Zimling et al. in malignant pleural mesothelioma patients treated with cisplatin/vinorelbine suggests that low ERCC1 expression, evaluated by immunohistochemistry, may predict longer progression-free survival, a result that warrants further validation [51].

7. Staging

Because of the lack of a universally accepted staging system, the International Mesothelioma Interest Group (IMIG) developed an internationally accepted staging system that was based on the available data correlating clinical and pathologic extent of disease with outcome [57]. The IMIG staging system has become universally accepted and adopted by the UICC and the AJCC. [17] This is based upon a TNM (tumour, node, metastasis) system (Tables 1 and 2) [57]. Information regarding the degree of visceral and parietal pleural involvement often requires the use of diagnostic thoracoscopy by means of VATS (Video Assisted Thoracic Surgery). Chest CT may also be helpful.

Cervical mediastinoscopy as a pre-operative invasive mediastinal staging tool remains still a debating issue. The high rate of false negative results or the presence of disease in lymph nodes inaccessible by mediastinoscopy, are the main reasons for its limited role in the staging algorithm [58]. Pilling et al. suggested the use of cervical mediastinoscopy as a selection tool in order to identify the patients who would benefit most from extrapleural pneumonectomy as nodal size on CT is an unreliable marker of malignancy [59]. Lately, it has been proposed that cervical mediastinoscopy should be used as routine method of prognostic staging in all patients undergoing radical surgery for malignant pleural mesothelioma [60].

Positron emission tomography (PET) scan has a crucial role in thoracic oncology due to its impact on diagnosis, staging and prognosis [61]. PET is useful diagnostic tool to identify and stage malignant pleural mesothelioma and differentiate it from benign pleural disease. Its impact in the prediction of survival, determination of mortality risk and detection of metastases and recurrent disease is considered valuable. However, the combination of PET-CT can produce superior diagnostic results than PET alone [62].

T1	T1a Tumour limited to the ipsilateral parietal pleura, including mediastinal and diaphragmatic pleura. No involvement of the visceral pleura
	T1b Tumour involving the ipsilateral parietal pleura, including mediastinal and diaphragmatic pleura. Scattered foci of tumour also involving the visceral pleura
T2	Tumour involving each of the ipsilateral pleural surfaces (parietal, mediastinal, diaphragmatic and visceral pleura) with at least one of the following features: Involvement of diaphragmatic muscle Confluent visceral pleural tumour (including the fissures) or extension of tumour from visceral pleura into the underlying pulmonary parenchyma
T3	Describes locally advanced but potentially resectable tumour. Tumour involving all of the ipsilateral pleural surfaces (parietal, mediastinal, diaphragmatic and visceral) with at least one of the following features: Involvement of the endothoracic fascia Extension into the mediastinal fat Solitary completely resectable focus of tumour extending into the soft tissues of the chest wall Non-transmural involvement of the pericardium
T4	Describes locally advanced technically unresectable tumour. Tumour involving all of the ipsilateral pleural surfaces (parietal, mediastinal, diaphragmatic and visceral) with at least one of the following features: Diffuse extension or multifocal masses of tumour in the chest wall with or without associated rib destruction Direct transdiaphragmatic extension of tumour to the peritoneum Direct extension of tumour to the contralateral pleura Direct extension of tumour to one or more mediastinal organs Direct extension of tumour into the spine Tumour extending through to the internal surface of the pericardium with or without a pericardial effusion, or tumour involving the myocardium
N	Lymph nodes
NX	Regional lymph nodes cannot be assessed
N0	No regional lymph node metastases
N1	Metastases in the ipsilateral bronchopulmonary or hilar lymph nodes
N2	Metastases in the subcarinal or the ipsilateral mediastinal lymph nodes including the ipsilateral internal mammary nodes
N3	Metastases in the contralateral mediastinal, contralateral internal mammary, ipsilateral or contralateral supraclavicular lymph nodes
M	Metastases
MX	Presence of distant metastases cannot be assessed
M0	No distant metastasis
M1	Distant metastasis present

Table 1. New International Staging System for Malignant Pleural Mesothelioma (IMIG): TNM staging (Rusch VW).

Stage	Description
Stage I	
Ia	T1aN0M0
Ib	T1bN0M0
Stage II	T2N0M0
Stage III	Any T3M0 Any N1M0 Any N2M0
Stage IV	Any T4 Any N3 Any M1

Table 2. New International Staging System for Malignant Pleural Mesothelioma (IMIG): Clinical staging (Rusch VW).

8. Surgical treatment

Malignant pleural mesothelioma is a disease that is difficult to be cured. But efforts made, combining various medical specialties such as thoracic surgery, oncology, radiotherapy and pulmonology, to the greatest possible therapeutic approach. In this chapter, the goal is, through the review of contemporary literature, to highlight the modern surgical strategy for treatment of malignant pleural mesothelioma.

Based on the clinical staging of disease and histological type, the treatment strategy should be decided. Specifically, for clinical stage I-III or epithelioid or mixed histology type, the proposed treatment is surgical or combined, whereas for clinical stage IV or sarcomatoid histology type, chemotherapy is suggested [63].

In case that surgical treatment has been chosen, the patient should undergo a careful preoperative evaluation, that includes the following selection criteria [64]:

- Performance status 0 – 1
- Predicted postoperative FEV1 > 1.0 L
- Room air PaO2 > 65 mmHg
- Room air PaCO2 < 45 mmHg

- Ejection fraction > 40%
- Mean pulmonary artery pressure < 30 mmHg

The aim of surgical treatment is to achieve the maximum cytoreduction and radical resection of macroscopic lesions of the disease and includes the following approaches [65]:

- Extrapleural pneumonectomy
- Pleurectomy - Decortication
- Pleurectomy - Decortication and Hyperthermic Pleural ChemoPerfusion / Photodynamic Therapy

9. Extrapleural pneumonectomy

The extrapleural pneumonectomy involves radical excision of the entire lung, en block with the parietal pleura, including the ipsilateral hemidiaphragm and pericardium and radical mediastinal lymph node dissection. The main goal of this surgical technique is to achieve complete exclusion of macroscopic disease [66].

The surgical technique is usually applied with posterolateral thoracotomy. In case of previous incisions (probably for biopsy), all scars should be excluded in order to avoid spreading the disease. Entry into the thoracic cavity is usually made through the sixth intercostal space. To achieve good surgical field, the sixth rib may be excised or a second thoracotomy must be performed below in order to facilitate better resection and reconstruction of the hemidiaphragm. After division of the intercostal space, an extrapleural plan is created separating the parietal pleura from endothoracic fascia, carefully, without entering the pleural cavity. Usually we begin with blunt and sharp dissection caudal-to-cephalad. Particular attention is required during the preparation of parietal pleura to the anatomical area of internal mammary vessels, azygos vein, aorta, esophagus, superior vena cava, inferior vena cava and mediastinum. The pericardium is opened and explored for possible metastases and eventually is resected. The hemidiaphragm is resected with very careful dissection from the peritoneum, without entering the peritoneal cavity. Then a complete mediastinal lymphadenectomy is carried out and ligation of major thoracic duct. Finally in order to complete pneumonectomy, pulmonary artery and veins as well as the main bronchus are ligated. The deficit of the pericardium is restored by placing bovine pericardium, while hemidiaphragm defect restored with synthetic mesh. Finally place a chest tube, followed by closure of the wound in accordance with the anatomical structures' class [64], [67].

The complications of this surgical procedure are represented in the table 3 below:

Common Complications	Unommon Complications
Hemothorax	Bronchopulmonary fistula
Atrial arrhythmias	Patch dehiscence
Cardiac tamponade	Empyema
Cardiac hernia	ARDS
Chylothorax	Pneumonia
Abdominal organs herniation	Septicemia
Postpneumonectomy	Vocal cord palsy
pulmonary edema	Horner's syndrome

Table 3. Complications of extrapleural pneumonectomy

Results obtained from the most recent studies show that the rate of perioperative complications ranges in 50 - 68 %, while the mean overall survival of patients receiving combination therapy which includes extrapleural pneumonectomy ranges 12,8 - 29,1 months (table 4) [68–74].

Surgical Technique	Study Group	Publication Year	Patient Population	Median Overall Survival (months)	Complications (%)
EPP	Bille et al	2012	25	12,8	68
EPP	Rena et al	2012	19	20	62
EPP	Nakas et al	2012	99	14,7	68
EPP	Buduhan et al	2009	46	24	
EPP	Hasani et al	2009	18	20,4	
EPP	Krug et al	2009	54	29,1	
EPP	Yan et al	2009	70	20	50

Table 4. Recent studies of extrapleural pneumonectomy (EPP) for the surgical treatment of mesothioma.

10. Pleurectomy - Decortication

Pleurectomy and decortication involves the surgical treatment with performance of dissection of parietal pleura from endothoracic fascia, diaphragm and mediastinum (including the pulmonary fissures down to the pulmonary artery and pleural reflections) and decortication of visceral pleura (visceral pleura is peeled away from the lung like the stripping away of a rind), with preservation of lung parenchyma (fig 1). The resection of the parietal and visceral pleura can be partial, radical or extensive (when included excision of the pericardium and / or hemidiaphragm) [75].

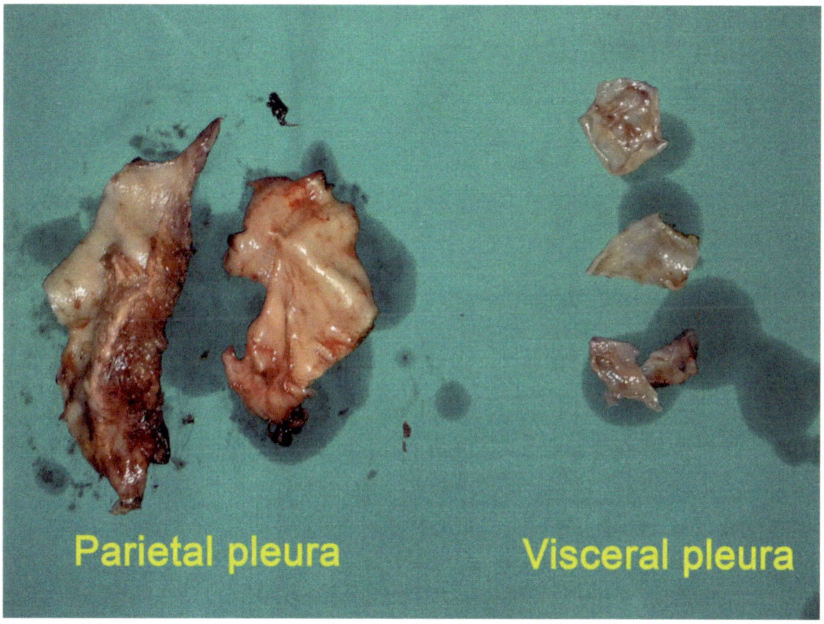

Figure 1. Parietal and visceral pleura after pleurectomy – decortication.

This surgical procedure is usually performed by posterolateral thoracotomy at the level of the sixth or seventh intercostal space. After opening the selected intercostal space, prepare the parietal pleura in all directions. We should mobilize the parietal pleura to dislodge it from the visceral pleura, where there are adhesions. In next step, visceral pleura is peeled gently away from the lung surface including the interlobar fissures, avoiding produce tears to the underlying lung. After the decortication, may proceed to parietal pleurectomy, carefully, preventing the injury of the brachial plexus, the vagus nerve, the subclavian artery and the sympathetic chain, the esophagus, the thoracic duct, the phrenic and recurrent nerves and hilar blood vessels. Finally place two chest tubes, followed by closure of the wound [67].

The complications of the procedure is primarily bleeding from the detachment of parietal pleura and the many air leaks from the detachment of visceral pleura. In recent studies, the complication rate fluctuates between 24 - 43 %, while the mean overall survival of patients with multimodality treatment including pleurectomy - decortication ranges 13,5 - 25 months (table 5).

Surgical Technique	Study Group	Publication Year	Patient Population	Median Overall Survival (months)	Complications (%)
P/D	Rena et al	2012	20	25	24
P/D	Nakas et al	2012	67	13,4	43

Table 5. Recent studies of pleurectomy - decortication (P/D) for the surgical treatment of mesothioma.

11. Pleurectomy - Decortication and hyperthermic pleural chemoperfusion / photodynamic therapy

The later and modern surgical therapy for the treatment of malignant mesothelioma is the combination of radical resection of parietal and visceral pleura (pleurectomy – decortication), by applying hyperthermic pleural lavage (40–41°C), using aqueous solution containing chemical agents such as povidone iodine or chemotherapeutic substances [76].

A newer and more advanced method is the combination of radical resection of parietal and visceral pleura (pleurectomy – decortication), followed by continuous (30min) chemoperfusion supported by extracorporeal circulation machine, for washing the pleural cavity with hyperthermic (40–41°C), aqueous solution containing chemotherapeutic substances (used also for systemic chemotherapy) [77].

Specifically after pleurectomy – decortication, place two chest tubes in the pleural cavity, ensuring that each is directed anteriorly and top and the other posteriorly and to diaphragm nearby. Usually, the first tube tube need for inflow and the second for outflow. The tubes are connected to a specific extracorporeal circulation machine and create a closed flow circuit, through which the hyperthermic solution circulate and washes the pleural cavity (fig 2-4).

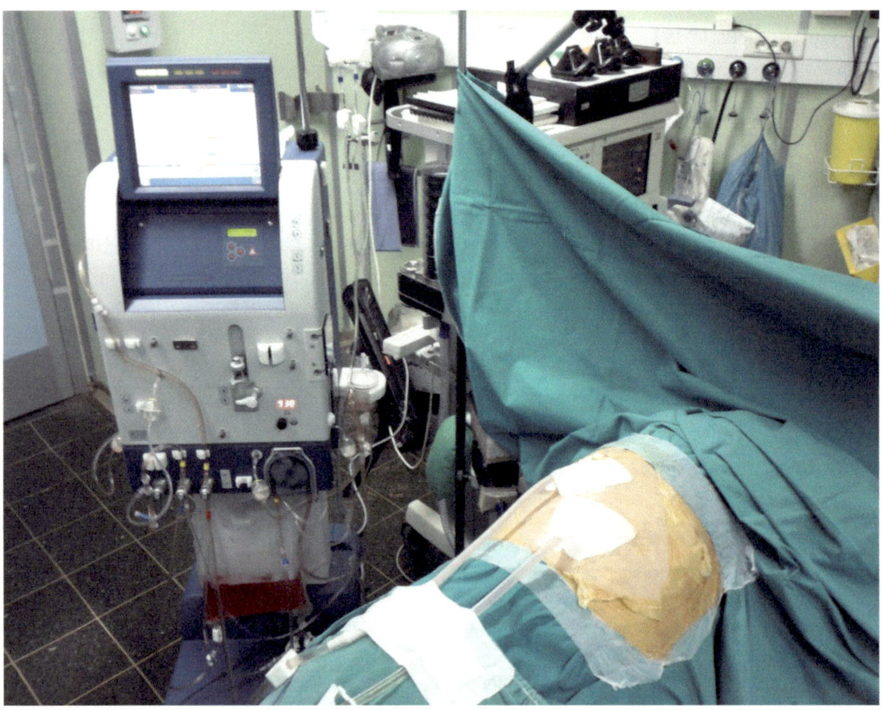

Figure 2. The patient is connected to the extracorporeal circulation circuit in order to apply hyperthermic pleural chemoperfusion.

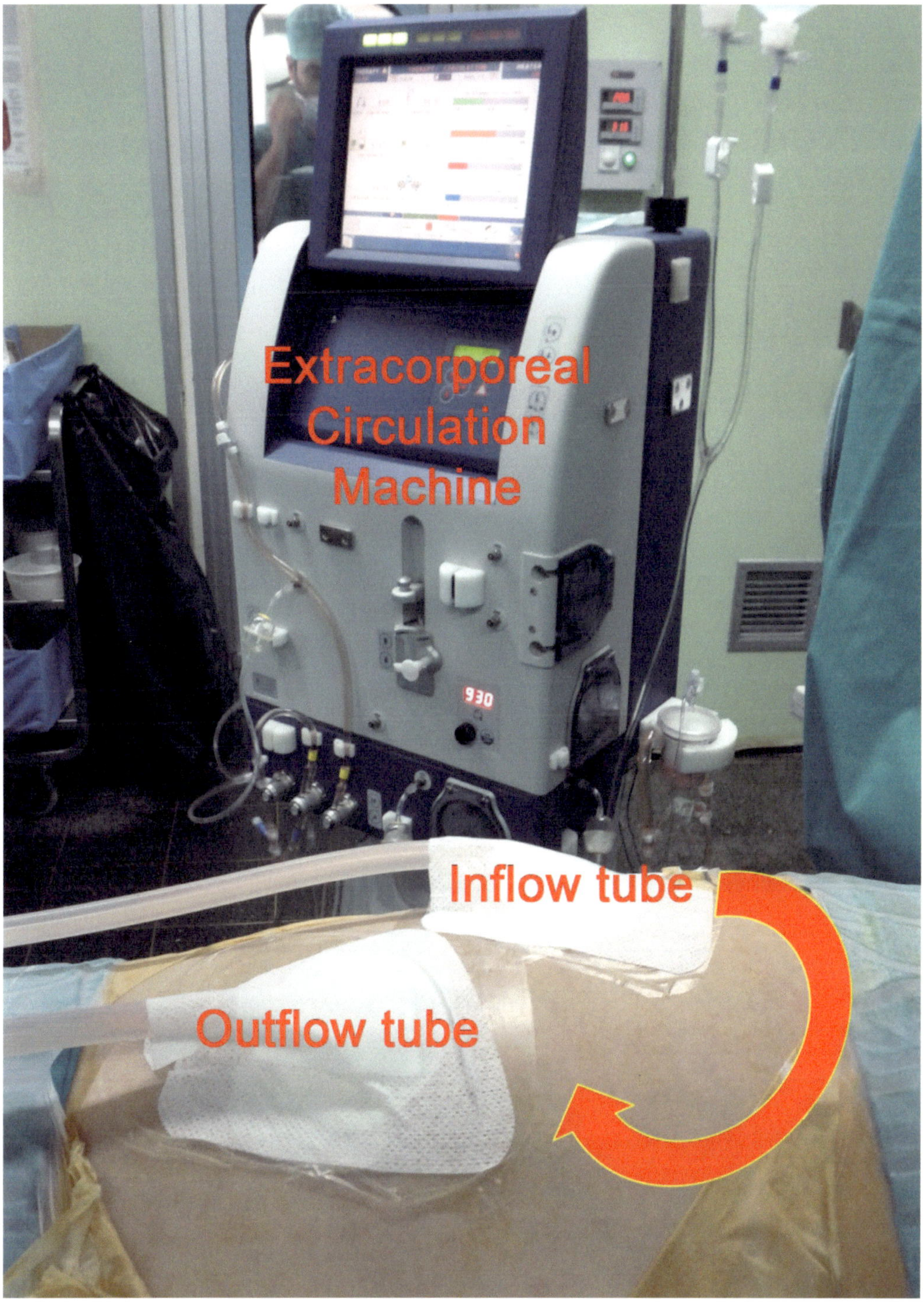

Figure 3. The arrow shows the direction flow of the hyperthermic solution inside the thoracic cavity.

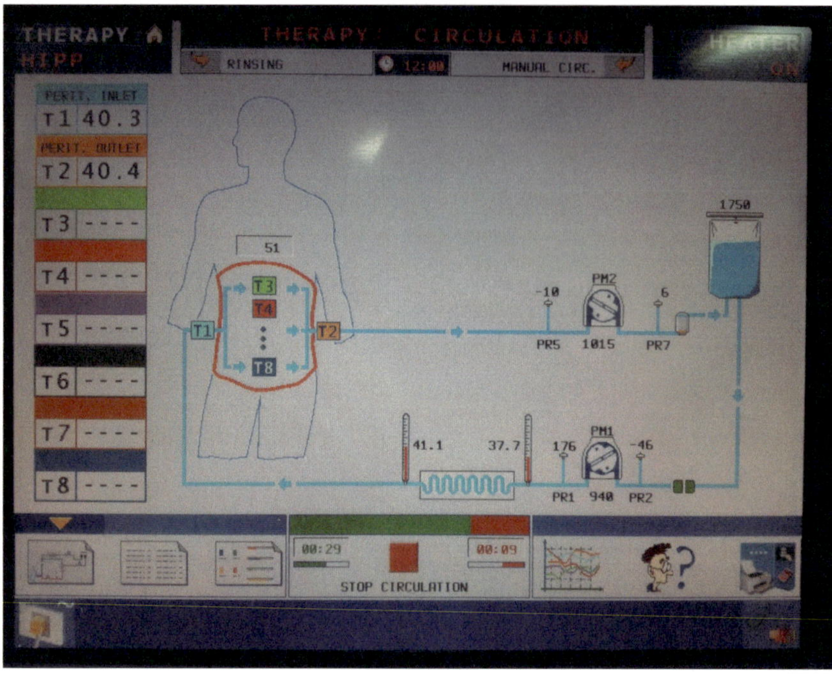

Figure 4. The screen of extracorporeal circulation machine showing in real time all parameters related to the procedure (temperature, flow-rate, time).

Hyperthermic pleural chemoperfusion can be combined with extrapleural pneumonectomy or with pleurectomy – decortication. Two recent studies suggest that the combination of hyperthermic pleural chemoperfusion after pleurectomy – decortication has a better median survival rate (23 VS 20 months) and fewer complications (27,7 VS 66 %) than the combination of hyperthermic pleural chemoperfusion after extrapleural pneumonectomy (table 6), [78], [79].

Surgical Technique	Study Group	Publication Year	Patient Population	Median Overall Survival (months)	Complications (%)
P/D and hyperthermic pleural lavage with povidone-iodine	Lang Lazdunski et al	2012	54	23	27,7
EPP and hyperthermic cisplatin perfusion	Zellos et al	2009	29	20	66

Table 6. Recent studies of extrapleural pneumonectomy (EPP) or pleurectomy - decortication (P/D) in combination with hyperthermic pleural chemoperfusion for the surgical treatment of mesothioma.

http://dx.doi.org/10.5772/53397

Futhermore, hypertermic intra-thoracic chemotherapy (HITHOC) can be used even in inoperable patients with clinical stage III-IV, with very good results, mean survival rate 30 months, because it increases the process of apoptosis [80].

Also the radical resection of parietal and visceral pleura (pleurectomy – decortication) can be combined with the application of intracavitary photodynamic therapy [81]. The latest, relevant studies are very few and come from the same center. They show very good median survival rate (25 - 31,8 months) and few complications (table 7) [82], [83].

Surgical Technique	Study Group	Publication Year	Patient Population	Median Overall Survival (months)
P/D - PDT	Friedberg et al	2012	38	31,8
P/D - PDT	Friedberg et al	2011	14	25

Table 7. Recent studies of pleurectomy - decortication (P/D) in combination with intracavitary photodynamic therapy (PDT) for the surgical treatment of mesothioma.

The main goal of all these combined techniques is the elimination of possible microscopic residual disease.

12. Discussion

Unfortunately, there are not too many recent studies to demonstrate clearly the most appropriate and effective surgical therapy in the treatment of malignant pleural mesothelioma. The latest studies regarding surgical treatment of malignant mesothelioma are presented in table 8.

However, some recent studies have tried to answer the question. Apparently, extrapleural pneumonectomy has achieved greater surgically induced cytoreduction and this method was the first surgical approach for many years [84]. Also, studies show that extrapleural pneumonectomy, when is not complicated, can have a significant and rapid, positive effect on resolution of symptoms and improve the quality of life in patients with malignant pleural mesothelioma [85]. It is claimed that co-removal of pericardium and hemidiaphragm should not be applicable to extrapleural pneumonectomy, because this fact increases very much the postoperative complications and the risk of disease seeding, without significantly increase in mean survival [86].

However, current studies, that compare extrapleural pneumonectomy and pleurectomy – decortication, showed that extrapleural pneumonectomy had more and larger postoperative complications with worse quality of life, disease recurrence was delayed a little longer, while the median survival did not show a statistically significant difference [69] [70] [87] [88]. Even more, recent studies demonstrated that patients with pleurectomy – decortication were superior therapeutically to extrapleural pneumonectomy because these patients were able to undergo even second-line chemotherapy [78].

Surgical Technique	Study Group	Publication Year	Patient Population	Radiotherapy	Systematic Chemotherapy	Median Overall Survival (months)	Complications (%)
EPP	Bille et al	2012	25	yes	yes	12,8	68
EPP	Rena et al	2012	19	yes	yes	20	62
EPP	Nakas et al	2012	99	yes	yes	14,7	68
P/D	Rena et al	2012	20	yes	yes	25	24
P/D	Nakas et al	2012	67	yes	yes	13,4	43
P/D and hyperthermic pleural lavage with povidone-iodine	Lang Lazdunski et al	2012	54	yes	yes	23	27,7
P/D PDT	Friedberg et al	2012	38	yes	yes	31,8	
MEPP	Friedberg et al	2011	14			8,4	
P/D PDT	Friedberg et al	2011	14	yes	yes	25	
EPP	Buduhan et al	2009	46	yes	yes	24	
EPP	Hasani et al	2009	18	yes	yes	20,4	
EPP	Krug et al	2009	54	yes	yes	29,1	
EPP and hyperthermic cisplatin perfusion	Zellos et al	2009	29			20	66
EPP	Yan et al	2009	70	yes	yes	20	50

Table 8. All recent studies of extrapleural pneumonectomy (EPP) or pleurectomy - decortication (P/D) or/and combination with hyperthermic pleural chemoperfusion or/and intracavitary photodynamic therapy (PDT) for the surgical treatment of mesothelioma

The results from the application of thoracic cavity lavage with hyperthermic solution and povidone iodide after pleurectomy – decortication, are promising and with fewer complications compared to extrapleural pneumonectomy [76]. In a small series of patients that chemotherapy perfusion was performed with cisplatin (100-150 mg / m) at 42 ° C for 1 h, very good results were observed. Specifically, the mean survival rate was 18 months (in combination with radiotherapy and chemotherapy), without serious perioperative complications [89].

In our department, the last three years, we have tried chemotherapy perfusion with pemetrexed (500 mg) at 42 ° C for 30 min, after pleurectomy – decortication in seven patients. Their overall treatment included radiotherapy and systemic chemotherapy (carboplatin and pemetrexed). The follow-up of patients continues until today and the results are very encouraging. Worth to mention the case of a patient who has completed three years after the start of treatment and continues with a very good performance status. Hopefully soon, after completion of these patients study (http://clinicaltrials.gov/ct2/show/NCT01409551), the final results will be published [77].

Photodynamic therapy is a therapeutic method based on the result of the reaction of a compound containing porphyrin to the effect of visible light. The result of this reaction is the direct cellular damage and the initiation of cell apoptosis [66]. A study showed that for unclear reasons, the mean overall survival of patients who have undergone pleurectomy – decortication plus photodynamic therapy, is much larger than the group of patients who received extrapleural pneumonectomy plus photodynamic therapy (8,4 VS 25 months) [83]. Reported that the combination of pleurectomy – decortication plus photodynamic therapy has comparatively much greater mean overall survival. Perhaps, this is potentially related to preservation of the lung or some photodynamic therapy -induced effect, or both [90].

Xenograft experiments has shown that low doses of photodynamic therapy can lead to a selective and strong uptake of a circulating macromolecular chemotherapeutic drug in human malignant mesothelioma xenografts, but not in normal tissue [91].

In a recent experimental study in pigs, showed that the use of cold-plasma coagulation may help in the treatment of mesothelioma. With this technique we can predetermine the depth of tissue damage (thermo necrosis) from the surface of the lung with the selection of the appropriate dose of energy [92].

13. Conclusion

As for any other type of cancer, the treatment options for malignant pleural mesothelioma include chemotherapy, irradiation, surgery, immunotherapy or some combination of these modalities. The choice of treatment is influenced by factors like the extensive nature of this tumor, its proximity to intrathoracic organs and the general medical condition of these patients who are usually older and often have underlying diseases. Most patients due to a lack of large prospective clinical trials are treated in a highly individualized manner. Most reported studies can at best be classified as phase I type. There are very few properly structured phase II studies and no phase III studies at all.

The limitations of chemotherapy and radiotherapy have made surgery an important part of multimodality treatment for MPM. Trimodality therapy has recently emerged as a new treatment strategy to improve prognosis. To improve resectability rate and local control, induction chemotherapy is combined with aggressive surgery and post-operative radiotherapy. Pemetrexed has been shown to be among the most active agents and is currently used in induction trials.

Operations for MPM can be divided into two categories – those performed for palliation and those performed with curative intent. Video-assisted thoracic surgery (VATS) with talc pleurodesis is an effective way to control pleural effusions in patients who are not candidates for further surgical resection. Thoracotomy and partial pleurectomy is necessary only in situations in which the pleural effusion has loculated and cannot be evacuated by VATS. The operations performed with curative intent are extrapleural pneumonectomy (EPP) and pleurectomy – decortication (PD). Surgical treatment can be combined with hyperthermic pleural chemoperfusion or intrapleural photodynamic therapy.

Author details

Christos Asteriou, Athanassios Kleontas and Nikolaos Barbetakis

Thoracic Surgery Department, Theagenio Cancer Hospital, Thessaloniki, Greece

References

[1] R. M. Rudd, "Malignant mesothelioma.," *British medical bulletin*, vol. 93, pp. 105–23, Jan. 2010.

[2] B. Price and A. Ware, "Time trend of mesothelioma incidence in the United States and projection of future cases: an update based on SEER data for 1973 through 2005.," *Critical reviews in toxicology*, vol. 39, no. 7, pp. 576–88, Jan. 2009.

[3] J. C. Wagner, C. A. Sleggs, And P. Marchand, "Diffuse pleural mesothelioma and asbestos exposure in the North Western Cape Province.," *British journal of industrial medicine*, vol. 17, pp. 260–71, Oct. 1960.

[4] I. J. Selikoff, J. Churg, And E. C. Hammond, "Relation Between Exposure To Asbestos And Mesothelioma.," *The New England journal of medicine*, vol. 272, pp. 560–5, Mar. 1965.

[5] W. E. Smith, L. Miller, J. Churg, And I. J. Selikoff, "Mesotheliomas In Hamsters Following Intrapleural Injection Of Asbestos.," *Journal of the Mount Sinai Hospital, New York*, vol. 32, pp. 1–8.

[6] F. Whitwell and R. M. Rawcliffe, "Diffuse malignant pleural mesothelioma and asbestos exposure.," *Thorax*, vol. 26, no. 1, pp. 6–22, Jan. 1971.

[7] M. T. Milano and H. Zhang, "Malignant pleural mesothelioma: a population-based study of survival.," *Journal of thoracic oncology®: official publication of the International Association for the Study of Lung Cancer*, vol. 5, no. 11, pp. 1841–8, Nov. 2010.

[8] J. Peto, A. Decarli, C. La Vecchia, F. Levi, and E. Negri, "The European mesothelioma epidemic.," *British journal of cancer*, vol. 79, no. 3–4, pp. 666–72, Feb. 1999.

[9] S. Altekruse, C. Kosary, M. Krapcho, N. Neyman, R. Aminou, W. Waldron, J. Ruhl, N. Howlader, Z. Tatalovich, H. Cho, A. Mariotto, M. Eisner, D. Lewis, K. Cronin, H. Chen, E. Feuer, D. Stinchcomb, and B. Edwards, "SEER cancer statistics review, 1975–2007," *National Cancer Institute*, 2010. [Online]. Available: http://seer.cancer.gov/csr/1975_2007/.

[10] R. Ismail-Khan, L. A. Robinson, C. C. Williams, C. R. Garrett, G. Bepler, and G. R. Simon, "Malignant pleural mesothelioma: a comprehensive review.," *Cancer control®: journal of the Moffitt Cancer Center*, vol. 13, no. 4, pp. 255–63, Oct. 2006.

[11] M. Carbone, B. H. Ly, R. F. Dodson, I. Pagano, P. T. Morris, U. A. Dogan, A. F. Gazdar, H. I. Pass, and H. Yang, "Malignant mesothelioma: facts, myths, and hypotheses.," *Journal of cellular physiology*, vol. 227, no. 1, pp. 44–58, Jan. 2012.

[12] C. Bianchi, L. Giarelli, G. Grandi, A. Brollo, L. Ramani, and C. Zuch, "Latency periods in asbestos-related mesothelioma of the pleura.," *European journal of cancer prevention®: the official journal of the European Cancer Prevention Organisation (ECP)*, vol. 6, no. 2, pp. 162–6, Apr. 1997.

[13] H. Yang, J. R. Testa, and M. Carbone, "Mesothelioma epidemiology, carcinogenesis, and pathogenesis.," *Current treatment options in oncology*, vol. 9, no. 2–3, pp. 147–57, Jun. 2008.

[14] S. C.-H. Kao, G. Reid, K. Lee, J. Vardy, S. Clarke, and N. van Zandwijk, "Malignant mesothelioma.," *Internal medicine journal*, vol. 40, no. 11, pp. 742–50, Nov. 2010.

[15] H. Yang, M. Bocchetta, B. Kroczynska, A. G. Elmishad, Y. Chen, Z. Liu, C. Bubici, B. T. Mossman, H. I. Pass, J. R. Testa, G. Franzoso, and M. Carbone, "TNF-alpha inhibits asbestos-induced cytotoxicity via a NF-kappaB-dependent pathway, a possible mechanism for asbestos-induced oncogenesis.," *Proceedings of the National Academy of Sciences of the United States of America*, vol. 103, no. 27, pp. 10397–402, Jul. 2006.

[16] A. Shukla, M. Gulumian, T. K. Hei, D. Kamp, Q. Rahman, and B. T. Mossman, "Multiple roles of oxidants in the pathogenesis of asbestos-induced diseases.," *Free radical biology & medicine*, vol. 34, no. 9, pp. 1117–29, May 2003.

[17] T. Shields, J. LoCicero, R. Ponn, and V. Rusch, *General Thoracic Surgery*, 6th ed. Philadelphia: Lippincott Williams & Wilkins, 2005.

[18] A. Churg and L. DePaoli, "Environmental pleural plaques in residents of a Quebec chrysotile mining town.," *Chest*, vol. 94, no. 1, pp. 58–60, Jul. 1988.

[19] J. C. McDonald, B. Armstrong, B. Case, D. Doell, W. T. McCaughey, A. D. McDonald, and P. Sébastien, "Mesothelioma and asbestos fiber type. Evidence from lung tissue analyses.," *Cancer*, vol. 63, no. 8, pp. 1544–7, Apr. 1989.

[20] M. Huncharek, "Changing risk groups for malignant mesothelioma.," *Cancer*, vol. 69, no. 11, pp. 2704–11, Jun. 1992.

[21] M. Andersson and J. H. Olsen, "Trend and distribution of mesothelioma in Denmark.," *British journal of cancer*, vol. 51, no. 5, pp. 699–705, May 1985.

[22] H. S. Malker, J. K. McLaughlin, B. K. Malker, B. J. Stone, J. A. Weiner, J. L. Erickson, and W. J. Blot, "Occupational risks for pleural mesothelioma in Sweden, 1961-79.," *Journal of the National Cancer Institute*, vol. 74, no. 1, pp. 61–6, Jan. 1985.

[23] A. D. McDonald and J. C. McDonald, "Malignant mesothelioma in North America.," *Cancer*, vol. 46, no. 7, pp. 1650–6, Oct. 1980.

[24] R. Doll and J. Peto, *Asbestos: Effects on Health of Exposure to Asbestos*. London: HMSO, 1985.

[25] A. Cavazza, L. B. Travis, W. D. Travis, J. T. Wolfe, M. L. Foo, D. J. Gillespie, N. Weidner, and T. V. Colby, "Post-irradiation malignant mesothelioma.," *Cancer*, vol. 77, no. 7, pp. 1379–85, Apr. 1996.

[26] M. R. Law, M. E. Hodson, and B. E. Heard, "Malignant mesothelioma of the pleura: relation between histological type and clinical behaviour.," *Thorax*, vol. 37, no. 11, pp. 810–5, Nov. 1982.

[27] British Thoracic Society Standards of Care Committee, "Statement on malignant mesothelioma in the United Kingdom," *Thorax*, vol. 56, no. 4, pp. 250–65, Apr. 2007.

[28] T. B. Crotty, J. L. Myers, A. L. Katzenstein, H. D. Tazelaar, S. J. Swensen, and A. Churg, "Localized malignant mesothelioma. A clinicopathologic and flow cytometric study.," *The American journal of surgical pathology*, vol. 18, no. 4, pp. 357–63, Apr. 1994.

[29] T. C. Allen, P. T. Cagle, A. M. Churg, T. V. Colby, A. R. Gibbs, S. P. Hammar, J. M. Corson, M. M. Grimes, N. G. Ordonez, V. Roggli, W. D. Travis, and M. R. Wick, "Localized malignant mesothelioma.," *The American journal of surgical pathology*, vol. 29, no. 7, pp. 866–73, Jul. 2005.

[30] H. F. Ojeda, K. Mech, and W. J. Hicken, "Localized malignant mesothelioma: a case report.," *The American surgeon*, vol. 64, no. 9, pp. 881–5, Sep. 1998.

[31] D. H. Yates, B. Corrin, P. N. Stidolph, and K. Browne, "Malignant mesothelioma in south east England: clinicopathological experience of 272 cases.," *Thorax*, vol. 52, no. 6, pp. 507–12, Jun. 1997.

[32] P. C. Elmes and J. C. Simpson, "The clinical aspects of mesothelioma.," *The Quarterly journal of medicine*, vol. 45, no. 179, pp. 427–49, Jul. 1976.

[33] P. Ruffie, R. Feld, S. Minkin, Y. Cormier, A. Boutan-Laroze, R. Ginsberg, J. Ayoub, F. A. Shepherd, W. K. Evans, and A. Figueredo, "Diffuse malignant mesothelioma of the pleura in Ontario and Quebec: a retrospective study of 332 patients.," *Journal of clinical oncology®: official journal of the American Society of Clinical Oncology*, vol. 7, no. 8, pp. 1157–68, Aug. 1989.

[34] K. Hollevoet, J. Van Cleemput, J. Thimpont, P. De Vuyst, L. Bosquée, K. Nackaerts, P. Germonpré, S. Vansteelandt, Y. Kishi, J. R. Delanghe, and J. P. van Meerbeeck, "Seri-

al measurements of mesothelioma serum biomarkers in asbestos-exposed individuals: a prospective longitudinal cohort study.," *Journal of thoracic oncology®: official publication of the International Association for the Study of Lung Cancer*, vol. 6, no. 5, pp. 889–95, May 2011.

[35] A. Cristaudo, A. Bonotti, S. Simonini, A. Vivaldi, G. Guglielmi, N. Ambrosino, A. Chella, M. Lucchi, A. Mussi, and R. Foddis, "Combined serum mesothelin and plasma osteopontin measurements in malignant pleural mesothelioma.," *Journal of thoracic oncology®: official publication of the International Association for the Study of Lung Cancer*, vol. 6, no. 9, pp. 1587–93, Sep. 2011.

[36] H. I. Pass and M. Carbone, "Current status of screening for malignant pleural mesothelioma.," *Seminars in thoracic and cardiovascular surgery*, vol. 21, no. 2, pp. 97–104, Jan. 2009.

[37] W. W. E. R. S. S. of T. S. T. F. 2010;35(3):479-495. Scherpereel A, Astoul P, Baas P, Berghmans T, Clayson H, de Vuyst P, Dienemann H, Galateau-Salle F, Hennequin C, Hillerdal G, Le Péchoux C, Mutti L,Pairon JC, Stahel R, van Houtte P, van Meerbeeck J, Waller D, "Guidelines of the European Respiratory Society and the European Society of Thoracic Surgeons for the management of malignant pleural mesothelioma.," *Eur Respir J*, vol. 35, no. 3, pp. 479–495, 2010.

[38] B. W. S. Robinson, J. Creaney, R. Lake, A. Nowak, A. W. Musk, N. de Klerk, P. Winzell, K. E. Hellstrom, and I. Hellstrom, "Mesothelin-family proteins and diagnosis of mesothelioma.," *Lancet*, vol. 362, no. 9396, pp. 1612–6, Nov. 2003.

[39] K. Iwahori, T. Osaki, S. Serada, M. Fujimoto, H. Suzuki, Y. Kishi, A. Yokoyama, H. Hamada, Y. Fujii, K. Yamaguchi, T. Hirashima, K. Matsui, I. Tachibana, Y. Nakamura, I. Kawase, and T. Naka, "Megakaryocyte potentiating factor as a tumor marker of malignant pleural mesothelioma: evaluation in comparison with mesothelin.," *Lung cancer (Amsterdam, Netherlands)*, vol. 62, no. 1, pp. 45–54, Oct. 2008.

[40] K. Chang and I. Pastan, "Molecular cloning of mesothelin, a differentiation antigen present on mesothelium, mesotheliomas, and ovarian cancers.," *Proceedings of the National Academy of Sciences of the United States of America*, vol. 93, no. 1, pp. 136–40, Jan. 1996.

[41] N. S. Fedarko, A. Jain, A. Karadag, M. R. Van Eman, and L. W. Fisher, "Elevated serum bone sialoprotein and osteopontin in colon, breast, prostate, and lung cancer.," *Clinical cancer research®: an official journal of the American Association for Cancer Research*, vol. 7, no. 12, pp. 4060–6, Dec. 2001.

[42] H. I. Pass, D. Lott, F. Lonardo, M. Harbut, Z. Liu, N. Tang, M. Carbone, C. Webb, and A. Wali, "Asbestos exposure, pleural mesothelioma, and serum osteopontin levels.," *The New England journal of medicine*, vol. 353, no. 15, pp. 1564–73, Oct. 2005.

[43] B.-D. Grigoriu, A. Scherpereel, P. Devos, B. Chahine, M. Letourneux, P. Lebailly, M. Grégoire, H. Porte, M.-C. Copin, and P. Lassalle, "Utility of osteopontin and serum

mesothelin in malignant pleural mesothelioma diagnosis and prognosis assessment.," *Clinical cancer research®: an official journal of the American Association for Cancer Research*, vol. 13, no. 10, pp. 2928–35, May 2007.

[44] F. E. E. G. W. G. Stahel RA, Weder W, LievensY, "Malignant pleural mesothelioma: ESMO Clinical Practice Guidelines for diagnosis, treatment and follow-up.," *Ann Onco*, vol. 21, no. November (suppl 5), pp. 126–128, 2010.

[45] C.-S. Wang and C.-F. Sun, "C-reactive protein and malignancy: clinico-pathological association and therapeutic implication.," *Chang Gung medical journal*, vol. 32, no. 5, pp. 471–82.

[46] B. L. Pierce, R. Ballard-Barbash, L. Bernstein, R. N. Baumgartner, M. L. Neuhouser, M. H. Wener, K. B. Baumgartner, F. D. Gilliland, B. E. Sorensen, A. McTiernan, and C. M. Ulrich, "Elevated biomarkers of inflammation are associated with reduced survival among breast cancer patients.," *Journal of clinical oncology®: official journal of the American Society of Clinical Oncology*, vol. 27, no. 21, pp. 3437–44, Jul. 2009.

[47] L. A. Hefler, N. Concin, G. Hofstetter, C. Marth, A. Mustea, J. Sehouli, R. Zeillinger, H. Leipold, H. Lass, C. Grimm, C. B. Tempfer, and A. Reinthaller, "Serum C-reactive protein as independent prognostic variable in patients with ovarian cancer.," *Clinical cancer research®: an official journal of the American Association for Cancer Research*, vol. 14, no. 3, pp. 710–4, Feb. 2008.

[48] C. O'Dowd, L. A. McRae, D. C. McMillan, A. Kirk, and R. Milroy, "Elevated preoperative C-reactive protein predicts poor cancer specific survival in patients undergoing resection for non-small cell lung cancer.," *Journal of thoracic oncology®: official publication of the International Association for the Study of Lung Cancer*, vol. 5, no. 7, pp. 988–92, Jul. 2010.

[49] S. P. K. Jagdev, W. Gregory, N. S. Vasudev, P. Harnden, S. Sim, D. Thompson, J. Cartledge, P. J. Selby, and R. E. Banks, "Improving the accuracy of pre-operative survival prediction in renal cell carcinoma with C-reactive protein.," *British journal of cancer*, vol. 103, no. 11, pp. 1649–56, Nov. 2010.

[50] B. Ghanim, M. A. Hoda, M.-P. Winter, T. Klikovits, A. Alimohammadi, B. Hegedus, B. Dome, M. Grusch, M. Arns, P. Schenk, W. Pohl, C. Zielinski, M. Filipits, W. Klepetko, and W. Berger, "Pretreatment serum C-reactive protein levels predict benefit from multimodality treatment including radical surgery in malignant pleural mesothelioma: a retrospective multicenter analysis.," *Annals of surgery*, vol. 256, no. 2, pp. 357–62, Aug. 2012.

[51] Z. G. Zimling, J. B. Sørensen, T. A. Gerds, C. Bech, C. B. Andersen, and E. Santoni-Rugiu, "Low ERCC1 expression in malignant pleural mesotheliomas treated with cisplatin and vinorelbine predicts prolonged progression-free survival.," *Journal of thoracic oncology®: official publication of the International Association for the Study of Lung Cancer*, vol. 7, no. 1, pp. 249–56, Jan. 2012.

[52] L. P. Martin, T. C. Hamilton, and R. J. Schilder, "Platinum resistance: the role of DNA repair pathways.," *Clinical cancer research®: an official journal of the American Association for Cancer Research*, vol. 14, no. 5, pp. 1291–5, Mar. 2008.

[53] Z. H. Siddik, "Cisplatin: mode of cytotoxic action and molecular basis of resistance.," *Oncogene*, vol. 22, no. 47, pp. 7265–79, Oct. 2003.

[54] H. Smeets, L. Bachinski, M. Coerwinkel, J. Schepens, J. Hoeijmakers, M. van Duin, K. H. Grzeschik, C. A. Weber, P. de Jong, and M. J. Siciliano, "A long-range restriction map of the human chromosome 19q13 region: close physical linkage between CKMM and the ERCC1 and ERCC2 genes.," *American journal of human genetics*, vol. 46, no. 3, pp. 492–501, Mar. 1990.

[55] L. Righi, M. G. Papotti, P. Ceppi, A. Billè, E. Bacillo, L. Molinaro, E. Ruffini, G. V. Scagliotti, and G. Selvaggi, "Thymidylate synthase but not excision repair cross-complementation group 1 tumor expression predicts outcome in patients with malignant pleural mesothelioma treated with pemetrexed-based chemotherapy.," *Journal of clinical oncology®: official journal of the American Society of Clinical Oncology*, vol. 28, no. 9, pp. 1534–9, Mar. 2010.

[56] P. A. Zucali, E. Giovannetti, A. Destro, M. Mencoboni, G. L. Ceresoli, L. Gianoncelli, E. Lorenzi, F. De Vincenzo, M. Simonelli, M. Perrino, A. Bruzzone, E. Thunnissen, G. Tunesi, L. Giordano, M. Roncalli, G. J. Peters, and A. Santoro, "Thymidylate synthase and excision repair cross-complementing group-1 as predictors of responsiveness in mesothelioma patients treated with pemetrexed/carboplatin.," *Clinical cancer research®: an official journal of the American Association for Cancer Research*, vol. 17, no. 8, pp. 2581–90, Apr. 2011.

[57] V. W. Rusch, "A proposed new international TNM staging system for malignant pleural mesothelioma. From the International Mesothelioma Interest Group.," *Chest*, vol. 108, no. 4, pp. 1122–8, Oct. 1995.

[58] M. de Perrot, K. Uy, M. Anraku, M. S. Tsao, G. Darling, T. K. Waddell, A. F. Pierre, A. Bezjak, S. Keshavjee, and M. R. Johnston, "Impact of lymph node metastasis on outcome after extrapleural pneumonectomy for malignant pleural mesothelioma.," *The Journal of thoracic and cardiovascular surgery*, vol. 133, no. 1, pp. 111–6, Jan. 2007.

[59] J. E. Pilling, D. J. Stewart, A. E. Martin-Ucar, S. Muller, K. J. O'Byrne, and D. A. Waller, "The case for routine cervical mediastinoscopy prior to radical surgery for malignant pleural mesothelioma.," *European journal of cardio-thoracic surgery®: official journal of the European Association for Cardio-thoracic Surgery*, vol. 25, no. 4, pp. 497–501, Apr. 2004.

[60] A. Nakas, D. Waller, K. Lau, C. Richards, and S. Muller, "The new case for cervical mediastinoscopy in selection for radical surgery for malignant pleural mesothelioma.," *European journal of cardio-thoracic surgery®: official journal of the European Association for Cardio-thoracic Surgery*, vol. 42, no. 1, pp. 72–6, Jul. 2012.

[61] L. Duranti, F. Leo, and U. Pastorino, "PET scan contribution in chest tumor management: a systematic review for thoracic surgeons.," *Tumori*, vol. 98, no. 2, pp. 175–84.

[62] S. Sharif, I. Zahid, T. Routledge, and M. Scarci, "Does positron emission tomography offer prognostic information in malignant pleural mesothelioma?," *Interactive cardiovascular and thoracic surgery*, vol. 12, no. 5, pp. 806–11, May 2011.

[63] Y. S. Ettinger DS, Akerley W, Borghaei H, Chang A, Cheney RT, Chirieac LR, D'Amico TA, Demmy TL, Ganti AK, Govindan R, Grannis FW, Horn L, Jahan TM, Jahanzeb M, Kessinger A, Komaki R, Kong FM, Kris MG, Krug LM, Lennes IT, Loo BW, Martins R, O'Malley J, Osarogia, "Malignant pleural mesothelioma - Clinical Practice Guidelines in Oncology," *JNCCN–Journal of the National Comprehensive Cancer Network*, vol. 10, no. 1, pp. 26–41, 2012.

[64] D. L.Miller, "Extrapleural Pneumonectomy," 2009. [Online]. Available: http://www.ctsnet.org/sections/clinicalresources/thoracic/expert_tech-7.html.

[65] D. Rice, V. Rusch, and H. Pass, "Recommendations for uniform definitions of surgical techniques for malignant pleural mesothelioma: a consensus report of the International Association for the Study," *Journal of Thoracic …*, vol. 6, no. 8, pp. 1304–1312, 2011.

[66] F. E. Mott, "Mesothelioma: a review.," *The Ochsner journal*, vol. 12, no. 1, pp. 70–9, Jan. 2012.

[67] L. M. Argote-Greene, M. Y. Chang, and D. J. Sugarbaker, "Extrapleural pneumonectomy for malignant pleural mesothelioma," *Multimedia Manual of Cardio-Thoracic Surgery*, vol. 2005, no. 0628, Jan. 2005.

[68] A. Bille, E. Belcher, H. Raubenheimer, D. Landau, P. Cane, J. Spicer, and L. Lang-Lazdunski, "Induction chemotherapy, extrapleural pneumonectomy, and adjuvant radiotherapy for malignant pleural mesothelioma: experience of Guy's and St Thomas' hospitals.," *General thoracic and cardiovascular surgery*, vol. 60, no. 5, pp. 289–96, May 2012.

[69] O. Rena and C. Casadio, "Extrapleural pneumonectomy for early stage malignant pleural mesothelioma: a harmful procedure.," *Lung cancer (Amsterdam, Netherlands)*, vol. 77, no. 1, pp. 151–5, Jul. 2012.

[70] A. Nakas, E. von Meyenfeldt, K. Lau, S. Muller, and D. Waller, "Long-term survival after lung-sparing total pleurectomy for locally advanced (International Mesothelioma Interest Group Stage T3-T4) non-sarcomatoid malignant pleural mesothelioma.," *European journal of cardio-thoracic surgery®: official journal of the European Association for Cardio-thoracic Surgery*, vol. 41, no. 5, pp. 1031–6, May 2012.

[71] G. Buduhan, S. Menon, R. Aye, B. Louie, V. Mehta, and E. Vallières, "Trimodality therapy for malignant pleural mesothelioma.," *The Annals of thoracic surgery*, vol. 88, no. 3, pp. 870–5; discussion 876, Sep. 2009.

[72] A. Hasani, J. M. Alvarez, J. M. Wyatt, S. Bydder, M. Millward, M. Byrne, A. W. B. Musk, and A. K. Nowak, "Outcome for patients with malignant pleural mesothelioma referred for Trimodality therapy in Western Australia.," *Journal of thoracic oncology®: official publication of the International Association for the Study of Lung Cancer*, vol. 4, no. 8, pp. 1010–6, Aug. 2009.

[73] L. M. Krug, H. I. Pass, V. W. Rusch, H. L. Kindler, D. J. Sugarbaker, K. E. Rosenzweig, R. Flores, J. S. Friedberg, K. Pisters, M. Monberg, C. K. Obasaju, and N. J. Vogelzang, "Multicenter phase II trial of neoadjuvant pemetrexed plus cisplatin followed by extrapleural pneumonectomy and radiation for malignant pleural mesothelioma.," *Journal of clinical oncology®: official journal of the American Society of Clinical Oncology*, vol. 27, no. 18, pp. 3007–13, Jun. 2009.

[74] T. D. Yan, M. Boyer, M. M. Tin, D. Wong, C. Kennedy, J. McLean, P. G. Bannon, and B. C. McCaughan, "Extrapleural pneumonectomy for malignant pleural mesothelioma: outcomes of treatment and prognostic factors.," *The Journal of thoracic and cardiovascular surgery*, vol. 138, no. 3, pp. 619–24, Sep. 2009.

[75] "Surgical Choices: Pleurectomy With Decortication," 2012. [Online]. Available: http://www.mesothel.com/asbestos-cancer/mesothelioma/surgery/pleurectomy-decortication/pd.htm.

[76] L. Lang-Lazdunski, A. Bille, E. Belcher, P. Cane, D. Landau, J. Steele, H. Taylor, and J. Spicer, "Pleurectomy/decortication, hyperthermic pleural lavage with povidone-iodine followed by adjuvant chemotherapy in patients with malignant pleural mesothelioma.," *Journal of thoracic oncology®: official publication of the International Association for the Study of Lung Cancer*, vol. 6, no. 10, pp. 1746–52, Oct. 2011.

[77] N. Barbetakis, C. Asteriou, A. Kleontas, C. Karvelas, I. Boukovinas, E. Stergiou, M. Lalountas, K. Avgitidis, and C. Tsilikas, "Cytoreductive surgery in combination with hyperthermic pleural chemoperfusion with pemetrexed for the treatment of malignant pleural mesothilioma.," Hellenic Journal of Surgery, vol. 82, no. 6, Supl. I, pp. 420-423, Dec. 2010.

[78] L. Lang-Lazdunski, A. Bille, R. Lal, P. Cane, E. McLean, D. Landau, J. Steele, and J. Spicer, "Pleurectomy/decortication is superior to extrapleural pneumonectomy in the multimodality management of patients with malignant pleural mesothelioma.," *Journal of thoracic oncology®: official publication of the International Association for the Study of Lung Cancer*, vol. 7, no. 4, pp. 737–43, Apr. 2012.

[79] L. Zellos, W. G. Richards, L. Capalbo, M. T. Jaklitsch, L. R. Chirieac, B. E. Johnson, R. Bueno, and D. J. Sugarbaker, "A phase I study of extrapleural pneumonectomy and intracavitary intraoperative hyperthermic cisplatin with amifostine cytoprotection for malignant pleural mesothelioma.," *The Journal of thoracic and cardiovascular surgery*, vol. 137, no. 2, pp. 453–8, Feb. 2009.

[80] Y. Matsuzaki, M. Tomita, T. Shimizu, M. Hara, T. Ayabe, and T. Onitsuka, "Induction of apoptosis by intrapleural perfusion hyperthermo-chemotherapy for malig-

nant pleural mesothelioma.," *Annals of thoracic and cardiovascular surgery®: official journal of the Association of Thoracic and Cardiovascular Surgeons of Asia*, vol. 14, no. 3, pp. 161–5, Jun. 2008.

[81] J. S. Friedberg, "Photodynamic therapy as an innovative treatment for malignant pleural mesothelioma.," *Seminars in thoracic and cardiovascular surgery*, vol. 21, no. 2, pp. 177–87, Jan. 2009.

[82] J. S. Friedberg, "Photodynamic therapy for malignant pleural mesothelioma: the future of treatment?," *Expert review of respiratory medicine*, vol. 5, no. 1, pp. 49–63, Feb. 2011.

[83] J. S. Friedberg, R. Mick, M. Culligan, J. Stevenson, A. Fernandes, D. Smith, E. Glatstein, S. M. Hahn, and K. Cengel, "Photodynamic therapy and the evolution of a lung-sparing surgical treatment for mesothelioma.," *The Annals of thoracic surgery*, vol. 91, no. 6, pp. 1738–45, Jun. 2011.

[84] S. Su, "Mesothelioma: path to multimodality treatment.," *Seminars in thoracic and cardiovascular surgery*, vol. 21, no. 2, pp. 125–31, Jan. 2009.

[85] V. Ambrogi, A. Baldi, O. Schillaci, and MineoTommaso Claudio, "Clinical Impact of Extrapleural Pneumonectomy for Malignant Pleural Mesothelioma," *Annals of Surgical Oncology*, vol. 19, no. July 2011, pp. 1692–1699, 2011.

[86] P. Bonnette, "Pleural mesothelioma: where are we with radical surgery and multimodal treatment?," *Revue de pneumologie clinique*, vol. 67, no. 4, pp. 184–90, Sep. 2011.

[87] G. Dimitrakakis, T. BinEsmael, A. Szafranek, and P. a. O'Keefe, "ERRATUM for a missing eComment 'Malignant pleural mesothelioma: a therapeutic challenge'," *Interactive CardioVascular and Thoracic Surgery*, vol. 13, no. 6, pp. 691–692, Dec. 2011.

[88] T. Treasure, L. Lang-Lazdunski, D. Waller, J. M. Bliss, C. Tan, J. Entwisle, M. Snee, M. O'Brien, G. Thomas, S. Senan, K. O'Byrne, L. S. Kilburn, J. Spicer, D. Landau, J. Edwards, G. Coombes, L. Darlison, and J. Peto, "Extra-pleural pneumonectomy versus no extra-pleural pneumonectomy for patients with malignant pleural mesothelioma: clinical outcomes of the Mesothelioma and Radical Surgery (MARS) randomised feasibility study.," *The lancet oncology*, vol. 12, no. 8, pp. 763–72, Aug. 2011.

[89] M. Ried, T. Potzger, N. Braune, R. Neu, Y. Zausig, B. Schalke, C. Diez, and H.-S. Hofmann, "Cytoreductive surgery and hyperthermic intrathoracic chemotherapy perfusion for malignant pleural tumours: perioperative management and clinical experience.," *European journal of cardio-thoracic surgery®: official journal of the European Association for Cardio-thoracic Surgery*, Aug. 2012.

[90] J. S. Friedberg, M. J. Culligan, R. Mick, J. Stevenson, S. M. Hahn, D. H. Sterman, S. Punekar, E. Glatstein, and K. Cengel, "Radical Pleurectomy and Intraoperative Photodynamic Therapy for Malignant Pleural Mesothelioma," in *Forty-seventh Annual*

Meeting of The Society of Thoracic Surgeons, 2011, vol. 93, no. 5, pp. 1658–65; discussion 1665–7.

[91] Y. Wang, J. Y. Perentes, S. C. Schäfer, M. Gonzalez, E. Debefve, H.-A. Lehr, H. van den Bergh, and T. Krueger, "Photodynamic drug delivery enhancement in tumours does not depend on leukocyte-endothelial interaction in a human mesothelioma xenograft model.," *European journal of cardio-thoracic surgery®: official journal of the European Association for Cardio-thoracic Surgery*, vol. 42, no. 2, pp. 348–54, Aug. 2012.

[92] M. Hoffmann, A. Ulrich, E. Schloericke, S. Limmer, J. K. Habermann, H. Wolken, H.-P. Bruch, and P. Kujath, "The application of cold-plasma coagulation on the visceral pleura results in a predictable depth of necrosis without fistula generation.," *Interactive cardiovascular and thoracic surgery*, vol. 14, no. 3, pp. 239–43, Mar. 2012.

Chapter 8

Thoracic Hydatid Cyst: Clinical Presentation, Radiological Features and Surgical Treatment

Ihsan Alloubi

Additional information is available at the end of the chapter

http://dx.doi.org/10.5772/53533

1. Introduction

Hydatid disease is caused by an infection with the cestode Echinococcus granulosus, It has been known since the time of Galen and Hippocrates, and was described by Thebesius in the 17th century [1, 2]. Rudolphy (1808) first used the term hydatid cyst to describe echinococcosis in humans [1]. It's frequently encountered in sheep- and cattle-raising regions of the world and has been observed most often in Australia, New Zealand, South Africa, South America, and Mediterranean countries. Adult worms mature in the intestine of dog (definitive host) and the eggs are released in the stool. Animals like sheep get this disease by via ingestion of contaminated vegetables. When local people living in contaminated areas (accidental host) accidentally ingest eggs after contamination of the hands by handling dogs, oncospheres hatch in the duodenum, penetrate the intestines and are carried via the bloodstream to various organs. (Fig1). About 70 per cent of hydatids lodge in the liver and develop there. Those that pass the liver are likely to travel *via* the right side of the heart to the lungs, which are second to the liver in frequency of involvement. Finally, a few embryos pass through the lungs and lodge in the systemic distribution, as in brain, bones, or kidneys. The presence of pulmonary hydatid disease should be considered in patients that present with a well-defined, spherical density of the lung, particularly in those who have lived or traveled in endemic areas.

2. Epidemiology

Annual incidence which is as high as 13-27 cases per 1, 00,000 population in certain countries of central Asia 2. The prevalence have been of pulmonary involvement is reported to be 10% to 40% in different reported series [3].

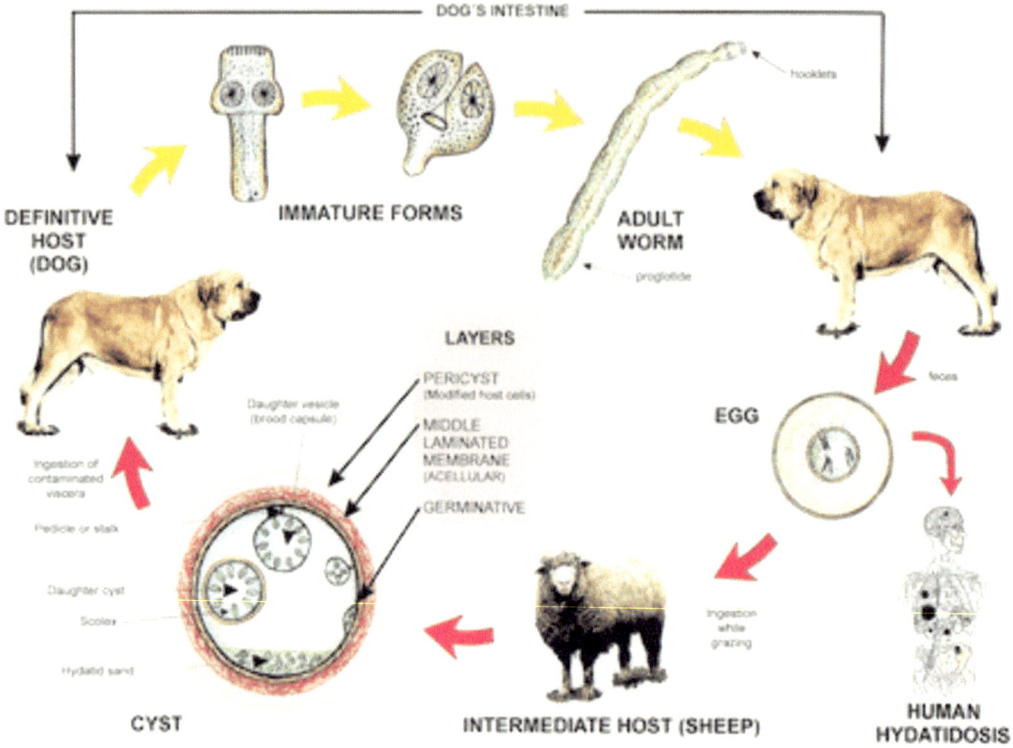

Figure 1. Life cycle (dog-sheep cycle) of *E granulosus.* Diagram shows the most prevalent life cycle of *E granulosus,* in which a dog and sheep serve as the definitive and intermediate hosts, respectively. Radiographics 2000; 20:795–817 (With permission)

3. Pathology

3.1. Cyst structure

Morphologically, hydatid cyst consists of three layers and hydatid fluid. The first is the avascular outer pericystic layer or adventitia which is the host tissue formed by the lung as a reaction to the foreign body (parasite) (Fig 2). The other two layers, the laminated membrane (external layer of the cyst) or the ectocyst laminated membrane is an acellular laminar mucopolysaccaride layer and the germinative layer (inner layer of the cyst), or endocyst layer that gives rise to larval scolices (Fig 3).

The cyst fluid resembles water in appearance which may contain daughter vesicles. The cysts exist in different forms: intact or ruptured, single or multiple, unilateral or bilateral, solely located in the lung or concomitantly in other organ lodgements (especially in the liver).

http://dx.doi.org/10.5772/53533

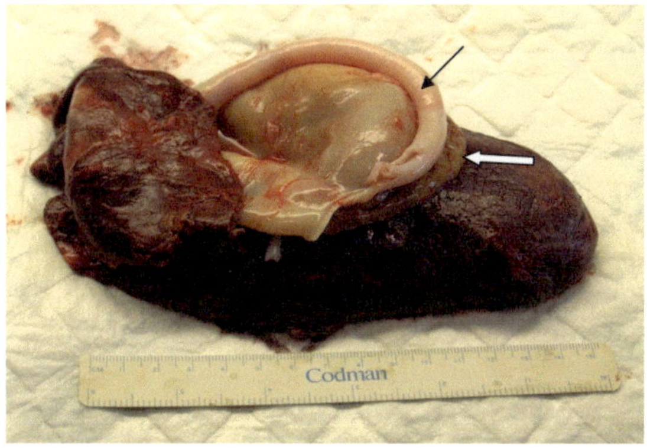

Figure 2. operative specimen: adventitia which is the host tissue formed by the lung as a reaction to the foreign body (white arrow) and de germinative membrane (black arrow); E Boeykens, A. M. Vints University Hospital of Antwerp (with permission)

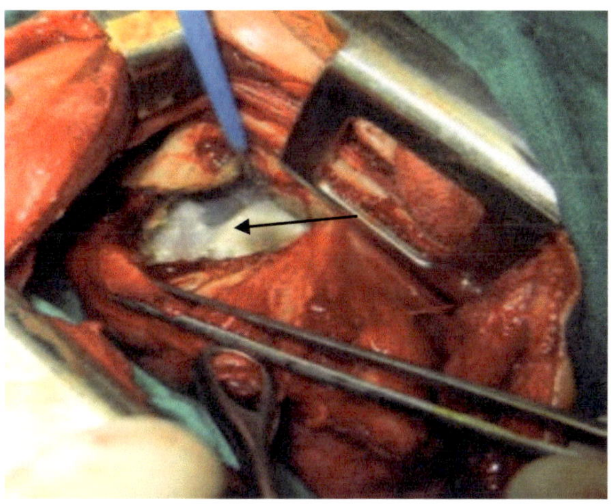

Figure 3. Operative view: endocyst layer that gives rise to larval scolices (arrow)

3.2. Cyst classification [4]

Based on morphology the cyst can be classified into 4 different types:

- **type I**: simple cyst with no internal architecture
- **type II**: cyst with daughter cyst(s) + matrix
  - **type IIa**: round daughter cysts at periphery
  - **type IIb**: larger, irregularly shaped daughter cysts occupying almost the entire volume of the mother cyst

  - **type IIc**: oval masses with scattered calcifications and occasional daughter cysts
- **type III**: calcified cyst (dead cyst)
- **type IV**: complicated cyst : e.g. ruptures cyst

4. Clinical presentation

Pulmonary hydatid disease (echinococcosis) does not present a constant clinical pattern, and consequently the clinical diagnosis tends to be inaccurate. As is so often the case, failure to think of the condition rather than lack of knowledge about it accounts for most of the misdiagnoses. It would appear, therefore, of some value to re-emphasize certain of the features of hydatid disease, more particularly from the radiological point of view.

Clinical manifestations varied widely depending on the status of the hydatid cyst. The most common presenting symptom of the patients was a cough, followed by chest pains of varying severity. Clinical presentation of pulmonary hydatid cysts depends on the size of the cyst and whether the cyst is intact or ruptured. Intact cysts are either incidental findings or present with cough, dyspnea or chest pain. If it ruptures into a bronchus, pleural cavity or billiary tree it is called complicated cyst and may present with expectoration of cystic contents, productive cough, repetitive hemoptysis, fever or anaphylactic shock in addition.

Patients come to the clinician's attention for different reasons, such as when a large cyst has some mechanical effect on organ function or rupture of a cyst causes acute hypersensitivity reactions. The cyst may also be discovered accidentally during radiographic examination, body scanning, surgery, or for other clinical reasons.

Physical findings are hepatomegaly when associated with liver involvement, a palpable mass if on the surface of the liver or other organs, and abdominal distention. If cysts in the lung rupture into the bronchi, intense cough may develop, followed by vomiting of hydatid material and cystic membranes.

5. Diagnosis

The combination of imaging and serology usually enables diagnosis. The standard diagnostic approach for cystic Echinococcosis is based on the clinical setting, imaging characteristics, predominantly ultrasonography, computed tomography (CT), X-ray examinations, and confirmation by detection of specific serum antibodies by immunodiagnostic tests.

In the detection of pulmonary echinococcosis very important role played by mass x-ray examination of the population. It allows preventive examination at the present time to identify the disease before any clinical symptoms. Differential diagnosis of conduct between the echinococcus, tuberculoma, peripheral carcinoma, between the diseases, giving the spherical formation in the lungs. Use the full range of special methods except for the puncture. End of

http://dx.doi.org/10.5772/53533

suspected unacceptable because of the possibility Echinococcus cyst rupture, risk of falling hydatid fluid in the pleura with the development of severe anaphylactoid reactions and colonization by the parasite. (Fig 4a, Fig 4 b)

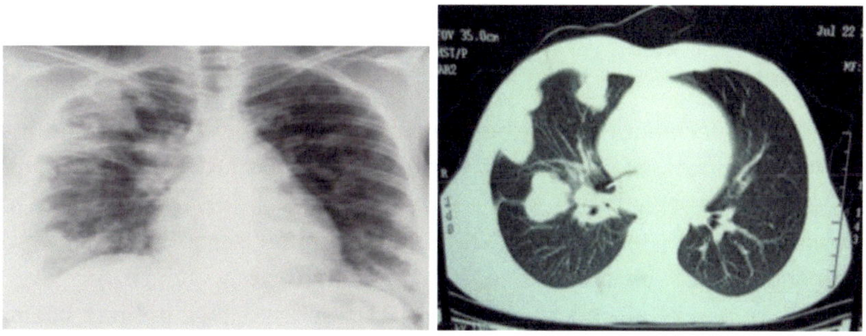

(a) (b)

Figure 4. (a) Chest radiograph demonstrates multiple peripheral round areas of soft-tissue opacity.(b) CT scan shows a clearly defined capsule with a relatively hypo attenuating center, a finding that reflects the cystic nature of the lesions.

Bronchoscopy is unnecessary in patients with a typical clinical and radiological picture but it can be performed for differential diagnosis in cases of atypical radiological appearance [5, 6]. When bronchoscopy was performed in thoracic hydatidosis, pathologic findings were revealed in 70%. Bronchoscopy detected a whitish endobronchial lesion imitating endobronchial tuberculosis with a caseous lesion. (Fig 5)

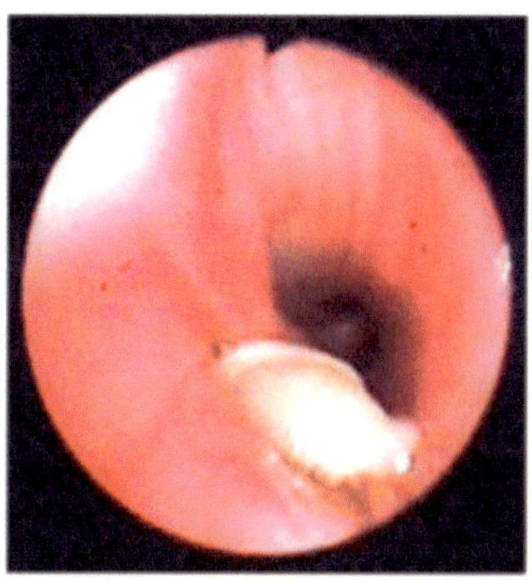

Figure 5. Flexible bronchoscopic image in a 42-year-old man with hemoptysis showing a white gelatinous membrane-like structure protruding from the medial basal segment of the right lower lobe; CMAJ (with permission)

When a cyst becomes infected or ruptures, the clinical and radiological profile can mimic diseases such as nonresolving pneumonia, tuberculosis, and abscess or tumor of the lungs. Direct bronchoscopic visualization with biopsy allowed to quickly clarifying the diagnosis, leading to effective treatment. On the other hand, one should bear in mind the possibility that carcinoma may rarely have clinical, radiological, and serological features, similar to those of a hydatid disease. It is uncommon for the diagnosis to be made from the microscopic discovery of hooklets in respiratory secretions, highlighting the value of close liaison with microbiological staff.

5.1. Laboratory tests

Most serodiagnostic techniques have been evaluated for diagnosis of cystic hydatid disease caused by Echinococcus granulosus. Formerly, the laboratory diagnosis of echinococcosis has been based chiefly on the results of the Casoni intradermal (ID) or the complement-fixation (CF) test. The CF test has a limited sensitivity, while the ID test may be unreliable since, once acquired, skin sensitivity may persist for life. After, the findings of Garabedian et al and Kagan et al [7,8] reported that indirect haemagglutination (IHA) was more sensitive to formers tests but there were some limitations with the practical aspect of IHA, for example false positive reactions with other helminthic infections, cancers and chronic immune complex disease.

Actually, the most sensitive technique in detecting pulmonary hydatid disease is immunoglobulin G enzyme-linked immunosorbent assay (ELISA) test, with a sensitivity of 85.3%; it's a quantitative serodiagnostic method that specific IgG ELISA kit was available commercially. It was a better test for initial screening of suspected cases of human hydatidosis and was more acceptable due to its higher sensitivity and simplicity in practice [9]. Our data showed that ELISA is more sensitive than IHA for initial screening of suspected cases of hydatidosis.

Serological tests are often helpful, but measurable immunological responses do not develop in some patients, essentially in lung hydatid cyst contrary to liver localization, where it seems that it has more supply antigenic stimuli to host tissues. Laboratory testing should be used either in highly suspicious cases or for postoperative follow-up of pulmonary hydatid cyst disease. Antibody production is elevated during the first 4 - 6 weeks after surgical intervention, followed by a decrease during the next 12 - 18 months. In patients who have a recurrence before 2 years, antibody production remains similar to pre-operative levels [8, 9]. Eosinophilia is 10-30% positive in hydatid cyst disease. Eosinophilia increases if cyst rupture and it is also high in countries where parasitosis is endemic [10].

6. Radiological features

The plain chest radiograph is very helpful in diagnosis of pulmonary hydatid cyst. In uncomplicated hydatid cysts, radiologic diagnosis is relatively easy and is identified on routine chest radiograph incidentally. Unruptured pulmonary hydatid cyst shows one or more homogenous round or oval wellshaped masses with smooth borders surrounded by normal lung tissue on chest radiograph. It can access large volumes and compress to the adjacent structures. (Fig 6, 7, 8)

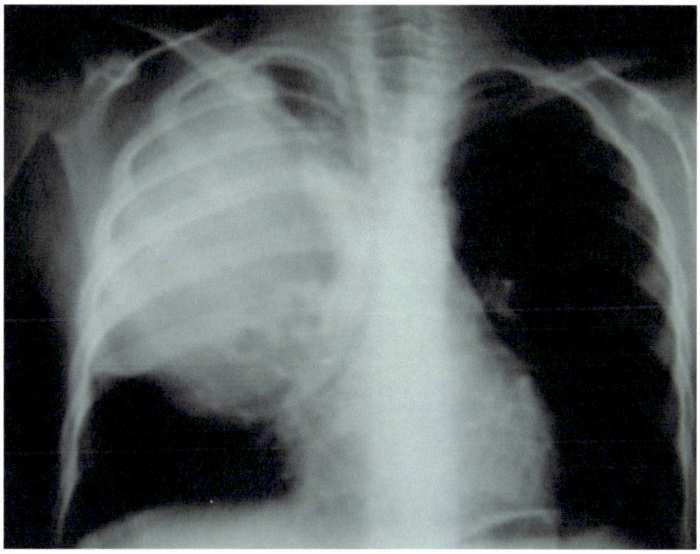

Figure 6. Chest radiograph showing large hydatid cyst right upper lobe causing mediastinal shift to opposite side

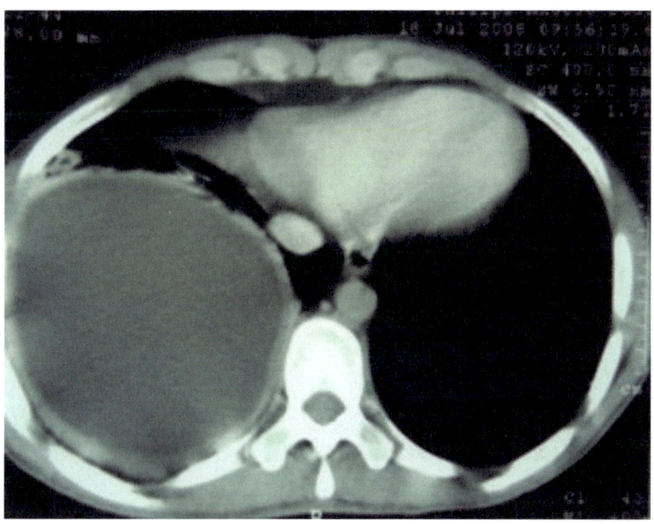

Figure 7. CT appearance of an uncomplicated giant hydatid cyst of the right lung.

If the hydatid cyst is infected or ruptured, the radiological appearance may become atypical and it may cause incorrect and delayed diagnosis.

Complicated, a variety of signs denoting different appearances of the hydatid cysts have been described. During enlargement, the cyst can erode into the bronchus and air can enter between the pericyst and endocyst leading to the thin crescent (meniscus) sign (fig 9)

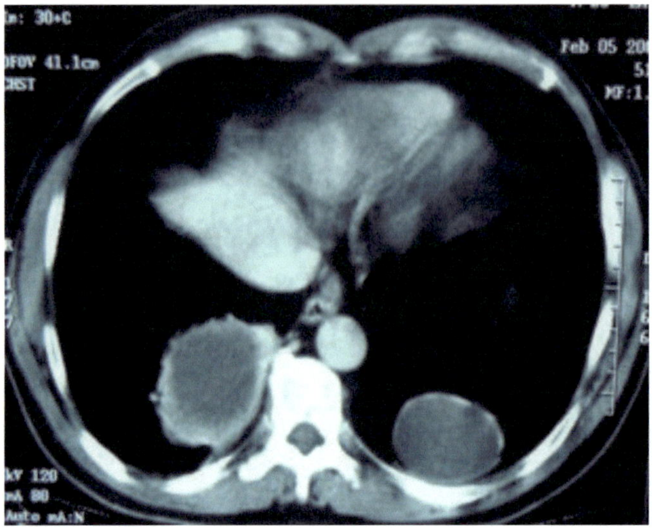

Figure 8. CT scan showing two well-circumscribed homogenous cysts over right and left lower lobes

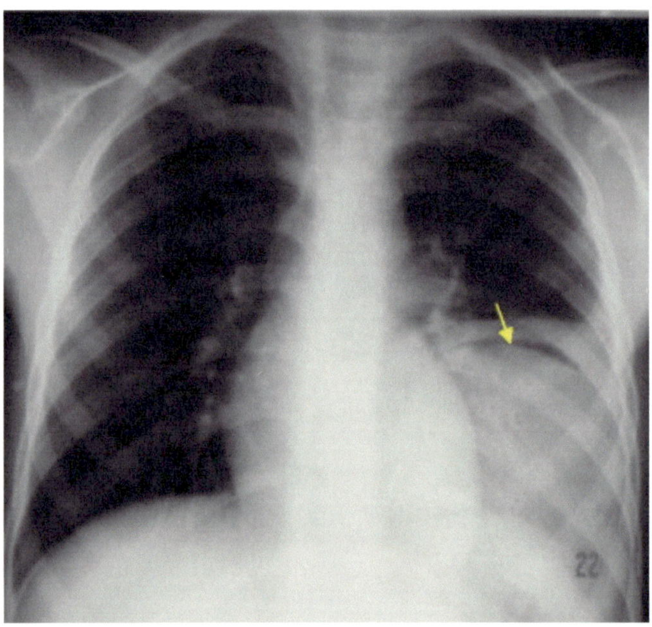

Figure 9. The pulmonary meniscus sign (arrow): crescent-shaped inclusion of air surrounded by consolidated lung tissue

As the air continues to enter this space, the cyst ruptures and air fills the endocyst. The air fluid level in the cyst and air like onion peel between pericyst and endocyst is called the Cumbo sign (Fig 10)

http://dx.doi.org/10.5772/53533

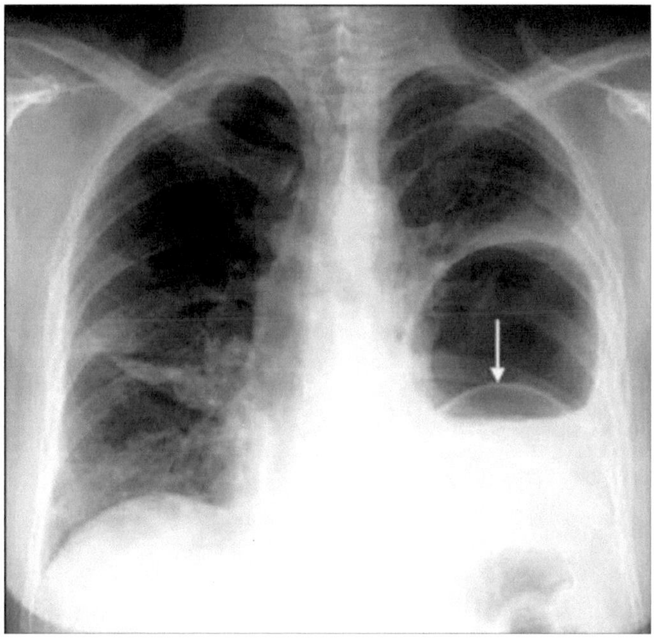

Figure 10. Combo sign (Double air layer appearances

After the contents of the cyst are partially expectorated, collapsed membranes inside the cyst form the serpent sign. (Fig 11)

Another pathognomonic sign is the water lily sign which occurs after the endocyst detaches completely and the layer caves into the cyst cavity, floating freely on the cyst fluid. (Fig 12, 13)

In pulmonary hydatid disease, the radiologial signs are usually precise contrary to the clinical presentation. The appearance of a pulmonary hydatid cyst may change secondary to perforation which necessitates further use of CT.

Rupture, with an incidence of 49%, is the most frequent complication of pulmonary hydatid disease. Communicating rupture occurs when the cyst contents escape via bronchial radicles which are incorporated in the pericyst. Rupture of the hydatid cyst into the bronchus occurs due to the degeneration of the membranes and manifests as coughing and expectoration of a large amount of salty sputum containing mucus, hydatid fluid, and rarely fragments of the laminated membrane. Thereby, solid remnants of the collpased parasitic membrane are left in the cavity. (Fig 14)

In the other hand, pulmonary hydatid cyst may mimic a variety of clinical and radiological problems including tuberculosis, primary and secondary tumors, lung abscess, bronchopulmonary infections, Wegener's granulomatosis, bronchiectasis, pneumothorax, pleurisy, and empyema.

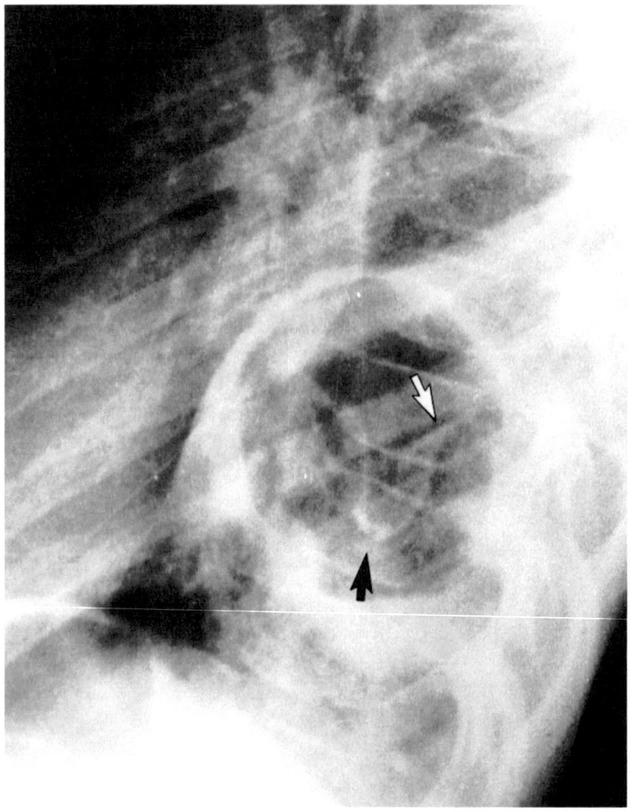

Figure 11. Lung involvement in a child with previous episodes of cough and expectoration. Collimated lateral chest radiograph shows an intracystic serpentine structure representing collapsed membranes (serpent sign) (arrows).

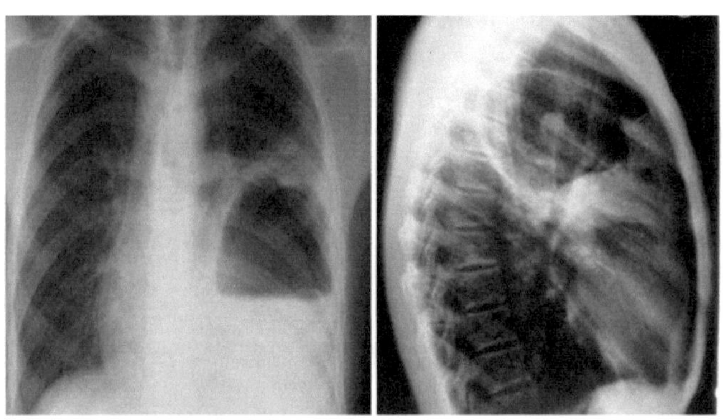

(a) (b)

Figure 12. (a) Postero-anterior and lateral (b) chest radiographs showing a cavitary lesion located at the left paracardiac region in the left hemithorax with an air-fluid level having a convex serpinginous margin with hetrogenous contents

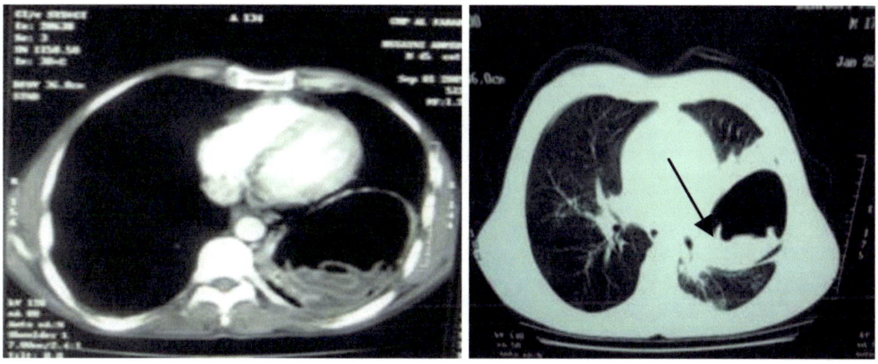

Figure 13. CT scan of thorax showing the torn germinal layer in the right hydatid cyst: the 'water-lily sign.'

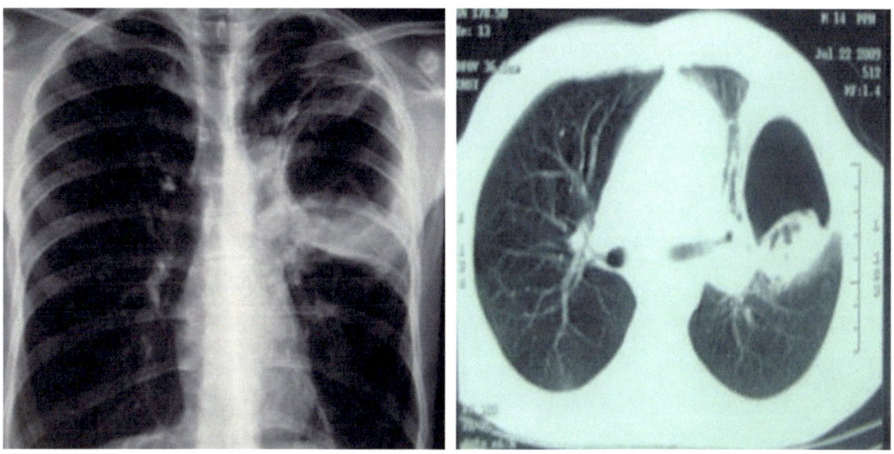

Figure 14. Chest X-ray showing a large cavity with a germinative layer in the left lung

However, CT scan can display the cystic appearance of a pulmonary mass lesion and help localize the cystic lesion for surgical purposes. CT provides further information in equivocal cases by revealing the fluid density of an intact cyst and the air-fluid density of a ruptured cyst. However, infection of the cyst may increase the attenuation values and a produce a solid appearance, which may hamper the correct diagnosis. Such a complicated cyst, in the absence of positive history, serologic tests and other radiologic signs, may simulate a malignant tumor, tuberculosis, abscess and other infected cystic lesions of the lung [11].

The "air bubble sign" was described in complicated cysts and reported to be an important clue in the differentiation of hydatid cysts from other disease processes. Air bubble sign is best demonstrated in mediastinal window settings as single or multiple small, rounded radiolucent areas with very sharp margins within solid media or pericystic areas. They should not, however, be mistaken as cavitations or pseudocavitations. (Fig 15)

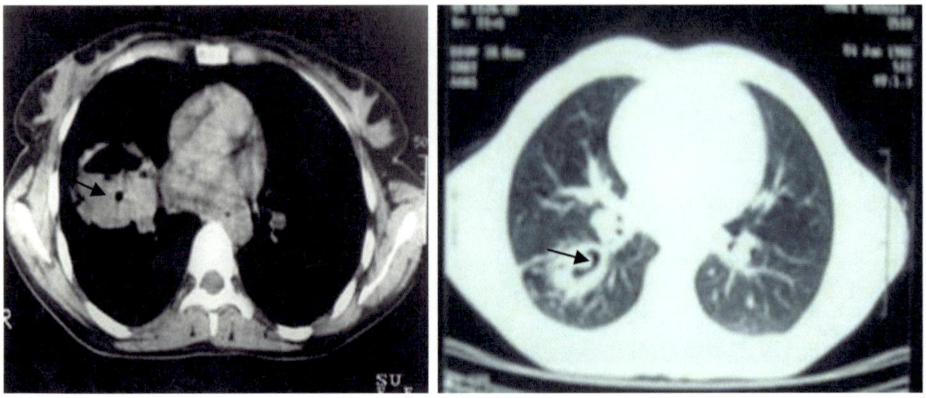

Figure 15. Mass with few air bubbles

The hydatid cysts can grow more easily and faster in the lungs because of the elastic structure of the lungs compared to the liver. For this reason, the growth rate of cysts in the lungs is estimated to be at least 5-fold higher than in the liver [12]. It has been noted that the percentage of pulmonary cysts larger than 10 cm (huge cyst) is 21.9%-25% [13, 14]. We also noted that huge pulmonary cysts occur more often in children than in adults.

Rarely, expectoration of the cystic fluid and germinative membrane may lead to spontaneous healing of the residual cavity in some of the small cysts. (Fig 16)

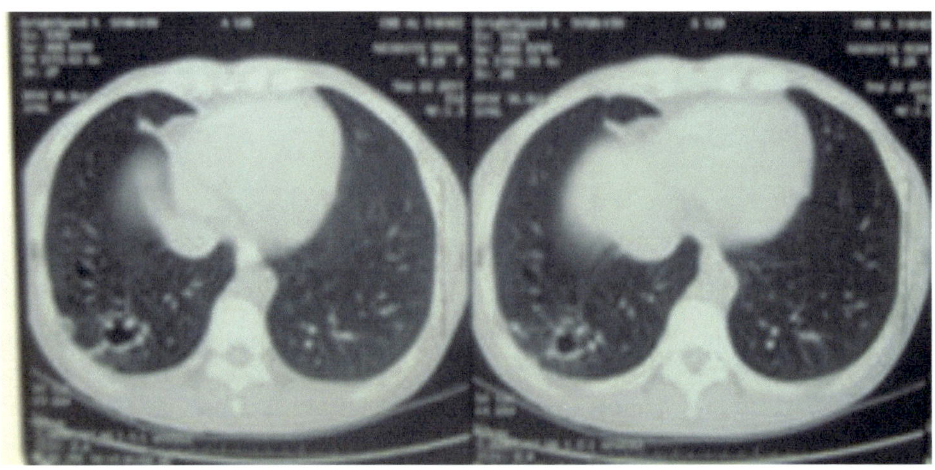

Figure 16. CT scan of the chest showing an empty cavity with thin walls after complete evacuation of hydatid membrane

The simultaneous involvement of the liver and lung is quite uncommon but when it occurs, the right lung is involved in 97% of the cases [15]. Transdiaphragmatic hydatid disease has been very seldom reported. (Fig 17)

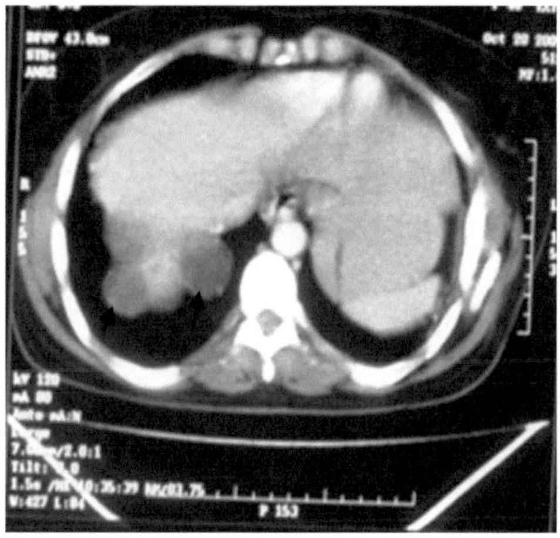

Figure 17. Contrast-enhanced CT scan obtained at the level of the dome of the diaphragm shows a partially calcified cyst originating in the posterior segment of the right hepatic lobe and growing through the diaphragm into the lung (arrows). The cyst has the characteristic hourglass shape.

7. Evolution

During the natural course of infection, the fate of the hydatid cysts is variable. Some cysts may grow (average increase: 1–30 mm per year) and persist without noticeable change for many years. Others may spontaneously rupture or collapse and can completely disappear. Calcified cysts are not uncommon. Spillage of viable protoscoleces after spontaneous or traumatic cyst rupture, or during interventional procedures, may result in secondary echinococcosis.

8. General principles of the treatment

8.1. Surgery methods

8.1.1. Conventional surgery

Initially, the surgical treatment of pulmonary hydatidosis involved the marsupialization of the cyst when it was attached to the wall, or an atypical pulmonary resection consisting of two stages: first pleurodesis was produced, followed by marsupialization in a second procedure. Evidently, these techniques have since been abandoned exceptly when the diagnosis of hydatid cyst rupture was carried later. We have treated young women with chronic pleuritis by marsupialization discovered one month after hydatid cyst rupture. (Fig 18, 19, 20)

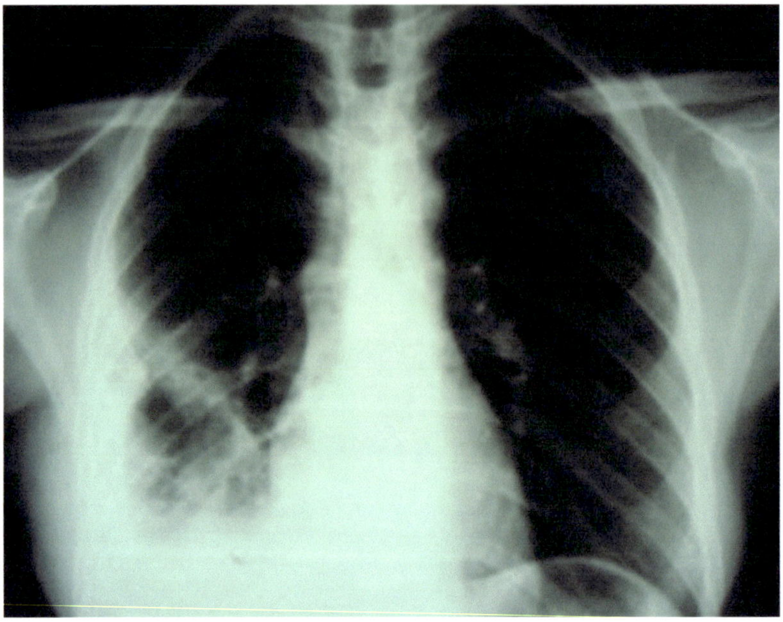

Figure 18. Complicated hydatid cyst with chronic pleuritis.

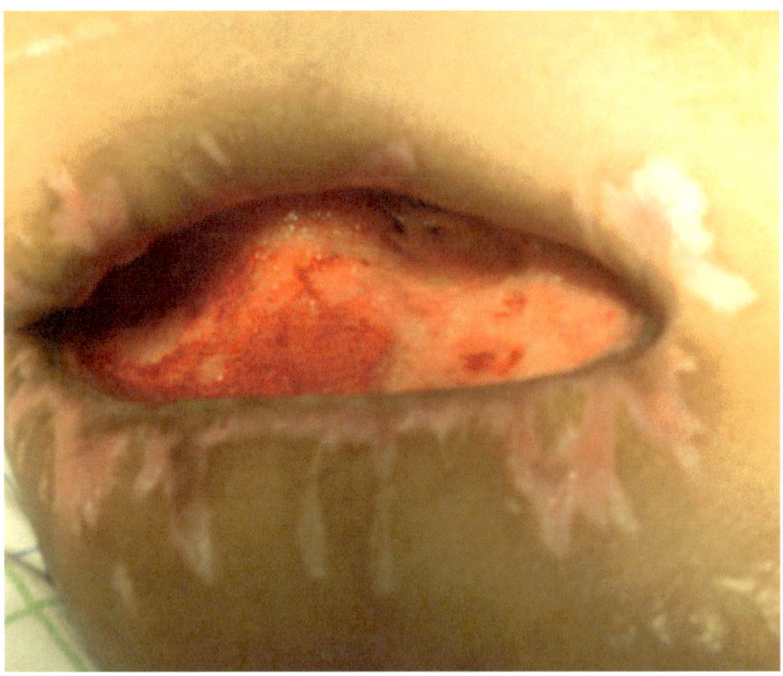

Figure 19. Marsupialization of the cyst

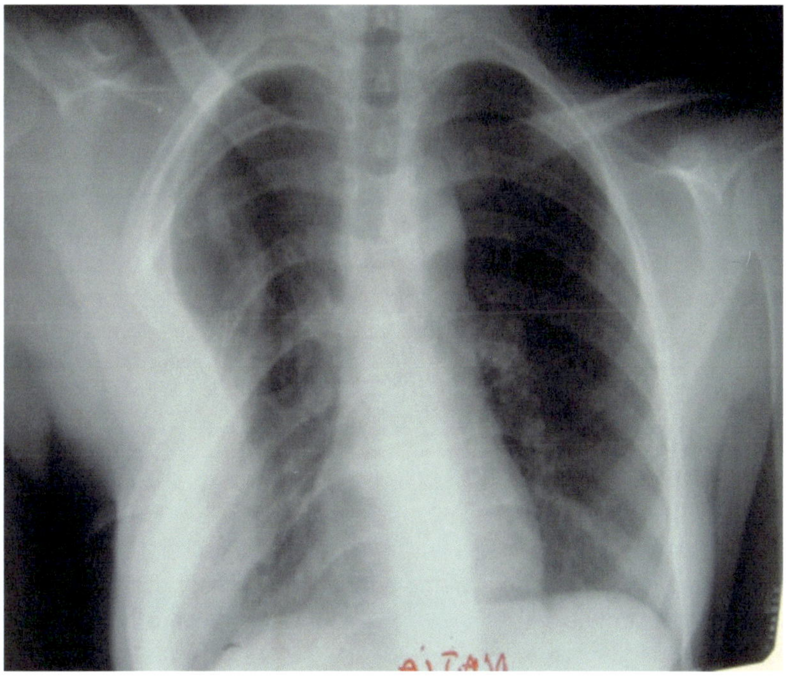

Figure 20. Outcomes of marsupialization after 1 year for complicated hydatid cyst

Actually the aim of surgery in pulmonary hydatid cyst is to remove the cyst completely while preserving the lung tissue as much as possible. Lung resection is performed only if there is an irreversible and disseminated pulmonary destruction. Careful manipulation of the cyst and adherence to the precaution to avoid the contamination of the operative field with the cyst content is the imperative part of the operation. Different surgical procedures have been described such as the enucleation of intact cyst, and needle aspiration for the evacuation of the cyst with serious risk by spillage of hydatid fluid around the puncture site. Cyst spillage may release a large number of viable scolices that implant elsewhere and produce secondary cysts [16]. Sood et al [17] reported a case of anaphylactic reaction following aspiration of a hydatid cyst in the liver during an operation under general anesthesia. The risks cited after fluid rupture by enucleation and needle aspiration are rare but serious, and prompted surgeons in endemic countries to develop a novel procedure to contain the cyst during surgery, preventing any spillage of hydatid fluid around the puncture; Santini et al [18] assembled a device using a transparent plastic cylinder used by nurses to perform venous blood harvesting. The top of the cylinder contains a hole that allows for the connection of two needles (Fig. 21). The base of the plastic cylinder was placed on top of the cyst. They penetrated the cyst using Needle A, and Needle B to create a negative depression in the plastic cylinder, thus allowing the tenacious adhesion of the cyst to the cylinder to eliminate the risk of extravasation of liquid during evacuation.

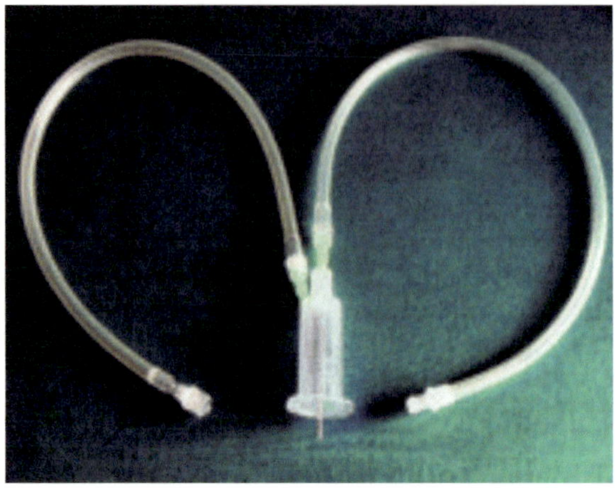

Figure 21. The photograph illustrates the home-made device of Mario Santini *Naples.*;With permission

Personally, Cystotomy and capitonnage, our preferred technique, was carried out in 95 % of our patients, we employed a trocar-suction device for needle aspiration (Fig. 22). The use of this instrument prevents the rupture of the cyst, eradicates the parasite and makes it possible to excise the residual cavity.

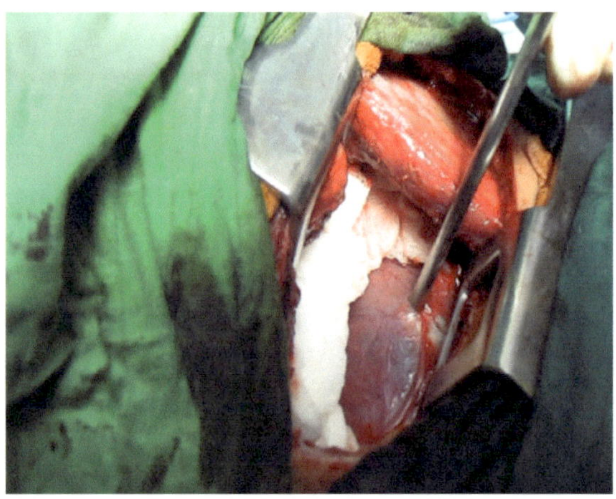

Figure 22. Trocar-suction device for needle aspiration

Thoracotomy was carried out under General anesthesia with double lumen endotracheal tubes for producing ipsilateral lung collapse during the procedure. After opening the chest wall and releasing the adhesions, we avoided any manipulation of the lung until evacuation of the cyst is not finished; the adjacent tissues were covered by towels soaked in 20% hypertonic saline solution (Fig. 23). We preferred sterilizing the cyst by aspiration of some fluid and its replacement with hypertonic saline for fifteen minutes before the cyst was aspirated by a trocar at a place and the contents of the cyst were evacuated by a powerful suction

http://dx.doi.org/10.5772/53533

through this trocar. There was another suction ready to be used by the assistant to remove any fluid leaking around the trocar. After evacuating the cyst contents, the cyst wall collapsed. Then the pericyst was incised and opened. All of the remaining contents including portions of the laminated membrane and the remaining fluid were removed under direct vision (Figure 24), followed by a partial resection of the pericystic area, the residual cavities were carefully treated with hypertonic saline solution, at this time, the anesthesiologist was asked to ventilate the operated lung to detect the exact location of all bronchial openings by observing air bubbles in the saline solution and all bronchial leaks found were closed individually with absorbable sutures (Fig 25). The cavity was obliterated with purse-string sutures of absorbable material (capitonnage).

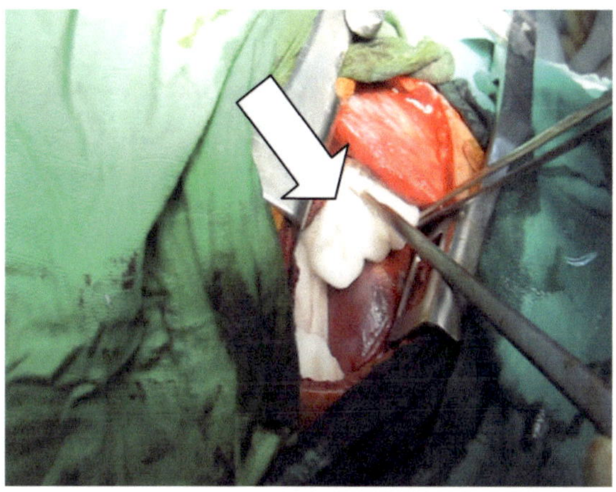

Figure 23. adjacent tissues were covered by towels soaked in 20% hypertonic saline solution (arrow)

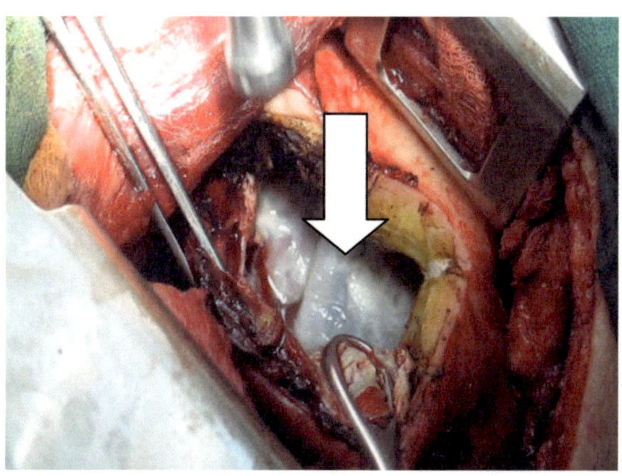

Figure 24. Simple cystectomy of germinative membrane (arrow)

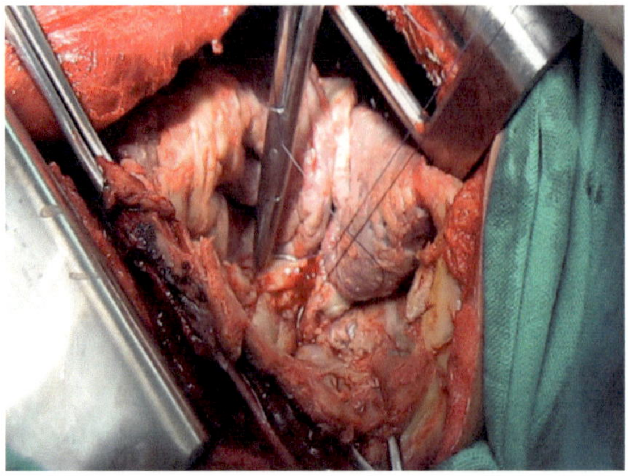

Figure 25. bronchial leaks found were closed individually with absorbable sutures

In our opinion, hypertonic saline solution 20% is effective to killing the ova (cyst injection) and for protection of the operation field with imbibed hypertonic saline pads. These precautions can limit disastrous complications of any spillage or per operative rupture.

Only 5 % of the patients with complicated cyst underwent wedge resection, segmentectomy, lobectomy, pneumonectomy or marsupialization.

8.1.2. Others conventional procedures [19, 20]

A number of methods have been described for the surgical removal of hydatid cysts of the lung.

The Barrett technique (Barrett and Thomas, 1952) which allows the removal of the parasite intact; the pericyst was incised and dissected carefully without rupturing the cyst. This procedure is eminently safe and free of risk of contamination of the pleural space, it's widely applicable, involves the loss of no appreciable pulmonary tissue or function. The technique is ideal for enucleation of all uncomplicated pulmonary hydatid cysts, even of the largest size, and after obliteration of the remaining cavity the inflated lobe looks normal

The Perez Fontana method: the cyst being removed with the pericyst (cystopericystectomy) and the residual cavity obliterated.

The Ugon technique: When the cyst is small and there is no risk of rupture', its complete removal can be attempted, aided by an increase in the airway pressure provided by the anesthetist.

However, the bronchial openings in the cavity must be closed by sutures in all techniques.

Capitonnage which is the folding of the pericystic zone by sutures for obliteration of the residual cavity is usually advocated to prevent air leak from residual bronchial openings. Without capitonnage, the wall of the pericystic cavity is supposed to be covered by epithelial cells for an uncertain length of time. On the other hand, capitonnage has the disadvant-

http://dx.doi.org/10.5772/53533

age of causing distortion of the pulmonary parenchyma, especially after removal of multiple or large cysts. However, there is no clear consensus on the use of capitonnage in surgical series of lung hydatid cyst. (Fig 26)

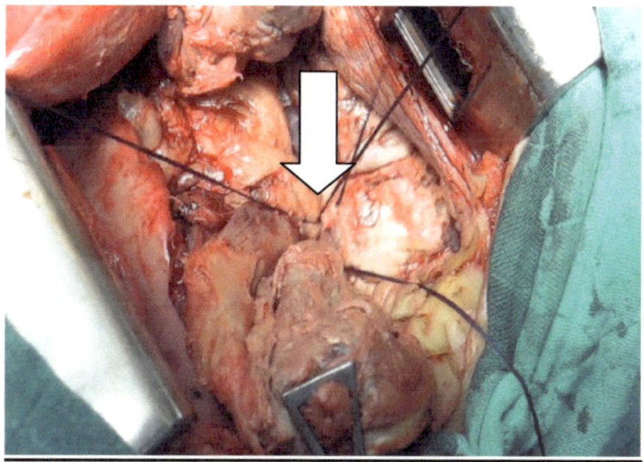

Figure 26. residual cavity after aspiration of hydatid cyst (capitonnage technique) (arrow)

Rarely, hydatid cysts can occur in other thoracic structures such as pulmonary artery, chest wall or diaphragm. (Fig 27, 28)

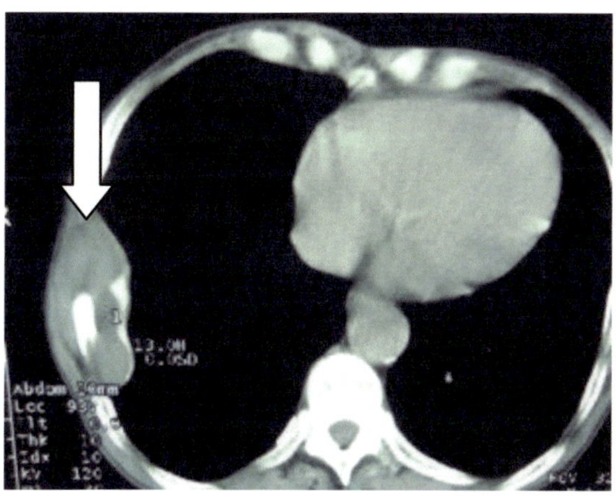

Figure 27. CT scan of rib hydatid cyst (arrow)

Most authors agree that the attempt should be made to remove as little lung tissue as possible and that resection of pulmonary parenchyma is only indicated when the adjacent tissue is seriously damaged or infected, when the atelectatic areas are presumably irrecoverable or when a big cyst or numerous cysts had destroyed a certain anatomical substrate [10].

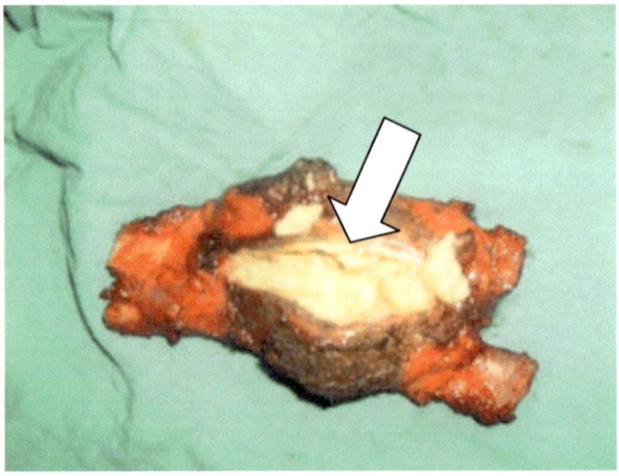

Figure 28. specimen of parietectomy for rib hydatid cyst with hydatid cyst material cotenant (arrow)

8.1.3. Video assisted thoracoscopic surgery

In adult, some authors [21] have reported the successful use of thoracoscopic procedures for the treatment of pulmonary hydatid disease. Sporadic cases were founded in the French and the other in the English literature. In our experience, we have treated three patients through this procedure. Postoperative course was uneventful in all cases. The thoracoscopic approach in pulmonary hydatid cysts must follows the same principles of the open technique, which include sterilization of the cyst with scolicidal agents (eg. hypertonic saline), complete excision of the endocyst, and closure of bronchial fistula, if present. The main advantage offered by thoracoscopy is less trauma and discomfort for the patient. The lack of intercostal muscle incision and the lower risk of rib fracture reduce the postoperative pain and when compared to thoracotomy, thoracoscopy reduces the chest tube duration and length of hospital stay. Conversion to thoracotomy is mainly related to major pleural adherences.

8.2. Medical therapy

Although surgery remains the treatment of choice for hydatid disease, the usefulness of drug therapy has been reported in many studies. Medical treatment is an alternative to surgery where a surgical approach is not recommended in risk patients, and in cases with small and multiple lesions in one or more organs, or proximity of cysts to major vascular structures. Antihelminthic agents, Mebendazole, and more recently albendazole, and praziquantal, reduce recurrence post-operatively, particularly where there has been spillage of cyst contents [22].

Many and substantial questions still remain unanswered, however. What is the optimum duration of treatment? Clearly, duration of treatment of < 3 months produces less than optimal response, whereas results of extension beyond 6 months have yet to be gauged because clinicians tend to adopt longer courses. We believe that the response of the therapy differs according to age (children and adults), cyst size, cyst structure (presence of daughter cysts inside the mother cysts and thickness of the pericystic capsule allowing penetration of the drugs), and localization of the cyst [23]. We think that selected pediatric patients with uncomplicated pulmonary hydatid cysts sized less than 5 cm, with thin pericystic capsule respond favorably to treatment. However a large pulmonary hydatid cyst should not be treated medically, because incomplete expectoration of the cyst contents after the parasite death may lead to infection through bronchial communication. Medical therapy may cause in some cases rupture of the lung cyst, and respiratory distress. We suggest that in patients with hydatid disease of the lungs associated with multiple organ involvement, medical treatment should not be given before the removal of hydatid cyst of lung.

We thought that medical treatment should be given after surgical therapy, patients surgically treated for complications following medical treatment are hospitalized twice as long as patients surgically treated in the first place. Postoperative Albendazole treatment (400 mg twice a day for the first 15 days of the month) was administered to patients for a period of 3 to 6 months.

9. Prevention

Necessary to strictly observe good personal hygiene when the content of the dogs and care for them, and be sure to wash your hands after contact with the dog, not to allow dogs to the food of man and his pot, limit direct exposure of children and dogs. Stray dogs are everywhere to be catching. In addition to current (and past) hydatid control campaigns, there have been significant technological improvements in the diagnosis and treatment of human and animal cystic echinococcosis, the diagnosis of canine echinococcosis, and the genetic characterization of strains and vaccination against *E. granulosus* in animals. Incorporation of these new measures could increase the efficiency of hydatid control programmes, potentially reducing the time required to achieve effective prevention of disease transmission to as little as 5 - 10 years.

10. Conclusion

We are of the view that surgical treatment of the lung cyst should be preferred firstly in cases of lung hydatid cyst disease. The diversity of the pathological process offers various tactics and approaches in the surgical treatment which must be individually tailored in each and every case. The goal of surgical therapy is to remove the cyst while preserving as much lung tissue as possible and medical treatment may be useful only in no operable patients.

Author details

Ihsan Alloubi*

Address all correspondence to: ialloubi@yahoo.fr

Thoracic surgery department, Centre Hospitalier Universitaire Oujda, Morocco

References

[1] Aletras H, Symbas PN: Hydatid disease of the lung. In: Shields TW, LoCicero J, Ponn RB (eds.), General Thoracic Surgery, 5th ed. Philadelphia: Lippincott Williams & Wilkins; 2000; 1113–22

[2] Torgerson PR, Oguljahan B, Muminov AE, Karaeva RR. The present situation of cystic echinococcosis in Central Asia. Parasitol Int. 2006; 55 Suppl: S207-12.

[3] CFraser RS, Muller NL, Coleman N, Pare PD. Protozoa, Helminths, Arthopods and Leeches. In: Fraser and Pare's Diagnosis of diseases of the chest. 4th ed. WB Saunders Philadelphia. 1999;1033-66.

[4] Santivanez S, Garcia HH. Pulmonary cystic echinococcosis. Curr Opin Pulm Med 2010;16(3):257-61.

[5] Yilmaz A, Tuncer LY, Damadoglu E, Pulmonary hydatid disease diagnosed by bronchoscopy: a report of three cases. Respirology 2009; 14:141–3.

[6] Saygi A, Otek I, Guder M, Sungun F, Arman B Value of fiberoptic bronchoscopy in the diagnosis of complicated pulmonary unilocular cystic hydatidosis. Eur Respir J (1997); 10: 811–814.

[7] Hiras PR, Shweiki H.. Counterimmunoelectrophoresis using an Arc -5 antigen for the rapid diagnosisof hydatidosis and comparison arison with the IHA test. Am J Tro Med Hyg 1987; 36(3): 592- 97.

[8] Porehi D, Felleisen E Differential immunodiagnosis between cystic hydatid disease and other cross- reactive pathologies Am J Trop Med Hyg 1999; 60: 193-198.

[9] Zarzosa MP, Orduña Domingo A, Gutiérrez P, et al. Evaluation of six serological tests in diagnosis and postoperative control of pulmonary hydatid disease patients. Diagn Microbiol Infect Dis 1999;35:255-262.

[10] Dogan R, Yuksel M, Cetin G, Süzer K, Alp M, Kaya S Surgical treatment of hydatid cysts of the lung: report on 1055 patients. Thorax 1989; 44: 192-9.

[11] Von Sinner WN. New diagnostic signs in hydatid disease; radiography, ultrasound, CT and MRI correlated to pathology. Eur J Radiol 1991; 12(2): 150-9

[12] Halezaroglu S, Celik M, Uysal A, Senol C, Keleş M, Arman B. Giant hydatid cysts of the lung. J Thorac Cardiovasc Surg 1997; 113: 712-7.

[13] Solak H, Yeniterzi M, Yüksek T, et al. The hydatid cyst of the lung in children and results of surgical treatment. Thorac Cardiovasc Surg 1990; 38(1): 45-7

[14] Saygý A, Öztek I, Güder M, et al. Value of fiberoptic bronchoscopyn the diagnosis of complicated pulmonary unilocular cystic hydatidosis. Eur RespirJ 1997;10(4): 811-4

[15] Yörük Y, Yalçýnkaya S, Çoþkun I, et al. Simultaneous operation for coexisting lung and liver hydatid cyst: a treatment modality. Hepatogastroenterology 1998; 45(23): 1831-2

[16] Ulku R, Onen A, Onat S. Surgical treatment of pulmonary hydatid cysts in children: report of 66 cases. Eur J Pediatr Surg 2004; 14: 255-9.

[17] Sood D, Sharma DR, Santoshi ID. Anaphylactic shock on aspiration of hydatid cyst of liver during operation: treatment with ketamine. Indian J Anaesth 1994 Jun;42:213–214.

[18] Santini M, Fiorello A, Vicidomini G, Perrone A. A home-made device for safe intraoperative aspiration of pulmonary hydatid cysts. Interactive CardioVascular and Thoracic Surgery 7 (2008) 365–367

[19] Anadol D, Gocmen A, Kiper N, Ozcelik U. Hydatid disease in childhood: a retrospective analysis of 376 cases. Pediatr Pulmonol 1998; 26: 190-6.

[20] [Safioleas M, Misiakos EP, Dosios T, et al. Surgical treatment for lung hydatid disease. World J Surg 1999; 23(11): 1181-5

[21] Mallick MS, Al-Qahtani A, Al-Saadi MM, Al-Boukai AA. Thoracoscopic treatment of pulmonary hydatid cyst in a child. J Pediatr Surg. 2005 Dec;40(12):e35-7

[22] Mahin Jamshidi, Minou Mohraz, Mehrangiz Zangeneh, Ali Jamshidi; The effect of combination therapy with albendazole and praziquantel on hydatid cyst treatment ; Parasitology Research Volume 103, Number 1 (2008), 195-199

[23] Stamatakos M, Sargedi C, Stefanaki Ch, Safioleas C, Matthaiopoulou I, Safioleas M. Anthelminthic treatment: an adjuvant therapeutic strategy against Echinococcus granulosus. Parasitol Int. 2009 Jun; 58(2):115-20.

Section 2

Cardiac Surgery

Chapter 9

The Basis of Management of Congenital Heart Disease

Krishnan Ganapathy Subramaniam and
Neville Solomon

Additional information is available at the end of the chapter

http://dx.doi.org/10.5772/53654

1. Introduction

1.1. Cardiac embryology — The development of the heart

1.1.1. Early heart development and the folding of the primitive tube

By the 3rd week of development the heart has developed from the cardiogenic region, a horseshoe-shaped structure, at the cranial end of the embryo, when it is about the size of a raisin. By day 21 the primitive heart tube has moved below the head region and by day 22 it fuses and moves into the future thoracic cavity and it is from this time that it begins to beat. The tube now starts to bend and twist and over the next 8 days, various chamber of the heart begin to develop and by the end of 2 months it bears a superficial resemblance to the fetal heart. [1]

The tube is anchored at one end by the arterial trunks and at the other end, by the various venous channels draining into it. Being fixed at both ends, the cardiac tube grows rapidly in length and begins to twist and bend. The embryonic ventricle is bent in to a loop to the right of the midline and the ventricle grows rapidly to cover the atrium and the great veins (figure 1). The sacculations projecting laterally will become the right atrium and the left atrium. The future left ventricle lies to the left of interventricular groove and the right ventricle or the bulboconus region communicates with the truncus arteriosus. A four chambered structure is formed from this convoluted tube by development of 3 septa which partitions the atria, ventricle and the truncus arteriosus. [2]

The septae develop simultaneously at about the same time between the 28 to 42nd day. The atria and ventricle are separated by a deep groove, the atrio-ventricular groove which appears like an invagination from inside.This forms the atrio-ventricular canal, which becomes divided

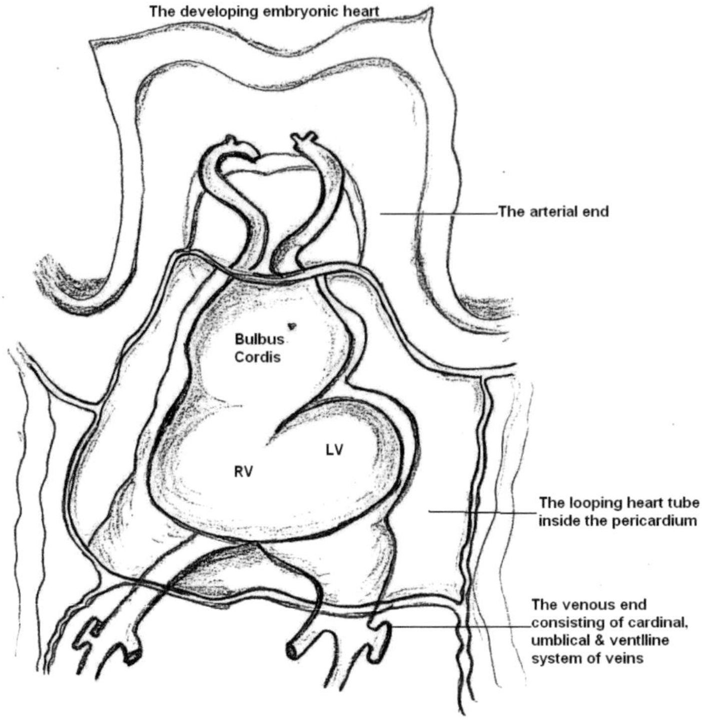

Figure 1. Development of the heart tube in the pericardial sac.

by the cushions which grow towards the junction. The endocardial cushions grow from opposite sides of the atrio-ventricular aperture and fuse to separate the atrium and ventricle.

From the interventricular ridge a proliferating muscular septum advances across the common ventricle towards the base of the heart. Simultaneously interatrial septum is formed by the septum primum growing rapidly towards endocardial cushions, leaving a foramen primum. Before the foramen primum becomes obliterated a new opening appears high on the interatrial septum- the foramen secundum-which allows shunting of blood from the right atrium to the left. The septum secundum develops from a ridge to the right of septum primum and grows like a curtain over the foramen secundum, the edge of the septum secundum forming the foramen ovale and the septum primum acting like a unidirectional valve, allowing blood to flow only from the right to the left.

The opening between the ventricular cavities -the interventricular foramen- persists, the closure of which depends on the development of a spiral septum which partitions the truncus and conus region into aorta and pulmonary artery.

The truncus arteriosus gives rise to the aortic arches, the 4th aortic arch forming the aorta and the 6th forming the origin of the pulmonary artery. A pair of ridges forms at the bifurcation which fuse and spiral down towards the interventricular foramen.

The interventricular foramen is obliterated by (a) masses of *endocardial tissue* at the interventricular septum, (b) masses of *'endocardial cushion'* tissue and (c) spiral septum. The partitioning of the heart is now complete. The aortopulmonary septum rotates 180 degree and fuses with the superior margin of the interventricular septum. This accounts for the manner in which the ventricular outflow tracts are aligned in a fully-developed heart- the aortic blood flowing posteriorly to anteriorly and the pulmonary blood flowing anterior to the aorta first and then posteriorly.

The events which occur during this period accounts for a majority of congenital heart disease. Atrial septal defect (which is most commonly a secundum defect) occurs due to defect of septum primum. Inadequate development of septum secundum (which forms by invagination of the developing superior vena cava and pulmonary veins) accounts for the sinus venosus type of defects.

The development of ventricular septum helps in understanding the predominance of perimembranous ventricular septal defects as three different regions have to fuse in a coordinated fashion to completely obliterate the interventricular communication. Uneven spiral partitioning of the outflow tracts can explain the occurrence of Tetralogy of Fallot (TOF) and double outlet right ventricle(DORV) and failure of the spiral pattern of aortopulmonary septum results in transposition of great arteries (TGA), when the aortopulmonary septum grows directly towards the interventricular septum. Failure of the septum to develop results in truncus arteriosus and the contribution of this septum to the interventricular septum explains the almost invariable association of truncus arteriosus defect with outlet VSD.

Failure of the endocardial cushions to develop properly results in the spectrum of endocardial cushion defects varying from ostium primum defects to partial and complete AV septal defects. [3]

1.1.2. Pulmonary venous development

Initially the blood coming from the lung buds drain into the splanchnic plexus which connects to the paired common cardinal and umbilicovitelline veins. The right common cardinal system forms the right SVC and azygous vein, the left common cardinal veins becomes the left superior vena cava and coronary sinus. The umbilicovitelline system becomes the inferior vena cava, ductus venosus and portal vein.

At 27 – 29 days the primitive pulmonary vein appears as an endothelial out pouching from superior left atrial wall and this joins the pulmonary venous plexus by 30 days. The common pulmonary vein enlarges and incorporates into the left atrium. The pulmonary venous part of the splanchnic plexus gradually loses its connection with cardinal and umbilicovitelline veins. Knowledge of the normal development of pulmonary venous pathway facilitates understanding of various types of anomalous pulmonary venous connections. [4]

1.1.3. Aortic arches

Aortic arches are series of six paired embryological structures connecting the ventral to the dorsal aorta.The ventral aorta at the level of 4- 6th arch fuses to form the truncus arteriosus which forms the distal end of the developing heart tube. The dorsal aorta on the right usually disappears and the dorsal aorta on the left forms the descending aorta.

The first arch disappears and the 2nd persists as stapedial artery which is not of clinical significance. The third arch forms the internal carotid artery on both the sides and is called the carotid arch. The 4th arch on the right forms the right subclavian artery as far as the origin of the internal mammary branch and the left 4th arch forms the arch of aorta between the left carotid artery and the termination of ductus arteriosus. The 5 th arch disappears on both sides. The proximal part of the right 6th arch forms the right pulmonary artery and the distal part disappears. The proximal part of the left 6th arch forms the left pulmonary artery and the distal part persists as the ductus arteriosus.(figure 2)

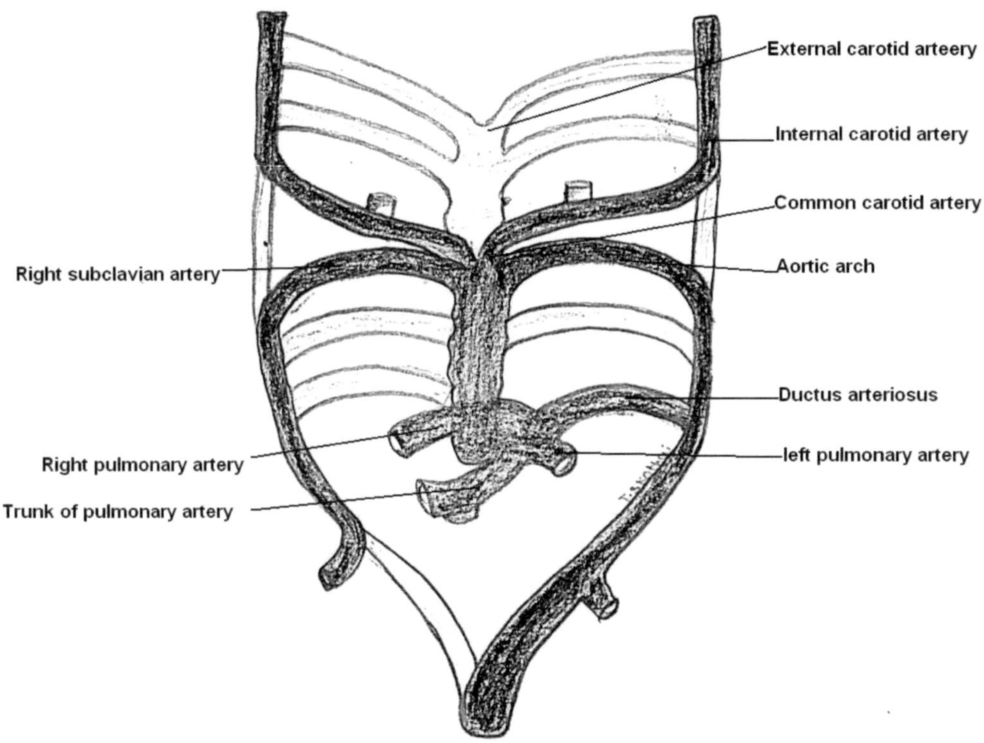

Figure 2. Development of aortic arches

Double aortic arch which is the commonest arch anomaly causing trachea and oesophageal compression occurs as a result of persistence of dorsal aorta. The recurrent laryngeal nerve loops around the 6th arch and hence goes around the ductus arteriosus on the left side and the subclavian artery on the right side. Persistence of the ductus arteriosus results in patent ductus arteriosus (PDA) and its excessive resorption can result in coarctation of aorta or stenosis of left pulmonary artery. [5]

http://dx.doi.org/10.5772/53654

The molecular mechanism behind the complex development is being now slowly unravelled. The consistent rightward looping of the heart suggests a highly conserved molecular control mechanism, The beating cilia on the node beats in a counter clockwise direction causing a leftward flow of fluid across the Hensen's node. The unidirectional movement is based on the inherent molecular chirality of the ciliary protein machinery. Pitx-2, a homeodomain containing protein plays a role in development of laterality. The Nkx2.5 and Tbx5 gene are expressed in atria and in conduction system. Irx4 is expressed only in ventricular chambers. The HAND 1 gene is expressed on the left ventricle and HAND 2 is expressed in the right ventricle.

The vertebral heart develops from precardiac mesoderm, anterior heart field and cardiac neural crest cells also play a critical part in myocardium and normal outflow tract development. The cardiac neural crest cell stabilizes the arch vessels and prevents their regression. A subpopulation of cardiac neural crest cells participates in the septation of outflow tract and contributes to the formation of semilunar valves. Retinoic acid is believed to have a role in signalling neural crest migration and cardiac development. Understanding the molecular and genetic mechanism may help in future fetal cardiac interventions. [6]

2. Surgical anatomy of the heart

The heart is enclosed in a pericardial sac. The pericardial cavity is the space between the inner lining of the fibrous pericardium and the surface of the heart.There are two recesses in the pericardial cavity lined by serous pericardium, the first is the transverse sinus behind the great arteries in front of the atria and is in free communication with the pericardial cavity on either side. The second is the oblique sinus, a blind ending cavity behind the left atrium.

The cardiac mass is 1/3rd to the right and 2/3rd to the left of midline. The ventricle is a three sided pyramid with diaphragmatic, anterior and left surfaces. The right sided margin is the acute margin and the left is the obtuse margin [7].

2.1. The morphological right atrium

The right atrium has 3 components-the appendage, venous sinus and the vestibule. (figure 3)The junction between the appendage and the venous sinus is marked by the prominent terminal groove. The groove internally corresponds to the crista terminalis, from which the pectinate muscle originates. The extensive array of pectinate muscles serves as one of the markers of the morphologic right atrium. Parallel and posterior to the groove is the second deeper groove between the right atrium and the right pulmonary veins. Dissection into this deep interatrial groove (Waterston's or Sondergaard's groove) permits incisions to be made into the left atrium (the *classic posterior approach* to the left atrium).

The sinus node lies in the subepicardial position at the cranial part of the terminal groove, and is a spindle-shaped structure which lies lateral to the superior cavoatrial junction. The artery to the sinus node arises from right coronary artery (55%) or cirumflex coronary artery (45%).

The septum between the right and left atria is formed by the floor of the oval fossa and its adjacent anteroinferior muscular rim. The superior rim or the septum secundum is formed by deep interatrial fold extending between the systemic and the pulmonary veins. Larger part of the anterior atrial wall is related to the aortic root (the torus aorticus). It is important to realize that the true atrial septum is rather small and it is easy to go outside the heart when attempting to gain access to the left atrium through the septal approach. Because of the infolding of the interatrial groove, access to the left atrium can be gained by approaching through the right atrium and incising superiorly within the fossa (*The septal superior approach*). [8]

The triangle of Koch which contains the atrioventricular (AV) node is an area of major surgical significance. The triangle is demarcated by the (a) the tendon of Todaro, (b) the attachment of the septal leaflet and (c) the orifice of the coronary sinus. The tendon of Todaro is formed by the fusion of the valve guarding the IVC (the Eustachian valve) and the coronary sinus (the Thebesian valve). This inserts into the central fibrous body and runs in the tissue separating the oval fossa from the mouth of the coronary sinus The trabeculated diverticulum found posterior to the coronary sinus is called the post-Eustachian sinus of Keith.

The node lies in the atrial muscle above the hinge point of the septal leaflet, and the bundle which arises from the node penetrates the interventricular septum at the apex of the triangle of Koch.

The central fibrous body is actually the area where the membranous septum and leaflets of the atrioventricular and the aortic valves join in fibrous continuity.

2.2. The morphological left atrium

Like the right atrium, the left atrium has a (a) venous sinus (b) appendage and (c) vestibule. The differences however are

a. The venous component of the left atrium is considerably larger than the appendage

b. the junction between them is NOT marked by a terminal groove or crest.

c. The pectinate muscles are confined within the appendage and do not extend around the vestibule

d. The appendage is long, tubular and finger like with a narrow end unlike the broad triangular appendage of the right atrium

Among these the confinement of the pectinate muscles within the appendage is the most reliable differentiating factor between the morphological right and left atrium.

2.3. The morphologic right ventricle

It has three components- the inlet, trabecular and outlet parts.

The inlet portion is limited by the tricuspid valve and its tension apparatus

The trabecular component extends to the apex, where it is thin and it is vulnerable to perforation by cardiac catheters and pacemaker electrodes.

http://dx.doi.org/10.5772/53654

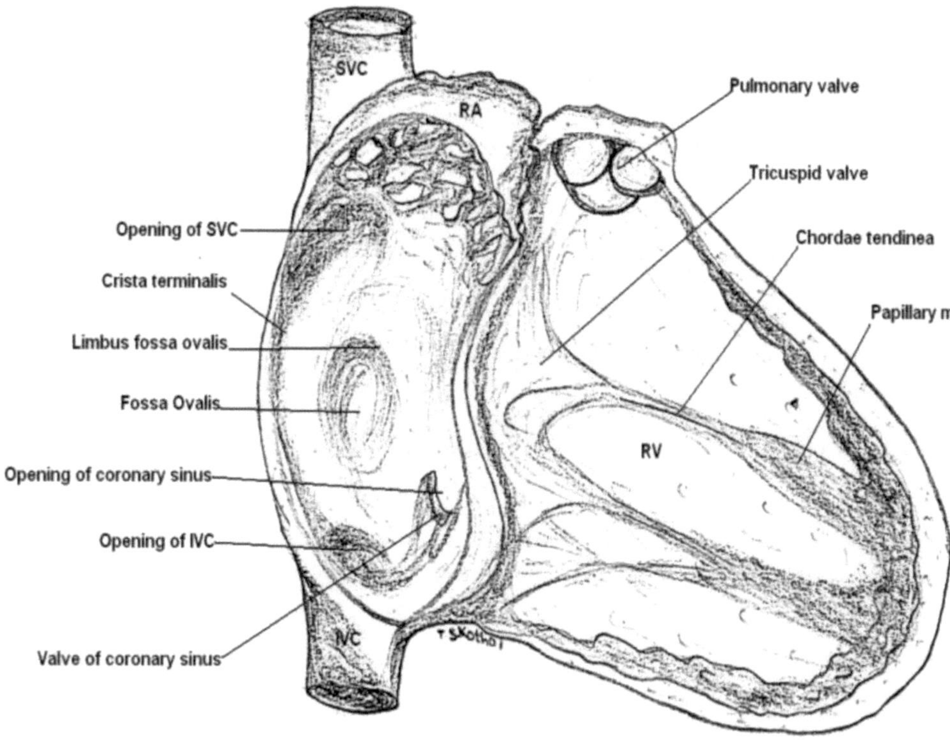

Figure 3. Right atrium and ventricle

The outlet component of the right ventricle is a complete muscular structure - the infundibulum- which supports the pulmonary valve.

The muscular shelf separating the tricuspid and the pulmonary valve is the supraventricular crest. Much of the crest is no more than the infolded inner heart curve and incisions and sutures deep in this area can jeopardize the right coronary artery. The distal part of the crest is continuous with the sub-pulmonary infundibulum, the presence of which permits the pulmonary valve to be removed and used as autograft during the Ross procedure.

The crest is cradled between two limbs of the prominent right ventricular trabecula called the septomarginal trabeculation, which has a superior limb, an inferior limb and a body.

The superior limb runs up to the attachment of the pulmonary valve.

The inferior limb gives rise to the medial papillary muscle (of Lancisi) and a line drawn from this muscle to the apex of the triangle of Koch marks the position of the atrioventricular conduction axis.

The body runs to the apex, and gives rise to the moderator band and the anterior papillary muscle.

The coarseness of the apical trabeculation is the most constant feature of the right ventricle. The other differences are the direct septal attachment of the tension apparatus of the atrio-ventricular valve, which is usually tricuspid in nature.

2.4. The morphologic left ventricle

The inlet component is limited by the mitral valve and its tension apparatus. The mitral valve has two leaflets, the aortic or the anterior leaflet which is in fibrous continuity with the aortic valve, which is short and square and the other leaflet which is connected to the wall of the left atrioventricular junction is called the mural or the posterior leaflet.

The leaflets do not have direct septal attachment unlike the right ventricle but instead attach through anterolateral and posteromedial papillary muscles.

The apical myocardium is thin like the RV. The septum is not completely muscular unlike RV, and it has a small membranous part which forms the subaortic outflow tract.

The muscular septal surface is characteristically smooth and the left bundle lies below the membranous septum corresponding to the zone of apposition between the right coronary and non-coronary leaflets.

The semilunar valves of the aortic and pulmonary valves are similar, the distal portion forms the sinotubular junction and the proximal part takes origin from the ventricular structure. The overall arrangement is like the crown, rather than forming an annulus. [9]

The aorta and pulmonary artery form the vascular pedicle. The aorta gives rise to the brachio-cephalic or innominate artery, the left common carotid artery and the left subclavian artery. The pulmonary artery arises anteriorly and courses posteriorly, and is a short vessel giving rise to the right and left pulmonary arteries. The left pulmonary artery lies superior to the left bronchi in front of the descending aorta. The right pulmonary artery is anterior to the left main bronchus and has a long mediastinal course beneath the aortic arch and behind the superior vena cava to reach the hilum of the right lung. Sometimes a early branching large upper lobar branch can be mistaken for the right pulmonary artery.

The coronary arteries arise from the aortic sinuses. According to Leiden convention the position is described in terms of an observer from the non-coronary sinus, the right hand of the person is called the sinus 1 and gives rise to the right coronary artery and left hand facing sinus is called the sinus 2 and gives rise to left coronary artery. The coronary artery arises beneath the sinotubular junction, and when it is displaced more than 1 cm from the ST junction it is considered abnormal which occurs in 3.5% of hearts.

The left coronary artery has a single orifice,while in 50% there are two orifices in the right sinus, one gives rise to the main RCA and the smaller orifice gives rise to the infundibular or sinus nodal artery. It is important while giving ostial cardioplegia for stopping the heart to perform cardiac surgeries to instill into the smaller orifices to protect the sinus node.

The epicardial course of the coronary arteries follows the atrioventricular and interventricular grooves. The RCA gives to the acute marginal branches, the sinus nodal artery (55%), and posterior descending artery (90%) at the crux which supplies the diaphragmatic surface. The LCA gives rise to the anterior interventricular (left anterior descending) and the circumflex branches. The anterior interventricular artery gives rise to the diagonal branches to the obtuse surface of the heart and the septal perforating branches. The circumflex artery gives rise to the obtuse marginal branches of the heart. [10]

The Coronary veins accompany the artery and drain into the coronary sinus.

The Great cardiac vein runs along the left anterior descending artery and encircles the mitral orifice, and at its left margin receives the oblique vein of the LA and forms the coronary sinus. The coronary sinus lies between the left atrium and left ventricle before joining the right atrium.

The Middle cardiac vein runs along the posterior descending artery and the small cardiac veins accompany the right coronary artery. The Thebesian valve guards the orifice of the coronary sinus.

3. Conductiion system and its surgical significance

3.1. The development

The heart develops from the mesoderm from fusion of vascular channels which forms the heart tube. The heart starts beating from the time the embryo is 22 days old. Even from the beginning there is a polarity and the peristaltic type of motion of the tube starts from the venous end and ends in the arterial end. This sequential contraction ensures that even in the absence of valves there is very little regurgitation of the blood, and an ECG similar to the adult ECG is recognized at the end of 1st month. It is believed that this primitive heart tube persists as the remnant of conduction tissue and the myocardium grows around this to form the atrium and the ventricle. The conduction system is one of the most primitive structures in the heart which forms even before the heart tube starts looping.

There is a circle of conduction tissue at the atrioventricular junction, which as the atrioventricular valves form and the great arteries are assigned to the respective ventricles gradually becomes restricted.The only area of electrical continuity between the atrium and the ventricles is the AV node and the penetrating bundle where the muscular septum comes in contact with the AV junction. This establishes connection with the Purkinje network in the ventricular myocardium, to ensure sequential contraction of atrium and ventricles. (figure 4)

This sequence of events occurs in the usual d-looping of the heart.If there is l-looping of the heart as in congenitally corrected transposition, where the right atrium joins the left ventricle, which then gives rise to the pulmonary artery and the left atrium joins the right ventricle which gives rise to aorta, the bundle can be extremely elongated bringing it under the pulmonary valve anteriorly. The conduction system is vulnerable to injury during surgery and otherwise Both congenital and spontaneous heart blocks can occur at the rate of 2% per annum in this condition. [11]

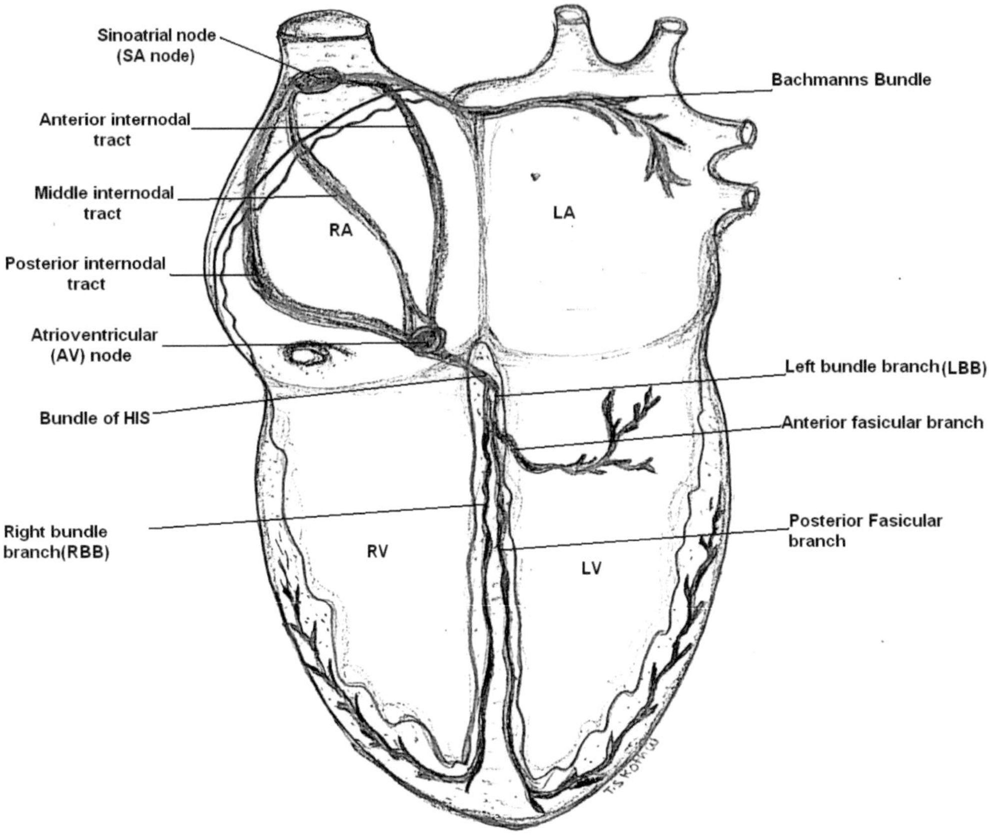

Figure 4. Conduction system

3.2. Surgical perspective

3.2.1. Sinoatrial (SA) node

SA node which is located at the lateral cavoatrial junction at the upper end of crista terminalis is the pacemaker which initiates contraction. This can be identified as a small oval shaped structure which is slightly more yellowish with SA nodal artery forming small ramifications over it.

This area is vulnerable during –

1. Glenn surgery – where the SVC is divided and anastomosed to the pulmonary artery end to side – the cavopulmonary anastomosis. Care has to be taken while clamping and dividing the SVC.
2. Sinus venosus atrial septal defect with partial anomalous pulmonary venous connection – some of the pulmonary veins can drain high into the SVC and during correction

sometimes it may be necessary to cut across the cavoatrial junction longitudinally which makes the SA node or the artery supplying this at risk.

3. Sennings procedure –the SA node is at risk during suturing the pulmonary venous baffle.

4. Superior septal approach to the mitral valve – which may put the artery supplying the SA node at risk. Injury is manifested by nodal rhythm during which the P wave is absent in the ECG. The distal portion of the conduction system gradually takes over or the SA node itself recovers, making the need for a permanent pacemaker rare in this setting.

3.2.2. Atrioventricular (AV) node

The AV node lies in the apex of the triangle of Koch, the penetrating bundle pierces the apex of the triangle and reaches the crest of the trabecular septum immediately beneath the membranous septum which is below the junction formed by the *right and noncoronary cusp*. It is in this area that the bundle is most vulnerable during surgical closure of ventricular septal defect. This corresponds to the commissure between the anterior and septal leaflets of the tricuspid valve which is usually supported by the medial papillary muscle.Sometimes there is a cleft in the septal leaflet which points to this area.

The penetrating bundle crosses from the atrial septum to the aortic outflow and then joins the muscular septum. In normal hearts with normal alignment the apex of the triangle is close to the crest of the interventricular septum.The length of the bundle is small in this setting and this length of the non-branching bundle can be excessive in the presence of VSD in the inlet portion of the ventricular septum.

It is only when the ventricular septum reaches the crux of the heart can a regular AV node join the AV conduction axis. The node and bundle is formed at the place where the ventricular septum joins the AV junction.

A few rules may help avoid heart block while closing VSD's

a. In perimembranous defects, which is also the type of defect usually seen in tetralogy of Fallot, the VSD patch should be sutured about 5 mm away from the posteroinferior margin, and in perimembranous defects with outlet extension the muscle protects the bundle and makes it more left sided and this makes the posteroinferior angle safe in VSD with outlet extension. It the perimembranous defects with inlet extension where the bundle is superficial and close to the posteroinferior angle of the defect, and hence is exposed to maximum risk of damage. The risk of damage to the node is minimal in cases of muscular and subpulmonic VSD's.

b. The base of the septal leaflet tissue is always safe to place sutures.

c. The fibrous tissue surrounding the VSD can be used to anchor the patch and this has to be differentiated from aneurysm of membranous septum which may sometimes harbour the bundle.

d. In AV canal defects the AV node and the coronary sinus are displaced inferiorly, and the AV node is placed in between the coronary sinus and the crest of interventricular septum at the so called 'NODAL triangle' rather than at the usual apex of the triangle of Koch. [12]

Transient damage to the conduction system can occur as a result of myocardial protection during cardiopulmonary bypass, which should usually recover in less than 7 days. A permanent pacemaker is usually needed if sinus rhythm does not return in 9-10 days

4. Fetal and neonatal circulation

The circulatory system evolved as the simple process of diffusion of nutrients from amniotic sac is no longer able to meet the metabolic needs of the growing embryo.

The placenta does the function of oxygenation in the fetus as the lungs are bypassed by presence of ductus. The arrangement of circulation in the fetus is such that the more oxygenated blood goes to the head and the less oxygenated blood goes through the ductus into descending aorta and into the umbilical arteries.

The umbilical vein brings the oxygenated blood which bypasses the liver through the ductus venosus and this blood coming into the IVC is preferentially streamed by the Eustachian valve into the left atrium through the foramen in the atrial septum and this oxygenated blood enters the left ventricle and from there to the aorta and arch vessels.

The more deoxygenated blood from the SVC goes into the right ventricle which is pumped by the RV into the PA and as the fetal lungs are collapsed with very high resistance in the pulmonary circulation, the blood bypasses the lungs and goes into the descending aorta through the ductus.

A few lesions provide insights, which can evolve into more complicated congenital heart pathologies. Absence of foramen is one such lesion, which has been linked to the development of hypoplastic left heart syndrome, the development of which can be prevented by dilating the foramen ovale.

Atresia of the pulmonary and aortic valve can also be intervened by ballooning to prevent the development of its sequel which can be hypoplastic left heart and RV dependent coronary circulation in cases of pulmonary atresia with intact ventricular septum.

Absence of ductus arteriosus is a condition which is associated with absent pulmonary valve The absence of ductus could be the primary condition which leads to RV output regurgitating back into ventricle due to high fetal pulmonary vascular resistance, with the VSD partially decompressing the right ventricle. The increased right ventricular output causes the main and the branch pulmonary arteries to dilate. This could extend into the lungs, compressing the airways, and thereby causing severe respiratory compromise in neonatal period as seen in extreme cases of TOF with absent pulmonary valve.

http://dx.doi.org/10.5772/53654

5. The transition from fetal to neonatal circulation

The first breath causes the lungs to expand and oxygen content in the blood to increase and this provides the impetus for the ductus to constrict and close. The right ventricular output goes to the lungs and reaches the left atrium, the increased pressure in the left atrium causing the flap valve to shut, closing the foramen ovale. The umbilical vein and ductus venosus regress to leave the vestigial ligamentum teres and the ligamentum venosum.

Maintaining the patency of ductus is critical to many potential fatal neonatal conditions. These can be any of the conditions in which the output of the heart through either the aorta or the pulmonary artery is critically reduced and the patent ductus maintains the flow from one great artery to the other. These are hypoplastic left heart syndrome, critical aortic stenosis and pulmonary atresia. The presence of ductus is also useful in mixing lesions like TGA though the degree of mixing is much better in the presence of atrial level communication. Patency of ductus can be maintained by Prostaglandin E1 infusion, the availability of which has enabled the stabilization of many sick neonates before subjecting them to surgery [13].

6. The pathophysiology of L->R shunt lesions

ASD, VSD and PDA are the main lesions which shunt from left to right.

In Atrial septal defect, the size of the shunt is determined by the size of the defect and the degree of pulmonary vascular resistance. Small shunts cause no enlargement of cardiac chambers, while large shunt cause significant RA and RV dilatation, mid- diastolic flow murmur though the tricuspid valve and ejection systolic murmur at the left upper sternal border due to increased flow across the pulmonary valve. The left chambers do not increase in size as the increased return to LA is decompressed into the RA through the defect.

The pathophysiology of the shunt in VSD and PDA are similar. The magnitude of shunt is determined by the size of the defect and the degree of pulmonary vascular resistance (PVR); PVR is more important in the large defects where it determines the degree of shunt. Since PVR is elevated at birth and falls by 6-8 wks, children with large VSD typically become symptomatic with signs of congestive heart failure (CHF) at this time.

A small defect causes no enlargement of cardiac chambers, the ECG and X-ray are normal, there is ejection systolic murmur and P2 is normal. For moderate sized defects, there is LA and LV enlargement unlike ASD and as the RV is contracting at the time of left to right shunt, it undergoes no volume load. However the increased blood pumped by the RV causes mid-diastolic murmur across the mitral valve.

Large defects and PDA cause CHF in infancy, especially if the PVR is low. This reflects in biventricular hypertrophy with increased saturations, pan systolic murmur and loud P2. As the PVR increases, the heart size becomes normal on Chest X-ray though the pulmonary segment remains prominent, the murmur is reduced, and there is pure RVH in ECG

In PDA in addition there is enlargement of aorta and transverse aortic arch, which is usually not very evident in on X-ray as the aortic arch does not form a part of cardiac silhouette. As the PVR increases, there can be differential cyanosis with lower limb saturations being lower than the upper limb reflecting right to left shunt at the level of PDA.

Endocardial cushion defects present with features of both ASD and VSD. The QRS axis is abnormal between -20 to -150 degree, which is due to the disposition of the His bundle and its branches intrinsic to the pathology and not due to hemodynamic consequence.

Obligatory shunts are those where the degree of shunting does not depend on the PVR, examples of which is Gerbode defect where is there is LV to RA shunt or ruptured sinus of Valsalva [14]

7. Stenosis and regurgitation of valves

If there is stenosis of atrioventricular valves, it causes systemic or pulmonary venous congestion, depending on the valves involved. Regurgitant lesions cause volume loading of both upstream and downstream chambers. Unlike stenotic lesions which cause pressure overload, regurgitation lesions cause volume overload.

Aortic regurgitation causes wide pulse pressure and the regurgitating jet causes diastolic flutter of mitral valve causing the Austin Flint murmur, and the jet also causes the mitral valve to close early and reduces the intensity of S1. Aortic regurgitation in children usually occurs as a part of ventricular septal defect when the leaflets either attempt to close the defect or get sucked in due to Bernouilli effect, or prolapse due to lack of support to the leaflets due to absence of continuity of media.

Pulmonary regurgitation is common after TOF repair and the significance of which depends on the diastolic distensibility of the right ventricle: patients with diastolic dysfunction of the RV tolerate PR better with less dilatation, and narrow QRS. TR causes prominent liver and neck pulsations.

7.1. Cyanotic heart defects pathophysiology – TGA and Truncus arteriosus

TGA is one of the common cyanotic conditions presenting in infancy where the aorta arises from the RV and PA arises from the LV. The systemic blood reaches the RV and from there to aorta and again back to RV,(the blood flow is parallel rather than in series). Such an arrangement is incompatible with life in the absence of atrial, ventricular or ductal level communication. In the presence of inadequate communication, they can present with very poor saturations (30-50%) with acidosis and hypoglycaemia in the first week of life. Of all the levels of communication the atrial septal defect provides the best area of mixing without streaming and atrial septostomy (Rashkind procedure) done for this purpose is the first palliative intervention for a congenital heart disease, which started off the practice of pediatric interventional cardiology.

http://dx.doi.org/10.5772/53654

Any newborn with deep cyanosis and cardiomegaly (egg on side appearance) and increased pulmonary vascular marking and no murmur can be diagnosed to have TGA. Patients with VSD present a little late with features of early CHF and these patients are prone to develop very early pulmonary hypertension, because they get relatively desaturated blood under high pressure. The unique feature of pulmonary circulation of 'hypoxic vasoconstriction ' accelerates the onset of pulmonary vascular disease.TGA, VSD and PS can occur and the presentation of which depends on the degree of reduction of pulmonary blood flow.

Truncus arteriosus has complete mixing of systemic and pulmonary blood and the level of saturation is proportional to the degree of pulmonary blood flow.

7.2. Pathophysiology of Tetralogy of Fallot

This is commonest cause of cyanosis in children in developing countries. Though classically supposed to have the features of a) VSD b) Aortic over-ride c) RV hypertrophy and d) Right ventricular outflow tract (RVOT) obstruction, the two important features are

a. A large VSD at least as big as the aortic annulus to equalise pressures in both ventricles.

b. Right ventricular outflow tract obstruction – which can be at any level infundibular, valvar, supravalvar or at branch PA level.

If a child presents clinically with signs of small VSD with RVH, it strongly suggests diagnosis of TOF, the probability of which increases in the presence of right aortic arch.

The intensity and the duration of heart murmur are inversely proportional to the severity of pulmonary stenosis. In pulmonary atresia or in cyanotic spells when there is critical reduction in pulmonary flow there may be no murmur at all due to absence of flow across the RVOT

There are no signs of CHF in TOF because no chamber is under volume overload and only RV is under pressure overload which is not suprasystemic and is well tolerated.

The degree of cyanosis depends on the balance between the systemic and pulmonary resistances, and decrease in SVR due to activities like crying and defecation can increase the degree of R-> L shunt.

The role of RVOT spasm in the development of cyanotic spell is controversial

Hyperpnoea plays an important role in the perpetuation of cyanotic spell as it increases the venous return and more desaturated blood enters the systemic circulation due to override.

Termination of a spell can be achieved by

a. By increasing SVR – by knee chest position, phenylephrine, ketamine

b. Reducing hyperpnoea by sedation – morphine, sodium bicarbonate which reduces respiratory stimulation, ketamine

c. Decreasing venous return – squatting

d. Stabilisation of vascular reactivity – propranolol prevents sudden decrease in SVR and its role in preventing RVOT spasm is controversial.

7.3. Pathophysiology of Tricuspid atresia and TAPVC

This is a single ventricle physiology where there is enlargement of RA, LA and LV and hypoplastic RV. 70% have normally related great arteries and 30% have transposed great arteries. In either of these situations the pulmonary blood flow can be increased or decreased. QRS axis is deviated leftward with LVH and the axis resembles endocardial cushion defect.

TAPVC – Total anomalous pulmonary venous connection can present as supracardiac, cardiac and infracardiac.The timing of clinical presentation depends on the presence of obstruction.

Non- obstructed TAPVC presents like large ASD. Obstructed variant can present with extremely sick child with pulmonary venous congestion causing ground glass appearance on chest X-ray, severe cyanosis, respiratory distress and severe pulmonary arterial hypertension. Murmur is usually soft or absent.

Any child with features of pulmonary oedema and ground glass appearance on chest X-ray with normal size cardiac shadow and no murmurs should be considered to have obstructed TAPVC. [15]

8. Chest X-ray

X-ray is integral part of the evaluation of a child with cardiac disease.

The x-ray helps in the evaluation of cardiomegaly, chamber size, and blood flow by looking at the pulmonary artery and venous markings. Lungs, spine, thorax and visceral situs are also evaluated using x-ray. For example the presence of aortic knuckle and gastric fundus on the same side is suggestive of corrected transposition.

The structures forming the margin of the heart on the right side are– SVC, aortic knuckle and RA and on the left side they are the pulmonary artery, left atrial appendage and LV.

Different conditions can have diagnostic X-ray features. TOF has a *' boot shaped'* heart, TGA has a *'egg on side'* heart and supracardiac TAPVC is associated with *'snow man sign'* the left vertical vein, the innominate vein and the right superior vena cava form the head of the snowman., Truncus, the dilated pulmonary artery particularly the right pulmonary artery produces the *' comma or the water fall sign'*. In Ebsteins anomaly there is cardiomegaly with a narrow pedicle, with *'Pencil line sharp'* cardiac borders.These classic appearances are not usually seen, though they are supportive evidences in broader clinical context.

8.1. The assessment of pulmonary arterial and venous pressure using X-ray

Pulmonary plethora – the presence of right descending pulmonary artery larger than the size of trachea is a sensitive sign of increased pulmonary blood flow. Other signs are prominent upper and lower zone vessels and vessels seen in the outer third of the lungs. Infants and children present with generalized mottling, due to increased pulmonary flow.

http://dx.doi.org/10.5772/53654

Pulmonary arterial hypertension: Is said to occur when the mean pulmonary artery pressure is > 20 mmHg,

In mild PAH – (20-29 mmHg) there is prominent pulmonary artery.

Moderate PAH- (30-49), the central vessels dilate further,

Severe PAH (50 mmHg) - there is central dilation with reduction in the calibre of peripheral vessels (peripheral pruning). The size of the pulmonary artery correlates with PAH, and it has been found that plethora correlates better with the degree of left to right shunt than cardiomegaly.

Pulmonary venous hypertension – normal 8-12 mm Hg, and gradual increase causes:

a. Redistribution of blood flow (10-20mm Hg) – Cephalization due to dilation of upper zone vessels and blurring of lower zone vessels

b. Interstitial oedema – (15-25 mm Hg) Kerley lines and peribronchial cuffing

c. Alveolar oedema- (25 – 35 mm Hg) causes the 'Bat's wing appearance' when the interstitial fluid accumulates at rate faster than it can be removed by lymphatics.

The presence of prominent aortic knuckle points to the presence of extra cardiac left to right shunt like PDA, Sinus of Valsalva rupture, Coronary arteriovenous fistula, or AP window. The absence points to intra- cardiac L-> R shunt like atrial septal defect and ventricular septal defect.

In addition to the above findings careful consideration should be given to lung parenchyma to look for any parenchymal patches and also the status of spine and bony thorax for complete preoperative assessment.

9. Echocardiography

Using ultrasound to visualize organs was first introduced in the 1970's and over the 1980's it transformed the field of imaging becoming the primary diagnostic modality for evaluation of congenital heart disease. During the 90's and 2000's steady progress has been made in the areas of 3D imaging, myocardial function assessment and trans-esophageal echocardiography(TEE).TEE is now routinely used intraoperatively for planning and performing cardiac procedures, TEE probes can now be placed in children as small as 3.5 kg.

Echo is non-invasive, has excellent spatial and temporal resolution, ability to see the anatomy and physiology in real time along with portability. Echo is now everywhere right from prenatal imaging, preoperative, intraoperative, postoperative and follow-up imaging.

A burst of ultrasonic energy is produced by the piezoelectric crystals placed on the transducer probe which passes through the tissue and the returning ultrasound is processed by amplification, filtering and is analysed to display in a moving real-time format.

The different modes of imaging are

a. M- Mode – uses a narrow ultrasound beam to provide a 'ice pick' image of the structure. It has good axial resolution. Used to measure the degree of movement of leaflets. Chamber thickness is measured using 2-D directed M-mode imaging.

b. 2-D mode –uses *phased array transducers* which are multiple piezoelectric crystals that both transmits and receives ultrasound simultaneously; used to provide an image of the 'section' of the heart.

c. 3-D mode *uses matrix array transducers* and sophisticated parallel array processing to provide real time image. With progressive miniaturization, real-time 3D Transesophageal images provide excellent images intraoperatively for planning valve repairs.

d. Doppler imaging – can be used to estimate the velocity and direction of blood flow to estimate the pressure gradient cross sectional flow area and prediction of intracardiac pressures.

e. Contrast Echocardiography – is based on the fact that any intravascular injection produces a contrast which can be detected by echocardiography. Used for intracardiac and great artery level shunts in patients with poor windows, for detecting pulmonary venous malformation and for detecting baffle leak following atrial switch procedures.

f. Fetal echocardiography – using trans abdominal screening majority of the cardiovascular malformations can be detected by 17- 20 weeks of life; by transvaginal window, heart and great vessels can be visualized at the end of 1st trimester. [16]

10. Magnetic Resonance Imaging

It is a imaging modality which uses magnetic fields and radiofrequency energy to stimulate hydrogen nuclei which emits radiofrequency waves that are used to construct images. Over the 1990's the field has evolved from a procedure which takes a long time to produce a series of static images to one in which real time 3-D visualization is possible. MRI uses magnetic field of strength 0.5 Tesla to 3 Tesla (1 Tesla is 10,000 Gauss; earth magnetic field is 0.5 G). MRI uses fields which are 5000 to 60000 more powerful than the earth's magnetic field.

Synchronisation or respiratory motion compensation is required as the heart is a moving object and 'gating' or ' synchronization' is required to return to the same point in the cardiac cycle in order to freeze the cardiac motion. Pulse oximetry, ECG signal or MRI navigator echoes can be used for gating. Advances in *gradient coil and parallel acquisition* methods can obviate the need for synchronization.

Two main modalities of MRI are:

a. Spin Echo – uses a radiofrequency pulse that tilts the hydrogen protons by 90 degrees followed by a second 180 degree pulse, which are used to generate images. Produces images in which the flowing 'blood is black'. This provides static anatomic information, with excellent blood myocardium contrast. Used for assessing cardiac tumours, pericardial disease and thoracic masses. Takes a relatively longer time

b. Gradient Echo - sequences uses radiofrequency pulses that are less than 90 degrees, that are faster than spin Echo images and used to produce images in which the flowing 'blood appears white'. 'Steady State free precession' MR sequences allow real time MR fluoroscopy, with shorter imaging times. Used to assess ventricular function and flow of blood in the cardiac pathways and for identifying stenotic or regurgitant jets.

Myocardial tagging – uses 'spatial modulation of magnetization' so that protons in selected volume are incapable of producing a signal. This produces stripes across the image, tagging the myocardium. As the heart moves the tags are followed and this allows calculation of myocardial strain

Velocity encoded Cine MRI- can be used to measure blood flow velocity and quantify blood flow rate.- can measure the regurgitation volume and can even calculate the shear stress exerted by the blood on the vessel wall.

Contrast enhanced MRI – Uses gadolinium chelate which produces bright blood signal used for clear delineation of spatial relationship and for imaging of baffles and outflow tracts. Hyper enhancement of myocardial regions observed 10-15 minutes after administration of gadolinium contrast is indicative of scar tissue and irreversible myocardial injury.

MRI in patients younger than 5-6 years would require sedation, Surgical clips, sternotomy wires, coils stents and occluding devices are MRI safe once the surrounding fibrous tissue grows over these implants and makes them immobile. Cardiac pacemakers, presence of intracranial, intra ocular or intracochlear implant are considered contraindication to MRI.

Cardiovascular MRI is fast becoming a tool which can provide us with anatomic and functional information not provided by echo or cardiac catheterization. [17]

11. Cardiac catheterisation and interventions

Catheterisation used to be the main diagnostic modality available when it was first introduced in 1946. The era of angiographic anatomic delineation is fading. Echocardiography is now preferred for evaluation of valvar and congenital cardiac defects with 3D echo promising real time surgical images of the valves for repair. MRI and CT angiography is fast replacing angiogram for delineation of complex relationship, volume estimation of chamber, extra cardiac vessels, aortic arches and venous anomalies. The field of MR imaging, has the potential to completely replace diagnostic angiography. The routine use of catheterization before single ventricle surgeries is being questioned, as the same information can be made available through non-invasive means

Angiogram still has a role in

a. Visualising branch PA anatomy beyond hilum- in case of tetralogy of Fallot with aorto-pulmonary collaterals

b. Coronary anatomy.

c. Measurement of flow, pressure, reactivity and resistance of pulmonary vasculature to various drugs in patients with elevated pulmonary artery pressure.

d. Estimation of cardiac output, Qp/Qs calculation for assessment of operability.

The cardiac output can be calculated by the thermodilution technique or the Fick's principle.

Fick's principle is based on the fact that

'The uptake or release of substance by an organ is equivalent to the blood flow to the organ multiplied by the arteriovenous difference of the substance'

O_2 is used as the indicator and all the systemic organs or lungs are considered as one organ to estimate the systemic or pulmonary output respectively.

We use the 0_2 consumption in ml/min/m2 and this divided by the arteriovenous difference would give the systemic or pulmonary flows. The consumption is made available through estimates based on age, sex and heart rate.

Systemic output would be the difference between the arterial oxygen content and mixed venous oxygen content (ideally measured in the middle of right atrium to average for the superior vena caval, inferior vena caval or coronary sinus venous blood whose oxygen content may be different)

Pulmonary output would be the difference between the pulmonary venous and pulmonary artery oxygen content.

Qp/Qs can be easily calculated even if we do not have the values of oxygen consumption. We need the systemic arterial, mixed venous and pulmonary arterial and pulmonary venous oxygen content (which is assumed to be 100% in the absence of pulmonary pathology).

Pressure measurements are based on fluid filled catheters, or large bore catheters with multiple side holes which would yield accurate description of intracardiac waveforms. The resistance is calculated using the Ohm's law, which is the difference in the pressure across the organ divided by the amount of blood flowing through it. PVR (Pulmonary vascular resistance) would be transpulmonary gradient (difference between the mean PA and LA pressures) divided by the pulmonary flow. Measured in mmHg/ L/min/m^2 or Wood units [18]

12. Interventions

With the availability of modified catheters and catheter delivery devices, the role of intervention in pediatric cardiology is increasingly becoming important

Catheter interventions can primarily do three things

1. Open things that are closed: Atrial septostomy – done in infants who need mixing of blood for maintaining saturation and cardiac output. Most common indication is transposition of great arteries with intact ventricular septum, other rarer indications are TAPVC with

http://dx.doi.org/10.5772/53654

restriction at the interatrial septum, tricuspid atresia, pulmonary atresia, mitral atresia. Septostomy with a blade would be required if the infant is > 6-8 weeks as the septum becomes thicker.

2. Widen things that are narrow – involving the blood vessels and heart valves, done using balloon catheters and stents to prevent recoil in case of vessels. The stent gets incorporated into the vessel wall. There can be neointimal proliferation causing restenosis, usually in the first 2 years The procedure uses special plastic polymer balloons which will not inflate beyond predetermined size even under high pressure. This needs a guide wire to be placed across the narrow area with balloon placed across so as to place the waist (middle of the sausage) in the narrow region which is dilated with dilute contrast.

Used commonly for

a. Pulmonary valvar stenosis- for gradients > 40 mmHg, has almost replaced surgery, except when the valve is very dysplastic or associated infundibular obstruction

b. Peripheral and branch pulmonary artery stenosis in the setting of postoperative tetralogy of Fallot, pulmonary atresia,- are surgical challenges and balloon dilatation with stenting has emerged as preferred alternatives with 60-80% success rate.

c. Aortic valve stenosis – used when gradient > 50-60 mm Hg in the absence of AR can be life-saving in small infants, can also be used for discrete subvalvar aortic stenosis but not for tunnel like subaortic stenosis.

d. Coarctation of aorta – preferred for re-coarctation or for coarctation in grown up children where it can be combined with stenting. Not for coarctation in infancy which has high rate of recurrence and surgery is better option.

e. Mitral valves – works well for rheumatic heart disease, not very successful with congenital MS. Heart block, tearing of leaflet and occurrence of MR are possible complications.

f. Prosthetic valves and conduits

g. Systemic vein stenosis in the setting of post- operative Mustard or Senning's procedure, does not work in the presence of pulmonary vein stenosis.

h. Close things that are open – this uses devices mounted on catheters that are passed through long and large sheaths after crossing the area to be closed.

ASD, VSD and PDA's – ASD's upto 32 mm diameter can be closed, the defect needs a rim of 4 mm for the device to be centred and placed. Amplatzer devices are FDA approved and have the longest track record.

Closure of VSD requires careful assessment to ensure that the device would not interfere with tricuspid or aortic valvar mechanisms. Arrhythmias, stroke, perforation, device embolization, incomplete closures are the risks involved.

Large PDA's > 5mm are closed with Amplatzer I device which has a single aortic rim and is mushroom shaped.

Coils – are metal wires coated with thrombogenic Dacron strands, suitable for vessels < 6-7 mm, with an area of narrowing. The thrombus formation around the coil plugs the vessel. Embolization, incomplete closure and hemolysis are possible risks.

Other defects which have been plugged are ruptured sinus of Valsalva especially the ones arising from the non-coronary sinus, aorta LV tunnels, veno-venous collaterals plugging following cavopulmonary connection. [19]

13. Pediatric anesthesia and critical care

The success of any pediatric cardiac surgical programme depends on a team effort and anesthetists and intensive care personnel are critical members of the team. The importance of effective communication between the various team members cannot be overemphasized.

Care of pediatric patients and care of the neonates in particular needs appreciation of the differences in **physiology** of the immature organ systems.

The neonate responds rapidly to any stressful situations which reflect in the sudden changes of various metabolic and hemodynamic parameters. The metabolic rate of neonates is 2-3 fold have increased compared to adults. The caloric requirement is between 100-150 Kcal/kg/day and neonatal gut is at risk of necrotizing enterocolitis with the use of hyperosmolar feeds.

The myocardium has only 30% contractile tissue as against 60% in mature myocardium. The myocardium has a reduced ability to respond to afterload stress and the compliance is reduced. Acute pressure afterload is poorly tolerated, and can lead to rapid ventricular dysfunction; chronic pressure load is longer tolerated than chronic volume load. Symptoms of CHF are rare unless the obstruction is severe and prolonged.

The stroke volume is relatively fixed and cardiac output is more heart rate dependent. They are more dependent on the trans-sarcolemma movement of calcium to initiate and sustain contraction as the sarcoplasmic reticulum and T-tubules are relatively underdeveloped.

Cardiorespiratory interactions and ventricular interdependence are particularly marked in infants. Positive pressure ventilation reduces the preload of both ventricles, increases the afterload of right ventricle and reduces the afterload of left ventricle. Implying that in situations where right ventricle is dysfunctional or in situations of single ventricle, early extubation with reduced afterload would be useful and in situations of left ventricular dysfunction, positive pressure ventilation would reduce the afterload of the heart and act as positive inotrope. This principle should be tempered against the background of ventricular interdependence where dysfunction of one ventricle can rapidly affect the other due to septal interactions.

Neonates rely on diaphragm as the main muscle of respiration. Only 25% of the diaphragm in neonates is made of type I fibre capable of slow and sustained activity against 55% by 8 months of age. Raised intra-abdominal pressure due to any cause like gastric distension, hepatic congestion and ascites can compromise its function. In neonates a larger portion of energy expenditure is used for ventilation and therefore they fatigue easily and have failure to thrive in the presence of increased work of breathing. They have increased closing capacity with airway closure occurring during normal tidal ventilation putting them at risk of developing hypoxemia and atelectasis. In addition dilated pulmonary arteries and left atrium can compress bronchi causing lobar collapse. [20]

Pulmonary hypertension both pre and postoperatively plays an important role in the planning of surgery, anesthesia and postoperative care.

Preoperatively it can be due to large left to right shunt lesions, or due to pulmonary venous obstruction, rarely due to pulmonary vascular obstructive disease.

Intraoperatively- light anesthesia, hypoxemia, hypoventilation, lung hyperinflation or hypoinflation, hypothermia, respiratory and metabolic acidosis, protamine, blood products, prolonged bypass with inflammatory response and capillary leak, compression and atelectasis of lung, pulmonary edema from inadequate venting of left atrium can all contribute to increased pulmonary vascular resistance (PVR).

Intravenous drugs can be used to reduce the PVR, but they lack selectivity and can cause systemic hypotension. Nitroprusside, glyceroltrinitrate, milrinone, Prostaglandin E1 and I2, tolazoline and isoproterenol have been used. Inhaled NO is most selective pulmonary vasodilator currently available; it is rapidly taken up and inactivated by haemoglobin as it diffuses from the alveoli. Oral drugs in the form of PDE type V inhibitor, sildenafil and endothelin I blocking drugs bosentan have shown encouraging results. [21,22]

Preoperative evaluation should keep in mind the physiology of defect, and the changes that the preoperative treatment could have caused (diuretics causing hypokalaemia) and the presence and severity of cyanosis and pulmonary hypertension. Haematocrit greater than 65% can exacerbate tissue hypoxia and can cause stasis and potential thrombosis. Avoiding dehydration is very important to avoid tissue hypoxia and to maintain renal function postoperatively.

Non-invasive monitoring using electrocardiography, pulse oximetry, capnography, non-invasive blood pressure is placed before induction, invasive arterial and central venous line should be planned according to procedure. Neurologic monitoring and cerebral protection is of concern during congenital heart surgery. Nasopharyngeal temperature, continuous EEG, transcranial Doppler, frontal lobe infrared spectroscopy and cerebral oximetry can be used to evaluate cerebral blood flow velocity and perfusion. Intraoperative echocardiography has achieved a significant role in repair of CHD. It helps in re-evaluation of anatomy before intervention, adequacy of surgical repair and de-airing after weaning from cardiopulmonary bypass and has become a integral part of monitoring in many units including ours.

Maintenance of diastolic pressure and coronary perfusion is important particularly in the setting of duct dependent lesions and in situations of altered coronary perfusion. There is a choice of induction techniques, inhalational, IV or IM.

Fentanyl (15-25 ug/kg), ketamine (1-3 mg/kg), Pancuronium (0.2mg/kg) or Suxamethonium (2mg/kg) in combination with glycopyrrolate (10ug/kg) allows prompt induction and airway control without significant increase in PVR. Midazolam (0.1-0.2mg/kg) is also a useful adjunct during narcotic induction but can cause hypotension in patients with high sympathetic drive. Isoflurane and midazolam can be used during bypass for maintenance and blunt awareness.

Reducing stress response using high dose opioid anesthesia and extending this to immediate postoperative period was considered important to reduce morbidity and mortality. With changes in surgical practice and particularly the timing of surgery, a strategy of using high dose opiod may be a less critical determinant of outcome. The main aim however is to maintain hemodynamic stability so that the team can focus on surgery without the distraction of side effects of anesthetic drugs.

14. Discontinuation of cardiopulmonary bypass and postoperative management

A co-ordinated approach must be used during weaning so that a smooth transition can be ensured - there should be close communication between surgeon, anesthesiologist and perfusionist. The need for vasopressors and inotropes is decided by close observation of the heart during re-warming period. Once adequate temperature is reached, ventilation is restarted after a good inflation of the lungs to prevent atelectasis and for deairing. Acid base status is normalized, adequate heart rate is ensured and the drainage from venous cannula is slowly reduced and CPB is stopped.

Myocardial edema and secondary fall in cardiac output by 20-30% is common in neonate in the first 6 – 12 hrs following surgery. Sternal closure is frequently delayed in neonates due to this reason. Avoiding hypothermia and hypoglycaemia, maintenance of optimal filling pressures, and preventing abdominal distension due to ascites by using catheter which can be used for peritoneal dialysis are important in the early postoperative period. An LA line and PA line may be inserted by the surgeons in the theatre in situations when LV dysfunction is anticipated or when pulmonary artery pressures are labile. This would help to fine tune management and help in decision making with regards to inotropes and ventilation management.

Postoperative management requires a precise knowledge about the anatomy, pathophysiology and details of the surgical and CPB technique. For most patients the recovery is uncomplicated and whenever the clinical progress does not follow the expected course possible residual or additional defects should be investigated.

14.1. Analgesia and sedation

Inadequate analgesia while the patient is on ventilator may be manifested by tachycardia, hypertension, pupillary dilation, diaphoresis etc, Changes in the respiratory pattern like tachypnea, grunting and splinting of the chest wall may also be seen. Fever, hypoxemia, hypercapnia, seizures, vasoactive infusions, early low cardiac output may also present in similar fashion and should be ruled out.

Opioid analgesics are the mainstay of pain management as they blunt hemodynamic response to procedures such as endotracheal suctioning. Morphine in intermittent or continuous infusion (50-100 ug/kg) is an excellent analgesic with sedative property. Disadvantage is that it can cause histamine release with systemic vasodilation and elevation of PVR.Fentanyl (5-10ug/kg/hr) is an alternative drug with less sedative action, and does not cause histamine release. There is wide variation in the metabolism of fentanyl, tolerance and dependence develops rapidly and chest wall rigidity can develop as a rare idiosyncratic reaction. It blocks the stress response and maintains systemic and pulmonary hemodynamic stability.

Dexmedetomidine (commonly called the dexmed) is alpha-2 agonist which is increasingly being used due to its sedative, anxiolytic, and its non-respiratory depressant property. This can cause hypotension and bradycardia and should be used with caution in children with CHD.

Recognition and early intervention for the management of low cardiac output is one of the pivotal roles of the intensivists. The following are some of the clues and the entire clinical picture should be considered rather than a isolated finding.

Physical examination: Core hyperthermia, tachycardia, cool peripheries with impalpable peripheral pulses, hypotension with narrow pulse pressure, ascites, hepatomegaly, oliguria, obtundation of sensorium.

Monitoring – Dampened arterial upstroke, narrow pulse pressure, elevated venous pressures (systemic or pulmonary – loss of sinus rhythm, residual outflow obstruction, tamponade, AV valve regurgitation should be ruled out)

Laboratory – Metabolic acidosis, low mixed venous oxygen saturation (or increased arterio-venous oxygen difference > 25 – 30%), increased arterial lactate, potassium, liver transaminases and Increased BUN and creatinine.

Strategies for management of Low CO should focus on optimizing the balance between oxygen supply and demand.

Demand – Maintaining adequate analgesia, sedation and paralysis when necessary, strict avoidance of hyperthermia and occasionally using mild hypothermia to reduce metabolic rate.

For optimizing delivery – Oxygen content can be optimized by managing Hemoglobin and fiO2, and the factors which determine output

Contractility – Dopamine (5-10ug/kg/min), dobutamine (5-10 ug/kg/min), epinephrine (upto 0.1ug/kg/min is considered acceptable. Requirement greater than 0.3 – 0.5ug/kg would make one assess the possibility of mechanical circulatory support. Calcium infusion may also be necessary especially in patients with diGeorge syndrome and 22q11 deletion.

Afterload – Milrinone (0.2- 0.75 ug/kg/min) has inotropic and peripheral and pulmonary vasodilating property and is useful for patients with ventricular dysfunction and increased afterload. Nitroprusside and GTN can be used in the setting of normal ventricular function. Norerpinephrine (upto -0.2ug/kg/min) and vasopressin (10-120 milliunits/kg/hr is a potent vasopressor) can be used in situations with low SVR ('warm' shock) [23]

Heart rate and sinus rhythm –temporary atrial and ventricular pacing wires are kept after any major cardiac procedure and can be used to optimize the heart rate, though a little trial and error would be required to find the best settings for the individual patient

Stress dose steroid – hydrocortisone (50mg/m2/day) has been demonstrated to increase systemic blood pressure and lower inotropic scores and should be used when the pressures are recalcitrant to inotropes. No consistent correlation has been found between the serum cortisol level and low cardiac output state. Due to risks of infection and poor wound healing its use should be restricted to 3- 5 days.

T3 at dose of 0.05ug/kg/hr has been shown to be beneficial in neonates due to sick euthyroid state when there is reduced conversion of thyroxine to active T3.

Fluid management – the first 24 hrs the maintenance fluids should be 50% of full maintenance and volume replacement should be titrated to filling pressures and hemodynamic response. Furosemide (0.2-0.3 mg/kg/hr is used after iv bolus of 1 mg/kg can provide consistent and sustained diuresis. Fenoldopam is a new selective dopamine DA1 receptor agonist with renal and mesenteric vasodilating properties (0.1-0.5 ug/kg/min).

Peritoneal dialysis, hemodialysis and continuous veno-venous hemofiltration provide renal replacement therapy for patients with persistent oliguria and renal failure. Besides helping in solute and water clearance, they help in nutritional support by allowing additional volume, and may also remove the inflammatory mediators. [24]

Weaning from ventilation and extubation should be possible once patients are hemodynamically stable and normothermic with good cardiac output. Patients after closed heart surgery like PDA ligation, ASD, small to moderate VSD, RV to PA conduit change, bidirectional Glenn shunt and Fontan procedure with fenestration are suitable for early extubation.Neonates undergoing surgery like TGA, Truncus, TAPVC, TOF would require elective ventilation for 48 hrs for the physiology to normalize.

Extubation of an infant after a major cardiac procedure is both an art and science.Upto to 25% of 1st extubation can end in reintubations, and if more than 3 attempts fail serious consideration should be given to the following conditions. Residual volume and pressure load, ventricular dysfunction. Phrenic nerve injury, bronchomalacia, retained secretions, vocal cord injury, Diuretic therapy with contraction alkalosis, Inadequate nutrition and an evolving sepsis are all factors to be considered for failed extubation. Early tracheostomy can sometimes help if there is no correctable lesions, and if predominantly retained secretions and nutrition are the major causes of failed extubation. [25,26]

14.2. Cardiopulmonary bypass and extracorporeal life support

Cardiopulmonary bypass machine essentially takes over the function of pumping and oxygenating the blood allowing surgery to be performed on arrested still heart.

Gibbon developed the first cardiopulmonary bypass machine used for closing an atrial septal defect in 1953, Throughout the 1960's the typical survival rate for open heart surgery remained around 50%. During the 1970's the mortality of CPB was reduced by using deep hypothermic circulatory arrest pioneered by Barrat- Boyes and Castaneda. Progressive improvement in circuit design and perfusion techniques has now brought the overall mortality to less than 5%. Even now the morbidity associated with the use of CPB is held to be the major limitation for completely successful outcomes.

Due to immature organ function, fetal contractile protein isoforms, immature calcium cycling, pulmonary dysfunction and exaggerated stress and inflammatory response the morbidity associated with CPB is more profound in infants and neonates.

The Cardiopulmonary bypass circuit consists of

1. Oxygenators - microporous membrane(0.05 – 0.25um) pores which allows more efficient oxygenation but lasts shorter are used for cardiac surgery, the nonporous folded sheet silicone membrane oxygenator is usually selected for longer term circulatory support applications.

2. Pumps – Roller pumps are used and the flow rate is governed by the revolutions per minute, occlusion produced by the rollers and the internal diameter of the tubing.

3. Tubing – usually ¼ inch tubing in used on arterial and venous limbs, the pump is situated close to the field to reduce the tubing length which contributes to the priming volume.

4. Venous reservoirs – Open rigid reservoirs are usually used to which the blood flows by gravity, the level of blood in the reservoir is an important safety mechanism – source of volume for arterial inflow and to judge adequacy of venous return. Malposition of venous cannulas and lost blood in the surgical field can reduce the venous volume which may need urgent attention. Collapsible venous reservoir with reduced air blood contact is increasingly being used. Vacuum can improve drainage through small venous cannulas and tubing which can theoretically reduce organ edema and improve organ function; venoarterial air embolism is a potential complication.

5. Arterial cannula – aorta is the usual site of cannulation, the location needs to be tailored according to surgery. Alternate sites are carotid artery in small infants and femoral artery in bigger children (> 10-15kg).

6. Venous cannula – SVC and IVC cannulas are used to maximize venous return and to minimize interference with the operative field, and optimally sited to prevent obstruction and kinking.

7. Filters – 0.2 um filters are used in gas inflow and for crystalloid and cardioplegia solutions. 40um filters are used in cardiotomy suction return lines to remove macro and micro aggregates and debris returning from the surgical field. Arterial filter (40um) may reduce microemboli, though some consider its use optional.

8. Prime – The fluid used to fill the oxygenator, minimum level required in the reservoir and the tubing is the priming volume. The prime consists of physiologic crystalloid solutions, packed red cells, colloids like albumin and FFP, and mannitol (used for its membrane stabilization, antioxidant and osmotic diuretic properties). The hematocrit during CPB should be maintained around 25 – 30 %. At low temperature and low flows, low hematocrit

may improve microvascular flow and oxygen delivery. For patients with myocardial dysfunction and complex prolonged surgeries a target of around 40% at the end of surgery may improve oxygen delivery.

14.3. Initiation, monitoring and termination of CPB

Heparin at a dose of about 4mg/kg is given to bring activated clotting time(ACT) of more than 400 seconds. ACT should be maintained between 400- 600 seconds to prevent activation of blood coagulation and clot formation. Inadequate concentration of heparin is believed to contribute to excess coagulation and fibrinolytic system activation.

Once the arterial and venous cannulae are in place, after confirming adequate anticoagulation and absence of air (especially at the arterial cannula and tubing) is confirmed, CPB is slowly initiated by beginning arterial inflow and unclamping the venous line. Any systemic to pulmonary shunts should be closed prior to, or immediately after CPB initiation. These can contribute to systemic runoff, contributing to organ malperfusion, increased left heart return, heart distension, and inadvertent rewarming. It is absolutely essential to prevent myocardial distension at all times after initiation of CPB.

The important CPB circuit variables that are monitored are:

1. Arterial line pressures (typically in the range of 200-250mm Hg to drive blood through the infant arterial cannula and tubing to maintain mean pressures around 40-60 mm Hg).

2. Pump flow rate - which is a calculated value in roller pumps based on rotation, internal tubing diameter and occlusion pressure.

3. Oxygenator gases – the flow rate ('sweep speed') and oxygen concentration controlled with blender and flow meter, usually started with 1: 1 ratio with the flow rates in membrane oxygenators.

4. Temperature- thermistors measure the temperature of the water bath, arterial and venous blood. The gradient between the patient and the perfusate should not exceed 10 degree C, especially during rewarming to prevent formation of gaseous bubbles.

Hypothermia delays loss of ionic hemostasis, slows consumption of ATP, decreases free radical generation, inflammatory cytokine production, white cell activation and leucocyte adhesion molecule synthesis, suppresses the release of excitatory amino acid neurotransmitters. It continues to be the mainstay for cerebral and other organ protection during CPB.

The important patient variables monitored are

1. Patient mean arterial and venous pressures – femoral arterial line preferred especially in small infants and in deep hypothermia.

2. Nasopharyngeal (reflecting brain temperature), rectal or bladder (core) and esophageal (aortic) temperatures are measured using appropriate thermistors, slow cooling over a period of 15-20 minutes- is necessary whenever deep hypothermic circulatory arrest (DHCA) is planned. Hct of 25% is favoured at this temperature.

3. Arterial and venous blood gases are measured every 15-30 minutes. Oxygen saturation of venous blood (SvO2) and blood lactates are an important index of tissue perfusion and SvO2 can also be measured continuously using calibrated inline monitor. Values < 60-70% should raise concerns of inadequate tissue oxygen delivery. At low temperature, due to increased affinity of Hb to oxygen, higher levels (90%) may have to be targeted

4. Blood glucose should be monitored frequently particularly in neonates and infants who are prone to hypoglycemia due to low glycogen reserves.

5. pH management – There are two methods –

6. Alpha stat - maintains electrical neutrality at lower temperatures, pH measured is 7.7 at 20° C. Advantages are better preservation of metabolic functions and buffering capacity, useful during **mild and moderate** hypothermia.

7. pH stat - Adds CO_2 to the circuit to correct pH for the fall of temperature, useful during **deep** hypothermia to increase cerebral blood flow and decrease metabolic rate, and also for management of aortopulmonary collaterals to increase pulmonary vascular resistance and to increase systemic flow.

15. Bleeding and organ injury

The coagulation factors reach the adult level at 6 – 12 months of age. The effects of CPB on blood activation and coagulation is far greater in neonates and infants because of hemodilution, hypothermia, greater shear stress, and more blood- air contact activation.

Platelets are the initial therapy for bleeding after adequate heparin reversal. 1 unit of platelets per 10 Kg raises the platelet count by approximately 50,000/mm^3. Cryoprecipitate which is a good source of fibrinogen is the next blood component usually used. Antifibrinolytic agents like aprotinin, e-aminocaproic acid, tranexamic acid have become popular to reduce bleeding after complex surgeries and in infants.

Lung, kidney and brain are at risk of injury during CPB. The stress and inflammatory response is 5-10 times greater in neonates and infants. High dose steroids have been used to mask the response and have been shown to be more beneficial in neonates and infants. Ultrafiltration, both conventional and modified are being used for hemoconcentration, removing inflammatory mediators, and decreasing total body water, with beneficial effects being shown for hematocrit, oxygenation, pulmonary vascular resistance and decreasing duration of mechanical ventilation.

16. Extracorporal life support

Modalities include extracorporeal membrane oxygenation (ECMO), intra-aortic balloon pump (IABP) counter pulsation and ventricular assist devices. Wide application in pediatric age group is limited by the need for miniaturization and ECMO is still the most common form of mechanical circulatory support for pediatric patients.

ECMO is now accepted modality of treatment in neonates with a variety of parenchymal and vascular lung disease (meconium aspiration, diaphragmatic hernia, persistent hypertension of newborn). The outcome irrespective of the indication depends *on early diagnosis, prompt institution and reversible nature of dysfunction.* The use of ECMO for respiratory indications has progressively decreased (due to increased availability of High frequency oscillatory ventilation, nitric oxide, and surfactant therapy) and there is a steady increase in its use after congenital cardiac surgery or as a bridge to transplantation to support failing circulation.

The cardiac indications for ECMO are in preoperative resuscitation (critical AS, pulmonary hypertension, obstructed TAPVC, transposition of great arteries), inability to wean from CPB, cardiomyopathy, myocarditis, after in- hospital cardiac arrest and CPR, and bridge to transplantation.

Venovenous ECMO is used in patients who need ventilatory support alone. Arteriovenous cannulation is used for cardiac ECMO. In the postoperative period single right atrial and ascending aortic cannula is preferred, internal jugular vein and carotid artery can be used in other settings. ACT is maintained around 180-200 seconds,flow rates between 100-150 ml/kg/min for children on full ECMO, hematocrit level between 35 -45% and platelet count > 100,000/ $mm^{3.}$

The daily management of ECMO needs assessment of cardiorespiratory function, end organ perfusion and evolving complications such as bleeding or sepsis. Assessing adequacy of flow and systemic perfusion is of paramount importance.

When instituted in post cardiac surgery setting, myocardial recovery should be anticipated in 2-3 days, failing which listing for transplantation or withdrawal of support must be considered. Patients with cardiomyopathies or with severe bronchiolitis due to viral infection may require longer period of support (1-2 weeks).

Weaning depends on the underlying indication. Inotropes are recommenced or increased, intravascular status is optimized and ventilator settings are adjusted, flows gradually decreased over a period of time and the circuit is clamped. ABG, serum lactated levels and mixed venous oxygen saturation levels are closely monitored and decannulation is done once patient has maintained stable circulation and acceptable gas exchange for upto 4hrs.

IABP (Intra-aortic Balloon Pump) has not been very successful in paediatric population because of a number of reasons, the usual right heart nature of pathology, rapid heart rate in children making timing difficult, distensible nature of aorta and collaterals making coronary flow augmentation and afterload reduction less. The smallest size available is 2.5ml and generally volume of 0.5ml/kg is recommended. Technical improvements including smaller sized consoles, catheters and M-mode echocardiography for timing may enhance its applicability in the future.

Ventricular assist devices require direct cannulation of heart. Reported indications are decompensated cardiomyopathy, ALCAPA (ischemic myocardium as a result of anomalous origin of coronary artery), and retraining of poorly prepared left ventricle after arterial switch procedure. They are simple in design and require less technical assistance once established. VAD are more suited as bridge to transplantation. Berlin Heart Excor VAD is the first extracorporeal pneumatically driven pulsatile VAD designed specifically for paediatric use and is available in 6 different sizes depending on stroke volume. Significant advances in the circulatory support technology for children are expected in the near future with various devices being in preclinical stages of development. [27]

17. Conduits in cardiac surgery

Allografts – tissues obtained from human body which are cryopreserved are used in repair of variety of congenital cardiac defects. Due to availability and preservation problems it fell into disrepute in 1980's only to re-emerge in 1990's mainly due to late complications of porcine valved Dacron conduits which became popular in 1980's and availability of better cryopreservation technology.

Allografts are currently available standards against which any conduit is compared. Factors which can reduce the longevity of allografts are – use of excessively large conduits (> +2 z score), aortic allografts which tends to calcify earlier probably because of higher elastin content (controversial) and immunogenicity due to blood and tissue incompatibility (controversial). No particular method is proven to enhance the longevity of allograft. Decellularisation process using anionic detergents and nucleases have been used to provide acellular matrix for the native tissue to repopulate and grow, but the long term structural impact of the decellularisation process is yet to be seen. Treating the decellularised tissue in a bioreactor using the recipient cells so as to repopulate the matrix is now in experimental stages.

Contegra which is made from Bovine jugular vein is one of the popular valved conduits in pediatric cardiac surgery; This conduit shows predictable function with survival approaching homografts over mid-term. The advantages are easy availability (12- 22mm sizes) and predictable quality. It is important to keep the conduit short and straight to prevent 'telescoping' and distal stenosis.

Alternative conduits have been used made of Polytetrafluoroethylene (PTFE) wall and leaflets, which has minimal tissue reactivity. Long term results are still awaited.

Conduits fashioned out of autologous pericardium with PTFE (0.1mm) leaflets are also increasingly being used, the disadvantages being non-availability in reoperations and limitation with respect to the length and diameter.

While a variety of choices are available for older children and adults, an ideal conduit for neonates and small children is still elusive. The availability of 'conduits which grow' using tissue engineering technology can potentially provide curative surgery for a number of conditions which require multiple reoperations for conduit replacements. [28]

18. Surgical approaches to the correction of congenital cardiac defects:

A simplified approach to such a variety of congenital cardiac defects is to broadly classify them as

1. left-to-right shunts
2. cyanotic conditions
3. single-ventricle physiology
4. valvular and coronary heart disease
5. tracheal and vascular rings

18.1. Left to right shunts

Left to right shunts are the most gratifying to treat as they are potentially life-saving and promote the growth of the child. The common lesions are atrial septal defect (ASD), ventricular septal defect (VSD) and patent ductus arteriosus (PDA).

The common variations of ASD [29] (figure 5) are ostium secundum, ostium primum, sinus venosus, coronary sinus and various combinations of these. Secundum ASD's are usually closed by the interventional cardiologists percutaneously provided parameters are satisfied including adequacy of rims and the safety of neighbouring structures. When these criteria are not met, surgery is via median sternotomy or right posterolateral or anterolateral thoracotomy (cosmetic), placing on cardiopulmonary bypass (CPB) and closure either directly or using the patient's own (autologous) pericardial patch. Ostium primum ASD is usually associated with abnormal mitral and sometimes tricuspid valves. Repair involves repair of the valves with closure of the ASD with a patch. Failure to close the cleft in the mitral valve increases reoperation rate for mitral regurgitation [30]. These patients require lifelong follow-up for mitral regurgitation and left ventricular outflow tract obstruction [31] Complete heart block is a potential complication due to the proximity of the bundle of His.

Sinus venosus ASD is usually superior vena cava (SVC) ASD with partial anomalous pulmonary venous connection (usually right upper lobe pulmonary veins draining anomalously to the right atrium instead of left atrium. Surgical options range from simple ASD closure (single-patch), two-patch technique and Warden's procedure which is more complex [32]. Complications range from SVC obstruction, pulmonary venous obstruction and sino-atrial nodal dysfunction. Coronary sinus ASD is rare and involves patch repair. Common atrium is complete absence of interatrial septum and surgery is partitioning of the atria. Autologous pericardial patch is the material of choice.

Ventricular septal defect (VSD) is deficiency of the interventricular septum. There are various classifications based on anatomy and embryology. The commonest classification is perimembranous VSD, muscular VSD, doubly commited subarterial VSD, inlet septal and multiple VSD's. [33] The majority close by one year, particularly perimembtranous and muscular. The doubly committed and inlet septal VSD's do not close spontaneously. Indications for surgery

http://dx.doi.org/10.5772/53654

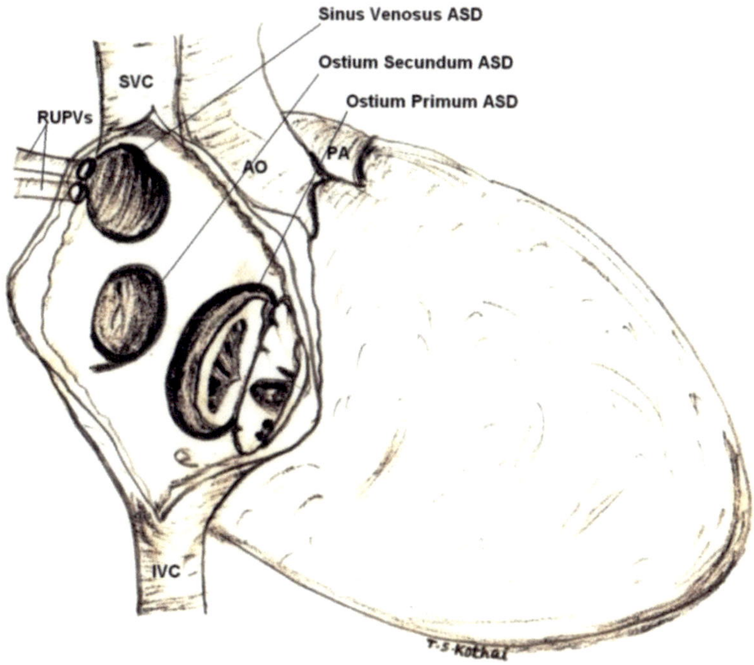

Figure 5. Atrial Septal Defects

are large VSD with congestive cardiac failure refractory to medical management, left atrial and left ventricular dilatation, aortic valve prolapse and aortic regurgitation and prevention of infective endocarditis [34] Open heart surgery entails closure directly (is small) or patch (Gore-tex, Dacron, bovine or autologous pericardium). (figure 6)

Patent ductus arteriousus (PDA) is the persistence of the fetal ductus arterious beyond two months after birth. This results in increased left heart return and failure to thrive with congestive cardiac failure. Most PDA's are amenable to closure by device (intervention) and surgery is done infrequently. Surgical approach is via left posterolateral thoracotomy. (figure 7) [35]

Aortopulmonary window (APW) is a communication between the aorta and pulmonary artery resulting in a large left-to-right shunt. This condition requires early surgical closure. This condition is rare and requires early surgery as there is steal from the systemic circulation. Surgical approaches vary but basically consist of division of the APW with suturing of a patch [36]

Double outlet right ventricle is a separate and complex entity wherein both great vessels arise predominantly from the right ventricle. When there is a VSD, this results in unrestricted pulmonary blood flow and physiologically is a left-to-right shunt. The classification of DORV by Lev is self-explanatory and the varying anatomy decides the clinical presentation which varies from simple left-to-right shunt, tetralogy of Fallot physiology, transposition of great

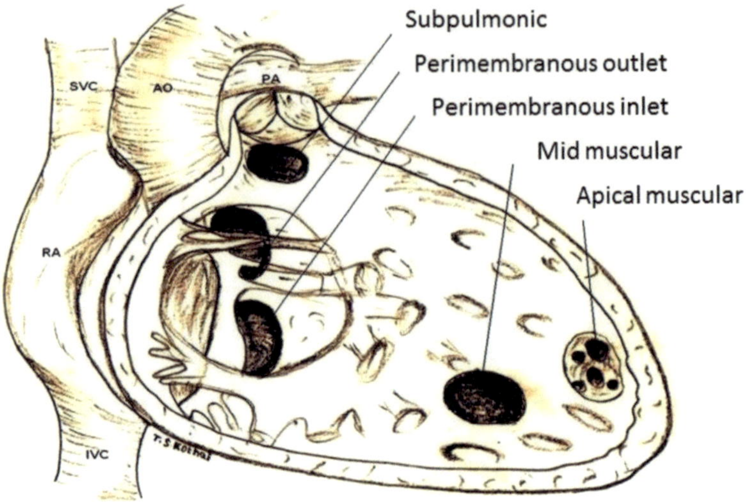

Figure 6. Ventricular Septal Defects.

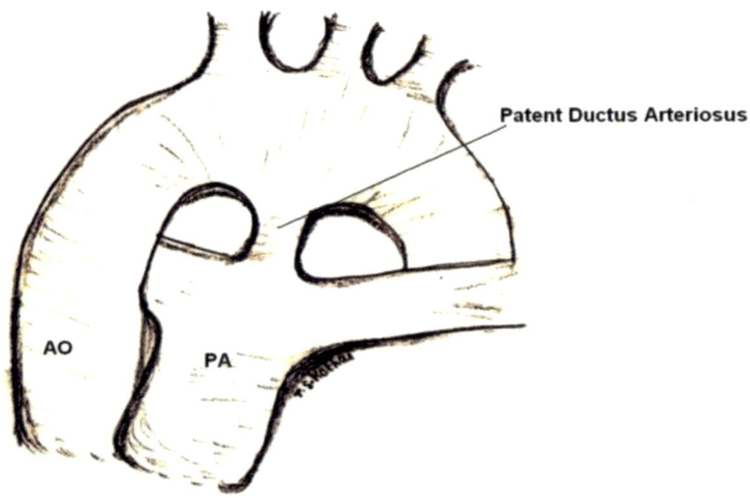

Figure 7. Patent Ductus Arteriosus

arteries physiology to single ventricle physiology. They occur with VSD which then presents as increased pulmonary blood flow. The treatment is surgical closure of VSD with routing of LV to drain into the aorta across the VSD. When they present with VSD and PS, the repair consists of VSD closure and relief of RVOTO with or without conduit. DORV with subpulmonic VSD Requires arterial switch and VSD closure [37]

Truncus arteriosus (figure 8) is a condition wherein the pulmonary arteries arise from the aorta directly. This results in torrential pulmonary blood flow and warrants early surgery in the neonatal period. The PA is detached from the aorta and reconnected to the right ventricle utilizing a conduit and closing of the VSD. Alternatives include direct connection of RV-PA utilizing neighbouring tissue. Mid-term and long-term results are determined by the fate of the RVOT- the presence of pulmonary regurgitation and the deterioration of the conduit. [38].

Coarctation of aorta is narrowing of the aorta near the insertion of the ductus arteriousus to the descending aorta This presents at various stages. Presentation in the neonatal period is usually as an emergency with closure of the ductus and sudden cessation of blood flow to the lower body. Treatment includes commencing prostaglandin to reopen the ductus, commencement of inotropes and correction of acidiosis. Emergency surgical repair of coarctation is warranted. Surgical techniques are varied and each has merits and demerits. The preferred technique is resection of the coarctation and end-to-end anastomosis [39] Alternatives include subclavian flap plasty and patch plasty. Interruption is total disconnection of the aorta and is usually associated with VSD. The classification is based on the location of the interruption (type A is distal to the left subclavian artery, type B is distal arch and type C proximal arch. Surgery is complex and involves disconnection of the PDA which supplies blood to the lower body and reconnection of the two ends of the aorta. The VSD is closed [40].

Pulmonary vein anomalies are rare and can present as stenosis of individual veins or as they enter the LA as a confluence. Prognosis is poor when all four pulmonary veins are involved [41] Surgery or balloon dilatation are both associated with high rates of restenosis.

18.2. Cyanotic congenital cardiac conditions

The congenital cardiac conditions are Tetralogy of Fallot (TOF), Transposition of Great Arteries (TGA), Total anomalous pulmonary venous connection (TAPVC), Tricuspid atresia (TA) and Truncus arteriosus.

Tetralogy of Fallot(figure 8) is the commonest cyanotic congenital cardiac condition. The condition described originally consists of four components- VSD, overriding of aorta, right ventricular outflow tract obstruction (RVOTO) and right ventricular hypertrophy. The extent and severity of RVOTO accounts for the variation in symptoms. Babies present early with cyanosis or cyanotic spells(due to infundibular spasm). Surgical strategies vary in different parts of the world. In the neonatal period, whenever the baby presents with symptoms, the tendency is surgical correction with closure of VSD and judicious relief of RVOTO. However, most centers follow the policy of performing Blalock-Taussig shunt if the baby presents with symptoms at less than 6 months of age or less than 5 kgs. If older, surgical correction is attempted [42].B-T shunt is still performed if the branch pulmonary arteries are hypoplastic or there are significant co-morbidities that preclude placing the baby on cardiopulmonary bypass. The postoperative course varies depending on the anatomically variations. Right heart failure is common due to the non-compliant RV and diastolic dysfunction.

B-T shunt is the connection of an artificial conduit between a branch of the aorta and one of the pulmonary arteries. This is a palliative surgery and is associated with complications such as blocked shunt precipitating cardiac arrest, low cardiac output, and pulmonary artery distortion. Historically, there have been several systemic-pulmonary artery shunts. These have

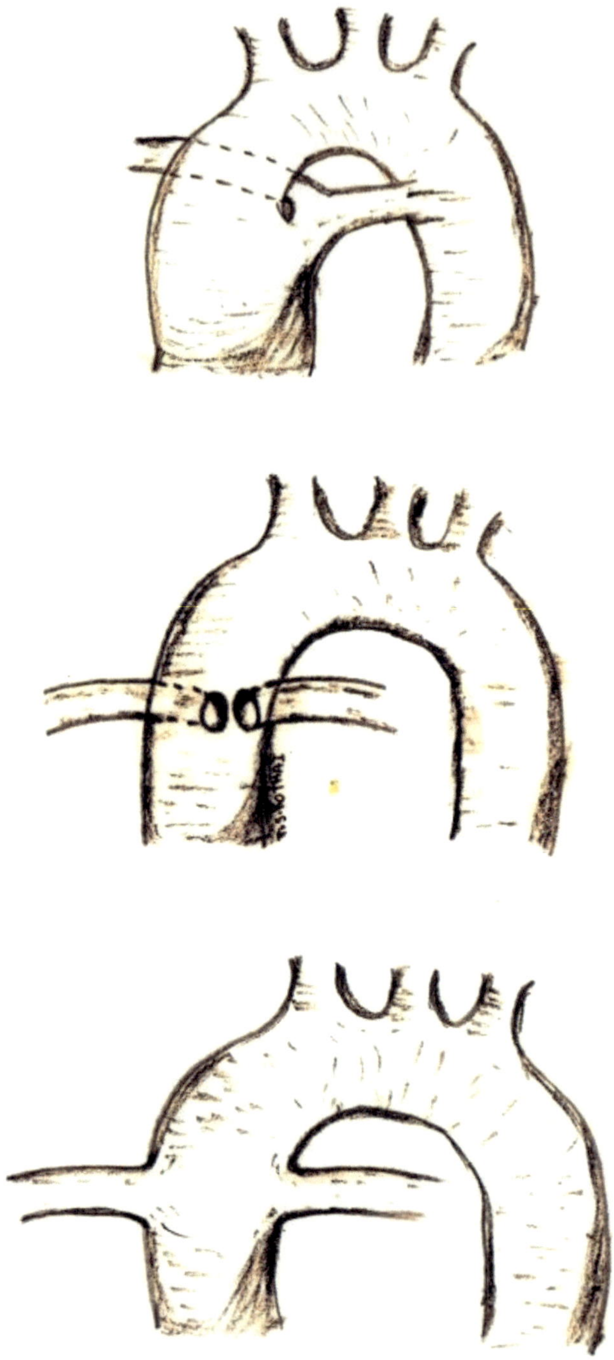

Figure 8. Types of Truncus Arteriosus

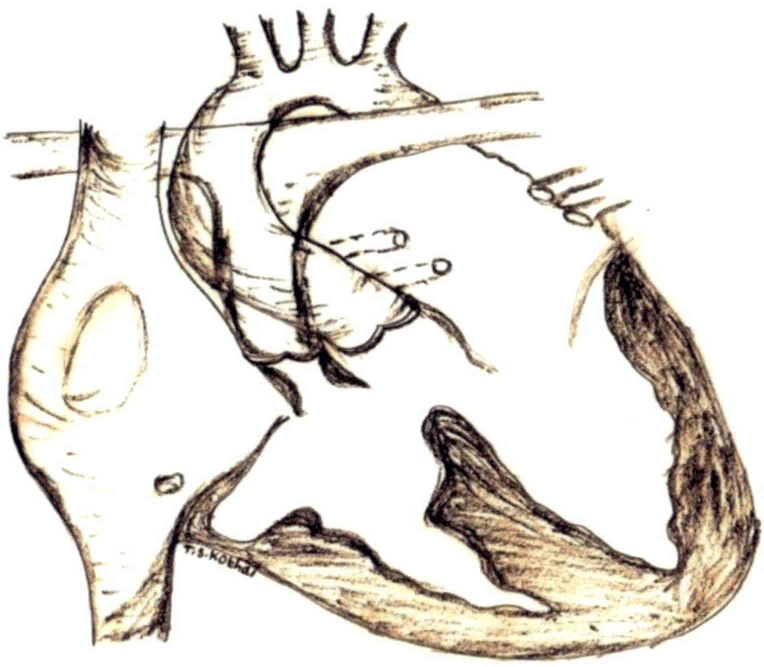

Figure 9. Tetralogy of Fallot showing a) VSD b) over ride of aorta c) Right ventricular hypertrophy and d) right ventricular outflow obstruction.

been anastomosis between ascending aorta and RPA (Waterston's) and descending aorta and LPA (Pott's). These shunts have resulted in uncontrolled pulmonary blood flow and gross distortion of pulmonary arteries.

Repair of TOF carries excellent results- less than 5% mortality in most centers. Potential complications are right heart failure, residual VSD, residual RVOTO and complete heart block. RVOTO relief varies from simple removal of obstructing muscle bundles to subannular patch to transannular patch. Transannular patch entails incising across the pulmonary valve annulus and results in free pulmonary regurgitation. This can cause right heart failure both acutely and in the long-term. Late pulmonary valve replacement is common in TOF repairs 10-15 years postoperatively. Surgeons are prophylactically placing bicuspid valves in the pulmonary position at the first surgery. [43] This improves immediate outcomes and as well as the long-term results.

Transposition of great arteries is the second ccommonest cyanotic condition. This presents in the neonatal period with the aorta arising from the right ventricle and pulmonary artery from the left ventricle. 50% are born with intact ventricular septum, 25% with VSD and 25% with VSD and PS. Senning's and Mustard's are procedures of historical importance. These are atrial switch procedures wherein the right atrium is directed to drain into the left ventricle and left atrium is directed to right ventricle. The disadvantage of this procedure is that the right ventricle is placed in the systemic circulation. The RV is not designed to sustain the systemic circulation for long periods and many of these patients develop heart failure later and are candidates for heart transplant. Arterial switch operation is the transfer of coronary arteries from aorta to the pulmonary arteries. This results in switching the left ventricle to the systemic circulation.

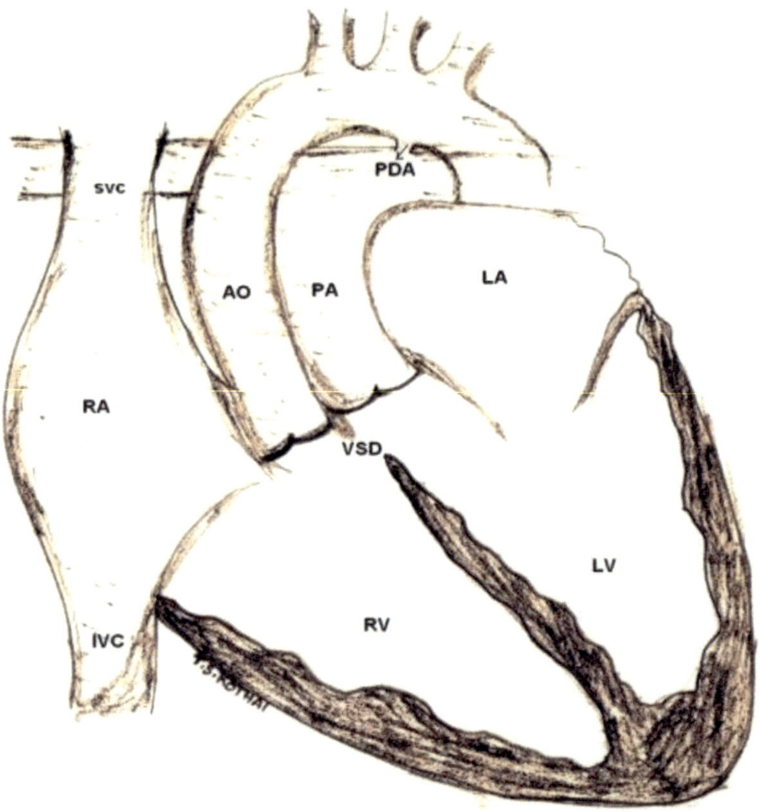

Figure 10. Transposition of Great Arteries

Babies with TGA and intact ventricular septum should ideally be operated within 2-3 weeks. The left ventricle loses its ability to sustain the systemic circulation beyond this as it adapts to the lower pulmonary artery pressures. When these patients present late, the options are to proceed with atrial switch which has lesser mortality and rapid two-stage arterial switch. The latter procedure is a staged procedure wherein the PA is banded and B-T shunt is created [44]. This creates the pressure and volume overload on the LV thereby retraining the LV to accept the systemic load. This is a relatively high-risk procedure. Serial echocardiographic assessment aids the surgeon to time the arterial switch once the LV is retrained.

Arterial switch is a worthwhile operation as the long-term results are excellent. Immediate postoperative complications are low cardiac output and myocardial ischemia due to coronary

http://dx.doi.org/10.5772/53654

insufficiency. Long-term complications are neoaortic regurgitation, neo-suprapulmonary stenosis and coronary ischemia [45] These occur in less than 10% of patients.

Total pulmonary venous connection (TAPVC) is a common congenital cardiac condition. Darling's classification divides TAPVC into 4 types- supracardiac, cardiac, infracardiac and mixed. The basic issue is that the pulmonary veins are not attached to the left atrium, form a common pulmonary venous chamber(CPVC) and drain via a communicating vein to some component of the systemic circulation. The commonest is supracardiac- the left vertical vein arising from the CPVC drains to the left innominate vein or less commonly, to the SVC just cranial to the SVC-RA junction. The cardiac variant usually joins the coronary sinus. The infracardiac type has a descending vertical vein draining vertically across the diaphragm to the portal vein or IVC. Mixed types are varying combinations of these. The presentation depends on whether there is obstruction in the pulmonary venous pathway or not. In supracardiac, the vertical vein may obstruct near the innominate vein or at the level of the ASD- this has to be completely unrestrictive or the child will present with obstructive pulmonary venous symptoms such as breathlessness, and even pulmonary edema. Cardiac type can have obstruction where the CPVC joins the coronary sinus or at the ASD. The infracardiac is the commonest type to present with obstruction as blood has to pass through the liver. This is one of the commonest neonatal cardiac emergencies. Surgery varies depending on the anatomy. Supracardiac TAPVC can be addressed by surgery - creation of anastomosis at the back of the heart between the Left atrium and CPVC. The creation of the anastomosis is dependent on the surgeon's preference- either working through the ASD, lifting the heart to the right, working lateral to the RA, working between the SVC and aorta or Shumacker's repair. Cardiac TAPVC is relatively simple- the coronary sinus is unroofed and pulmonary veins are committed to the LA after partitioning of the atria. The infracardiacTAPVC is again by creation of anastomosis between the LA and CPVC with disconnection of the descending vertical vein.

Immediate postoperative complications are low cardiac output, pulmonary hypertensive crisis and pulmonary vein restenosis- either early or late, at the anastomosis or in the individual pulmonary veins.

Tricuspid atresia is the absence of the tricuspid valve. ASD is mandatory for survival. They can present unrestricted pulmonary blood flow (PBF), in which case they need pulmonary artery band, followed by Glenn followed by Fontan. If the neonate presents with decreased PBF, the first operation is a B-T shunt followed by Glenn and Fontan. At each stage, before the Glenn and Fontan operations, the baby undergoes cardiac catheterization and angiography. The Glenn operation consists of dividing SVC and suturing this to the RPA. This unloads the single ventricle. The Fontan operation consists of a conduit being placed between the IVC and RPA. The single ventricle is thus unloaded of the pulmonary circulation and pumps blood to two circulations in series instead of two ventricles pumping blood to two circulations in parallel. Low cardiac output may occur and long-term complications include protein-losing enteropathy, plastic bronchitis and cardiac failure.

There are variations in univentricular physiology. The treatment protocol is similar to the one followed for tricuspid atresia. The common variant of this is hypoplastic left heart syndrome (HLHS) wherein the aorta is hypoplastic and a complex operation called Norwood is performed in the neonatal period. The PA is disconnected and reconnected to the systemic circulation to enhance the arch. The pulmonary circulation is provided by a B-T shunt. The patient subsequently undergoes Glenn and Fontan procedures.

Corrected transposition of great arteries (CCTGA) or l-TGA consists of atrio-ventricular and ventriculo-arterial discordance. The child may present with intact ventricular septum. The disadvantage lies in the fact that the RV is in the systemic circulation and will fail over a period of time. The child may present with VSD and with or without pulmonary stenosis. There are two approaches- anatomic and physiologic repairs. The physiologic approach consists of addressing the various lesions- VSD and PS thereby leaving the RV in the systemic circulation with doubtful long-term outcomes. The anatomic repair consists of double switch. The procedure consists of performing atrial switch and arterial switch. This eventually results in the LV being in the systemic circulation. If there is a VSD, this is surgically closed. The chances of complete heart block requiring a pacemaker is high as the A-V node and Bundle of His are in an abnormal position. If there is a PS, the procedure is an atrial switch-Rastelli- the RV is connected to the PA via conduit. These are complex procedures carrying significant morbidity and mortality [46] These children present with left A-V valve regurgitation as well. This is the tricuspid valve functioning as the systemic valve. A simplified approach to this condition is to perform Glenn followed by Fontan procedure if they present with VSD with significant PS. This carries lesser mortality than the above procedures. However, the Fontan circulation is an imperfect state and has its own disadvantages.

18.3. Congenital lesions of valves, aorta and coronary arteries

The four valves are prone to various congenital anomalies:

1. Tricuspid valve- Ebstein's anomaly is the commonest congenital anomaly of the TV. There is apical displacement of the septal and postero-inferior leaflets with a sail-like anterior leaflet. This results in severe TR. The RA is dilated with RV dilatation and dysfunction. This condition is associated with accessory conduction pathways which predispose to supraventricular arrhythmias. This is diagnosed from the presence of delta waves in the ECG. Criteria for surgery are presence of dyspnoea NYHA III-IV, cardiomegaly (CTR ratio > 0.65) and cyanosis in the presence of ASD. LV dysfunction is noted when cases present late due to RV dysfunction causing LV to be affected by the phenomenon-of ventricular interdependence. Neonatal Ebstein's is a particular difficult subset to treat and the Starne's operation has been described- elective closure of the tricuspid valve and B-T shunt followed by staging to Glenn and Fontan.(figure 10).

Children and adults with Ebstein'sanomaly require tricuspid valve repair. There are various techniques described such as Danielson's [47], Carpentier's, Cone [48] and Stanford [49] technique and variations on these with proponents for each. The repair aims to achieve tricuspid competence, without compromising RV cavity if possible. Some techniques aim to obliterate the atrialised RV and others ignore it. Complications include severe RV dysfunction, arrhythmias, low cardiac output. Glenn is performed by the surgeon if he feels the RV will not be able to cope. If tricuspid regurgitation is significant, the tricuspid valve is electively

http://dx.doi.org/10.5772/53654

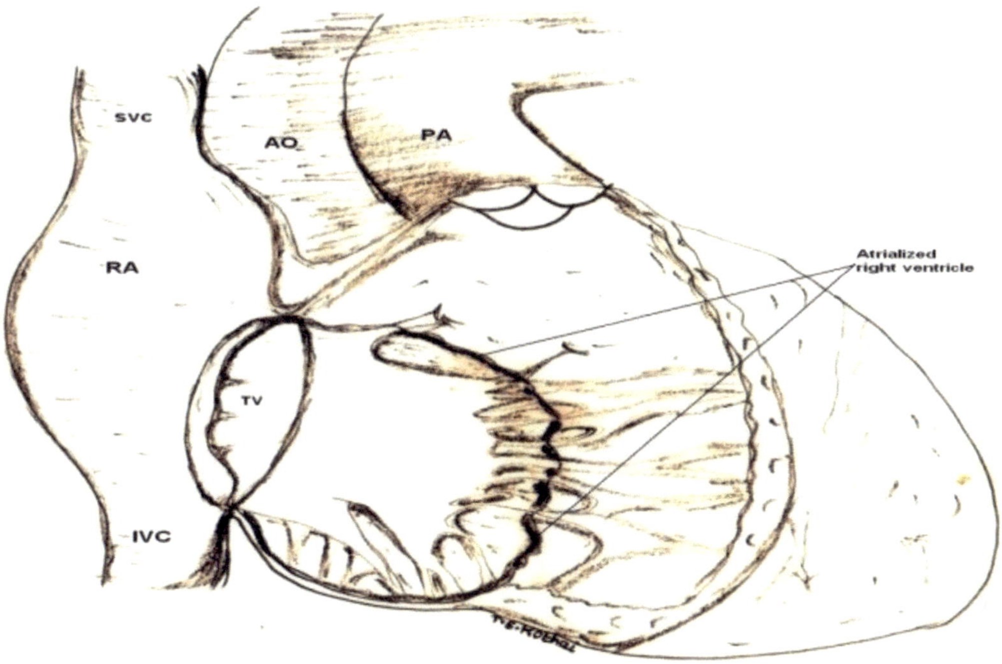

Figure 11. Ebsteins anomaly of tricuspid valve showing atrialised RV and displaced tricuspid leaflets.

replaced. Bioprosthetic valves are preferred in the tricuspid position as the circulation is sluggish compared to the left heart and mechanical valves in this position are prone to clotting and there have been reports of sudden death. Bioprosthetic valves require reoperation as they deteriorate over a period but reoperations are not associated with increased mortality.

Other causes of congenital TR are due congenital dysplastic leaflets. Various standard valve repair strategies are employed such as artificial Chordae, closure of clefts and commissures, and leaflet enhancements with commissural annuloplasty or ring annuloplasty.

2. Pulmonary valve- Congenital anomalies of the PV present as pulmonary stenosis. Intervention is indicated when the gradient > 50 mm Hg. This is usually performed by the interventional cardiologist. Most cases are amenable to balloon valvuloplasty. Surgery is only indicated if there is supra-annular narrowing, annular hypoplasia or dysplastic leaflets. Surgical relief is by open pulmonary valvotomy with or without transannular patch. Patients can present with isolated infundibular obstruction. This requires open heart surgery- either resection of RVOT muscle bundles and if necessary, subannular patch.

When patients present with free pulmonary regurgitation following TOF repair, reoperation is indicated if children are symptomatic, the RV dilates or the patient presents with ventricular tachycardia. Surgical options include pulmonary valve replacement with pulmonary or aortic homografts, bovine jugular vein conduits and bioprosthetic valves. These valves are of limited durability and will require re-replacment. Percutaneous deployment of pulmonary valves has clinically employed with limited success.

2. Mitral valve- Congenital anomalies MV can be either mitral stenosis (MS) or mitral regurgitation (MR). Variants of MS include commissural fusion, parachute MV (single papillary muscle), hammock MV and variations in anomalies of the annulus, leaflets, chordae and papillary muscles. Congenital MR is due to the following mechanisms: Carpentier's classification- type 1-normal leaflets, type 2-leaflet prolapsed, type 3-leaflet restriction. If there is perforation in the leaflet, this is closed with a patch. If the annulus is dilated, this is reduced either by suture annuloplasty, commissural annuloplasty or ring annuloplasty. In leaflet prolapsed, the use of artificial chordate is gaining popularity. Contrary to the belief that this is contraindicated in children as they may outgrow their chordae, this has not been found to be the case as corresponding growth of the papillary muscle compensates. Chordal transposition or chordal shortening are described with good results. Leaflet restriction is addressed by releasing tethering secondary and tertiary chordae and leaflet enhancement with pericardial patch. Repair is always preferable in children at the expense of residual MS/MR as mitral valve replacement carries high risk in children due to their small annulus. Bioprosthetic valves degenerate rapidly due to the accelerated calcium metabolism of adolescence and mechanical valves require anticoagulation which is difficult to manage in children. Small valves are quickly outgrown by the child.

3. Aortic valve- Commonest AV lesion is congenital bicuspid aortic valve. This usually presents with stenosis. The optimal treatment when obstruction is significant is balloon valvuloplasty. This is associated with greater recurrence but delaying surgery is always preferable till the child is bigger and the annulus is larger. Congenital AS may present as unicuspid valve as well. Open aortic valvotomy is a simple procedure wherein the surgeon splits the valve judiciously at the commissures. Bicuspid valve can present with AR as well. Repair is still preferable and various valve preservation techniques are described. Residual AR is preferable to aortic valve replacement in infants and children. AVR in children varies from mechanical valve replacement in older children, Ross procedure wherein the patients PV is placed in the aortic position and conduit placed in the pulmonary position and aortic homograft root replacement. Anticoagulation is not required for Ross and homografts with the former carrying the advantage of increased durability of the aortic autograft. Mechanical valves, particularly if small, are fraught with problems particularly outgrowth.

Children, particularly those with Marfan's and other connective tissue disorder, can present with aneuysmal dilatation of the aorta. The indications for surgery are similar to those for adults with the aim being to prevent rupture. Surgical options include replacement of the ascending aorta with an interposition graft and Bentall procedure wherein the whole aortic root is replaced with composite graft including a mechanical valve and reimplantation of the coronary arteries if there is associated AR. Current concepts are to preserve the native valve whenever possible and hence, further surgical options are to replace ascending aorta and repair the AV or root-preserving surgery.

Coronary artery anomalies are uncommon and include anomalous origin of the left coronary artery from pulmonary artery (ALCAPA), coronary arterio-venous fistula and coronary artery aneurysms. ALCAPA characteristically presents with severe LV dysfunction and mitral regurgitation. The problems are two-fold: connection of the left coronary artery to the PA which results in myocardial ischemia and the left-to-right shunt ensuing. Ideal procedure is urgent surgery and re-implantation of the left coronary to the aorta. Takeuchi repair or its modifications to baffle the left coronary to the aorta has also been described. Less than ideal is to tie off the left main and leave the patient on a single coronary. Adults have been managed by ligation of left main and coronary artery bypass grafting.

18.4. Congenital tracheal anomalies and vascular rings

These are rare conditions. Congenital tracheal stenosis consists of localised or long-segment stenosis of trachea due to presence of complete tracheal rings. These are associated with cardiac lesions such as TOF. The patients present with stridor. Surgery is the treatment of choice. These include slide plasty,resection and end-to-end anastomosis, homograft replacement and patch plasty of trachea simultaneous with the cardiac repair.

The two common vascular anomalies that present are double aortic arch and left pulmonary artery sling. Double aortic arch [50] is due to the persistence of both right and left dorsal aortic arches. Symptoms are related to the compression of the trachea and esophagus by the relevant vascular structures. Surgery for double arch is via left thoracotomy, division of the PDA/ ligamentumarteriosum and surgical division of the smaller arch distal to the corresponding subclavian artery. LPA sling is associated in 50-65% of cases with tracheal stenosis due to complete rings. Surgery is by reimplantation of the LPA onto the MPA either via left thoracotomy or median sternotomy on cardiopulmonary bypass [51]

18.5. Adult congenital cardiac surgery

Children who grow into adults with congenital heart disease come under this category.

Left-to-right shunts: Atrial septal defect of all types can present in adulthood and are usually operable. A small percentage present with irreversible pulmonary hypertension. Operations on adults provide a survival benefit upto 25 years of age, but beyond that, the main indication is improving quality of life, prevention of paradoxical embolism and most importantly, prevent the onset of atrial fibrillation.

Ventricular septal defect rarely present in adulthood as they are operable only as children. The only odd case maybe the rare ones with large VSD that have not become Eisenmenger's and the one who present with aortic valve prolapse or along with aortic regurgitation and/ or ruptured sinus of Valsalva aneurysm. The latter characteristically present in middle age. The other common subset is those adults who present with VSD and RVOT obstruction (double chamber right ventricle or adults with closing VSD and acquired RVOT obstruction-gazzulization.)

Adults do occasionally present with PDA- the large ones are rarely still operable and the small ones can be occluded by the interventional cardiologist. Surgery in PDA with pulmonary hypertension is high-risk as they are fragile and prone to catastrophic tears during surgery- they may be calcified. Surgery is more complex- requiring cardiopulmonary bypass.

Coarctation is not uncommon in presentation as an adult, either as a primary coarctation or re-coarctation. Surgery is high-risk, particularly with tight coarctation with multiple collaterals. Entry into the chest is associated with significant bleeding and very often, the coarct segment has to be excised and replaced with an interposition graft. The aortic tissue is usually friable and is prone to tear. A bypass graft from the left subclavian artery to the descending aorta may then be preferable. Recoarctation is better dealt with balloon plasty and stenting. Adults with coarctation may be managed with covered stents.

Tetralogy of Fallot may present in adulthood. They are amenable to corrective surgery provided criteria are met such as adequacy of pulmonary arteries and there are no significant collaterals. They may need preoperative embolization of collaterals and intraoperative RV-PA conduit as they may not tolerate free pulmonary regurgitation in the event of transannular patch. The children who underwent repair as children may present in adulthood with RV dysfunction due to free PR. They require redo sternotomy and insertion of RV-PA conduit. A subset of these patients presents as adults with aortic regurgitation and/or ascending aortic aneurysm and require AVR with or without ascending aorta replacement.

Patients may present de novo with RVOT obstruction at various levels. These are amenable to surgery or intervention based on various criteria.

Children who underwent Senning's or Mustard's procedure from transposition of great arteries (TGA) present in adulthood with residual defects such as baffle leaks or with cardiac failure as the RV in the systemic position is prone to failure. These patients require heart transplant or conversion to arterial switch following PA banding to retrain the LV. These are high-risk procedures.

Children with single ventricle physiology present in adulthood requiring Fontan procedure. Some have had atriopulmonary Fontan and require conversion to an extracardiac Fontan if the former surgery fails.

Ebstein's anomaly, cor triatriatum sinister (membrane in the left atrium obstructing pulmonary veins), ALCAPA and TAPVC with unrestricted ASD are conditions with which patients may present as adults for surgery. Congenital corrected transposition of great arteries, with VSD and PS may also present late.

Children who have undergone arterial switch as infants present as adults with coronary issues, neo-pulmonarysupravalvular stenosis, and neoaortic regurgitation. These patients require stenting of their coronary artery obstructions, coronary artery bypass grafting, patch plasty of supravalvular obstruction and replacement of the aortic valve.

http://dx.doi.org/10.5772/53654

19. Arryhtmias, pacemakers and defibrillators

The congenital population is prone to postoperative complete heart block and even nodal arrhythmias are not tolerated by the population with single ventricle physiology. These children will require to be under the care of the electrophysiologist. They will need lifelong pacemaker changes and lead changes. Arrhythmias are common such as atrial fibrillation and those related to accessory bundle pathways. Children with dilated RV/LV are prone to malignant ventricular arrhythmias such as ventricular tachycardia and ventricular fibrillation. These require monitoring and insertion of AICD (automatic internal cardioverter-defibrillator). Patients with chronic atrial fibrillation may benefit from the Maze procedure (antiarrhythmic surgery). This procedure may involve either right atrium or left atrium or both.

20. Future of congenital cardiac surgery

1. **Rise of interventional cardiology:** The interventional cardiologists have taken over many of the procedures formerly done exclusively by the surgeons. These include atrial septal defect (ostium secundum), and patent ductus arteriosus closure. Certain VSD's are being closed by the cardiologists. Open pulmonary valvotomy is a procedure of historical importance and open aortic valvotomy is rarely undertaken as a primary procedure. Procedures which will be undertaken with increasing aggressiveness by the interventionalist include ductal stenting, and RVOT stenting as a substitute for B-T shunt, and percutaneous pulmonary valve replacement. Percutaneous maze procedures, percutaneous mitral valve repairs, and percutaneous completion Fontan are on the anvil. Lesions such as aortopulmonary window, aorto-cameral tunnel and coronary a-v fistulae are amenable to interventional strategies. This will result in a change in the spectrum of surgeries done- surgeries will become more complex and the number of simple surgeries will dwindle. Hybrid procedures will rise wherein the cardiologist and cardiac surgeon will work together.

2. **Fetal echocardiography:** Antenatal diagnosis of congenital cardiac conditions is possible at 18-20 weeks of gestational age. This will empower parents with the option of medical termination of pregnancy. This will reduce the number of children requiring heart surgery.

3. **Robotic cardiac surgery/ thoracoscopic surgery:** Certain operations may be performed by the surgeon sitting at the console or maybe even in another part of the world utilising computer-controlled robotic arms. Thoracoscopic surgery may be an alternative for PDA.

4. **Disappearance of valve replacements:** Surgeons will become increasingly skilled at preserving the patient's own valve by mastering the skill of repairing rather than replacing with substandard alternatives.

5. **Genetic engineering:** Valves manufactured from the patient's own genetic material will demonstrate greater durability and biocompatibility and may become available off the shelf.

6. **Heart and heart-lung transplant:** There is a huge population of patients with Eisenmenger's syndrome who will eventually require transplant. Transplant restrictions such as availability of organs (genetically manufactured) and rejection will be overcome.

7. **Advancements in perfusion, anaesthesia and intensive care:** Better perfusion technology and techniques to avoid cardiopulmonary bypass with its deleterious effects on children will improve results of cardiac surgery. Pharmocological advances and newer drugs will provide for better outcomes via improved anaesthesia and postoperative strategies.

21. Quality improvement and risk stratification in congenital cardiac surgery

There are various risk-stratification scores in congenital cardiac surgery such as RACHS-1 and Aristotle Comprehensive Complexity Score. This places into perspective the mortality and morbidity rates of the hospital relative to the complexity of the cases they accept.

Databases exist such as the Society of Thoracic Surgeons database (STS) and EACTS congenital database which allows surgeons to compare the results of their surgery on various diagnoses with those of various others across the world.

22. Conclusion

Pediatric cardiac surgery is a noble pursuit, the healing of a sick heart by surgery in a fragile child. The future remains exciting with many anticipated developments. Many complex conditions will disappear as antenatal diagnosis becomes a norm and medical termination of pregnancy the rule. There will be an explosive growth in the number of adults presenting with congenital heart disease. This would present a huge stress on the healthcare providers and we must be prepared for this.

Surgeons will have to sharpen their skills as simple conditions will disappear from their operating list, which would be dealt with by interventional cardiologist. It would be replaced by complex conditions, adolescents and adults with congenital problems, requiring reoperations. They will have to accept fresh challenges- a surgeon cannot just replace a valve, but figure out strategies and surgical techniques to repair the patient's valve. The bar is thus raised.

In the late 1990's and early part of this century, mortality rate was the parameter by which a surgeon or unit was judged. This will be replaced by tougher parameters- complication rates and success rates with the more complex congenital cardiac conditions. Genetic engineering and transplant technology will have the greatest impact on the future of congenital cardiac surgery. Emphasis will be on the quality of life of survivors and normalizing their lives as much as possible. The future is indeed exciting and full of wonderful possibilities!

Author details

Krishnan Ganapathy Subramaniam* and Neville Solomon*

*Address all correspondence to: ganapathysubramaniamk@gmail.com

*Address all correspondence to: nevillesolomon@gmail.com

Apollo Children's Hospital, Chennai, Tamil Nadu, India

References

[1] DeHaan RL. Morphogenesis of the vertebrate heart.in: DeHaan RL, Ursprung H. editors. Organogenesis. New York: Rinehart and Winston ; 1965 p 377-420.

[2] Srivastava D, Baldwin HS. Molecular determinants of cardiac development. In: Allen HD, Gutfesell HP, Clark EB, Driscoll DJ, editors Moss and Adams Heart Disease in infants children and Adolescents Including the Fetus and Young Adult. Philadelphia: Lippincott Williams and Wilkins ; 2001

[3] Mjaatvedt CH, Yamamura H, Wessels A, Ramsdell A, Turner D, Markwald RR. Mechanisms of segmentation,septation and remodeling of the tubular heart: editors. Heart development. San Diego: Academic Press ; 1999.

[4] Webb S, Brown NA, Wessels A, Anderson RH. Development of the muringe pulmonary vein and its relationship to the embryonic venous sinus.Anat Rec 1998 Mar ; 250 (3); 323-34.

[5] Harvey RP, Rosenthal N, editors Heart Development. San Diego: Academic Press 1999 p 180-182.

[6] Dees E, Baldwin HS. New Frontiers in molecular pediatric cardiology.CurrOpinPediatr 2002; 14: 627-633.

[7] Wilcox BR, Anderson RH.Surgical Anatomy of the Heart. Ed 2 Lonton: Gower Medical ; 1992.

[8] Sweeney LJ, Rosenquist GC. The normal anatomy of thte atrial septum in the human heart. Am Heart J 1979; 98: 194-9.

[9] Anderson RH, Devine WA, Ho SY et al. The myth of the aortic annulus: the anatomy of the subaortic outflow tract. Ann ThoracSurg 1991; 52: 640-46.

[10] Anderson RH, Becker AE. Cardiac anatomy: an Integrated Text and Colour Atlas ed1London ; Gower Medical ; 1980.

[11] Van mierop LHS. Location of pacemaker in chick embryo heart at the time of initiation of heart beat. Am J Physiol1996; 212: 407-15.

[12] Stark, M de Leval, V T Tsang. Surgery for Congenital Heart Defects. 3 Ed. John Wiley and Sons, 2006.

[13] Berman W. The hemodynamics of shunts in congenital heart disease. Cardiovascular shunts: Phylogenetic, ontogenetic, and clinical aspects. In KJ, WW B, EditorNewYork: Raven Press ; 1978 p 399-410.

[14] Hoffman JI, Rudolph AM, Heymann MA. Pulmonary vascular disease with congenital heart lesios ; pathologic features and causes. Circulation 1981 ; 64: 873-7.

[15] Myung K Park. Pediatric Cardiology for Practitioners.5 Ed. Mosby Elsevier, 2008.

[16] Marx GR. Advances in cardiac imaging in congenital heart disease. CurrOpinPediatr 1995; 7(5); 580-6.

[17] Prakash A, Powell AJ, Krishnamurthy R, Geva T. Magnetic resonance imaging evaluation of myocardial perfusion and viability in congenital and acquired pediatric heart disease. Am J Cardiol 2004; 93950: 657-61.

[18] Freedom RM, Mawson JB, Yoo S, Benson LN. Congenital heart disease: textbook of angiocardiography. Armonk NY ; Futura Publishing ; 1997.

[19] Sharma S, Kothari SS, Krishnakumar R, Saxena A, Sharma R, Taneja K et al. Systemic to pulmonary artery collateral vessels and surgical shunts in patients with cyanotic congenital heart disease ; Treatment by transcatheter embolization. AJR Am J Roentgenol 1995; 164960 ; 1505-10.

[20] Baum VC, Palmisano BW. The immature heart and anesthesia. Anesthesiology 1997; 87: 1529-48.

[21] Heymann MA. Control of pulmonary circulation in the perinatal period. J DevPhysiol 1984; 6: 281-90.

[22] Rosenzweig EB, Barst RJ. Pulmonary arterial hypertension in children: a medical update. CurrOpinPediatr2008 ; 20: 288-93.

[23] Hoffman TM, Wernovsky G, Atz AM, Kulik TJ, Nelson DP, Chang AC et al. Efficacy and safety of milrinone in preventing low cardiac output syndrome in infants and children after corrective surgery for congenital heart disease. Circulation 2003; 107: 996-1002.

[24] Fiuffre RM, Tam KH, Williams WW, Freedom RM. Acute renal failure complicating pediatric cardiac surgeru: a comparison of survivors and nonsurvivors following acute peritoneal dialysis. PediatrCardiol 1992; 13: 208-213.

[25] Lister G, Talner N. Management of respiratory failure of cardiac origin New York, Churchill – Livingstone; 1981.

[26] Jenkins J, Lynn A, Edmonds J, Barker G. Effects of mechanical ventilation on cardiopulmonary function in children after open – heart surgery. Crit Care Med 1985; 13: 77-80.

[27] Laussen PC, Thompson FF. Surgical approaches, cardiopulmonary bypass, and Mechanical Circulatory Support in Children. In Frank W..Sellke, Pedro J.delNdio, Scott J. Swanson. Sabiston and Spencer Surgery of the Chest, 8th Editions Saunders Elseviers, 2010.

[28] Stark J. The use of Valved Conduits in Pediatric Cardiac Surgery.PediatrCardiol 1998; 19: 282-288.

[29] Corno AF, Festa P. Congenital Heart Defects vol. 3, Decision making for cardiac surgery, 35. Springer 2009.

[30] MuralidharPadala, Nikolay V. Vasilyev, James W. Owen, Jr., Jorge H. Jimenez, Lakshmi P. Dasi, Pedro J. del Nido, and Ajit P. Yoganathan. Cleft closure and undersizingannuloplasty improve mitral valve repair in atrioventricular canal defects.J. Thorac. Cardiovasc. Surg., November 2008; 136: 1243 - 1249.

[31] A. TayfunGurbuz, William M. Novick, Connie A. Pierce, and Donald C. Watson. Left ventricular outflow tract obstruction after partial atrioventricularseptal defect reapir. Ann. Thorac. Surg., Nov 1999; 68: 1723 - 1726.

[32] Jennifer L Russell, Jacques G LeBlanc, Margaret L Deagle, James E Potts, and PhD. Outcome Following Repair of Sinus Venosus Atrial Septal Defects in Children. Asian CardiovascThorac Ann, Sep 2002; 10: 231 - 234.

[33] Mary S Minette, DavidSahn. Congenital Heart Disease for the Adult Cardiologist. Ventricular septal defects. Congenital Heart Disease for the Adult Cardiologist. Ventricular septal defects. Circulation 2006; 114: 2190-2197.

[34] BolRaap G, Meijboom FJ. Long-term follow-up and quality of life after closureof ventricular septal defect in adults. Eur J Cardiothorac Surg. 2007; 32: 215-219.

[35] ShuSen Li, Si AnXu, You RenZheng, and Xi Wu Zhao. Surgical interruption of Patent DuctusArteriosus in Children. Asian CardiovascThorac Ann 1998; 6: 34-36.

[36] KhawarAizaz, Howaida Al Qethamy, Khalid Al Jubair, Yahya Al Faraidi and Mohammed R Al Fagih. Aortopulmonary Window Repair: 15- year Surgical Experience. Asian CardiovascThorac Ann, Jun 2001; 9: 111 - 114.

[37] John W. Brown, Mark Ruzmetov, Yuji Okada, Palaniswamy Vijay, and Mark W. Turrentine. Surgical results in patients with double outlet right ventricle: a 20-year experience. Ann. Thorac. Surg., Nov 2001; 72: 1630 - 1635.

[38] GeorgiosKalavrouziotis, Manoj Purohit, Giovanna Ciotti, Antonio F. Corno, and Marco Pozzi. Truncusarteriosuscommunis: early and midterm results of early and primary repair. Ann. Thorac. Surg., December 2006; 82: 2200 - 2206.

[39] Carl L. Backer, Constantine Mavroudis, Elias A. Zias, Zahid Amin, and Thomas J. Weigel. Repair of coarctation with resection and extended end-to-end anastomosis. Ann. Thorac. Surg., Oct 1998; 66: 1365 - 1370.

[40] Stark J, de Leval M, Tsang VT. Interruption of aortic arch. John Wiley & sons ltd. 3rded 2006. 299-305.

[41] Eric J. Devaney, Andrew C. Chang, Richard G. Ohye, and Edward L. Bove. Management of Congenital and Acquired Pulmonary Vein Stenosis. Ann. Thorac. Surg., Mar 2006; 81: 992 - 996.

[42] Hamad F. Al Habib, Jeffrey Phillip Jacobs, Constantine Mavroudis, Christo I. Tchervenkov, Sean M. O'Brien, SiamakMohammadi, and Marshall L. Jacobs. Contemporary Patterns of Management of Tetralogy of Fallot: Data from the Society of Thoracic Surgeons Database. Ann. Thorac. Surg., September 2010; 90: 813 - 820.

[43] Miguel A. Maluf, Domingo M. Braile, Célia Silva, Roberto Catani, Antônio C. Carvalho, and ÊnioBuffolo. Reconstruction of the pulmonary valve and outflow tract with bicuspid prosthesis in tetralogy of Fallot. Ann. Thorac. Surg., Dec 2000; 70: 1911 - 1917.

[44] Howaida O Al Qethamy, KhawarAizaz, Saber AR Aboelnazar, Samina Hijab, and Yahya Al Faraidi. Two-stage Arterial Switch Operation: is late ever too late? Asian CardiovascThorac Ann, Sep 2002; 10: 235 - 239.

[45] SerbanStoica, Esther Carpenter, David Campbell, Max Mitchell, Eduardo da Cruz, Dunbar Ivy, and Francois Lacour-Gayet. Morbidity of the Arterial Switch Operation. Ann. Thorac. Surg., June 2012; 93: 1977 – 1983.

[46] David W. Quinn, Simon P. McGuirk, ChetanMetha, Peter Nightingale, Joseph V. de Giovanni, Rami Dhillon, Paul Miller, Oliver Stumper, John G. Wright, David J. Barron, and William J. Brawn. The morphologic left ventricle that requires training by means of pulmonary artery banding before the double-switch procedure for congenitally corrected transposition of the great arteries is at risk of late dysfunction. J. Thorac. Cardiovasc. Surg., May 2008; 135: 1137 - 1144.

[47] Umar S. Boston, Joseph A. Dearani, Patrick W. O'Leary, David J. Driscoll, and Gordon K. Danielson. Tricuspid Valve Repair for Ebstein's Anomaly in Young Children: A 30-year experience. Ann. Thorac. Surg., Feb 2006; 81: 690 - 696.

[48] Qingyu Wu and Zhixiong Huang. A new procedure for Ebstein's anomaly. Ann. Thorac. Surg., Feb 2004; 77: 470 - 476.

[49] Sunil P. Malhotra, Ed Petrossian, V. Mohan Reddy, Mary Qiu, Katsushide Sam Sulema n, Malcolm MacDonald, Olaf Reinhartz, and Frank L. Hanley. Selective Right

Ventricular Unloading and Novel Technical Concepts in Ebstein's Anomaly.Ann. Thorac. Surg., December 2009; 88: 1975 - 1981.

[50] Ganesh Shanmugam, Kenneth Macarthur, and James Pollock. Surgical repair of Double Aortic Arch: 16-year Experience. Asian CardiovascThorac Ann, Mar 2005; 13: 4 - 10.

[51] Shu-Chien Huang, En-Ting Wu, Ching-Chia Wang, Chun-An Chen, Chien-Yi Chen, Shyh-Jye Chen, and Mei-Hwan Wu. Repair of Complex Tracheobronchial Stenosis with Left Pulmonary Artery Sling and bridging bronchus. Ann. Thorac. Surg., October 2010; 90: 1379 - 1381.

Chapter 10

Veno-Arterial Extracorporeal Membrane Oxygenation for Refractory Cardiogenic Shock and Cardiac Arrest

Francesco Formica and Giovanni Paolini

Additional information is available at the end of the chapter

http://dx.doi.org/10.5772/54719

1. Introduction

Cardiogenic shock (CS) following acute myocardial infarction (AMI) occurs in 7% to 9% of patients affected by AMI with a high mortality rates. Despite all recent advanced treatments such as use of inotropes, vasoconstrictors and intra-aortic balloon pump (IAPB) therapy, revascularization techniques and application of different systems of mechanical circulatory support, CS is still the most common cause of hospital mortality ranging between 60%-70% compared to patients with AMI without advanced CS whose hospital mortality is about 10% [1]. Cardiac arrest is a major cause of unexpected death and complicates about 22% of patients with acute myocardial infarction [2]. Cardiac arrest has a poor prognosis, and despite conventional cardiopulmonary resuscitation (CPR) maneuvers, only a few patients can fully return to a normal lifestyle. The main reasons for very poor outcome and prognosis in CA are a lack of return of spontaneous circulation (ROSC), a long time of CPR [3],[4], re-arrest from hemodynamic instability after ROSC, hypoxic encephalopathy [5], out-of-hospital CA [6-8]. In both refractory CS and CA secondary AMI, which are very critical circumstances, Veno-Arterial Extracorporeal Membrane Oxygenation (V-A ECMO) has been proposed and utilized during the last decades to obtain rapid resuscitation, stabilization, and subsequent triage to a more permanent treatment strategy.

The aim of this chapter is to describe the more recent indications, techniques and results in the usage of the V-A ECMO in patients with refractory cardiogenic shock and cardiac arrest secondary to acute myocardial infarction.

2. Definition of V-A ECMO

Extracorporeal membrane oxygenation is essentially a modification of the cardiopulmonary bypass circuit, which is used routinely in cardiac surgery. Blood is removed from the venous system, oxygenated by an oxygenator and then returned back to the body by a pump. ECMO provides both full cardiac and respiratory support. In brief, every ECMO system is basically a closed tubing loop with the interpolation of a blood pump (centrifugal or roller) and an oxygenator. Two vessel cannulas complete the system. Technically the ECMO system is more complex and several configurations have been developed according to the primary etiology.

The veno-arterial ECMO configuration is a tubing loop with a venous arm connected to a venous cannula to allow the venous blood drainage and an arterial arm to return back the oxygenated blood inside the patient's circulatory system. This mode provides both cardiac and respiratory support and can be achieved by either peripheral or central cannulation (Figure1).

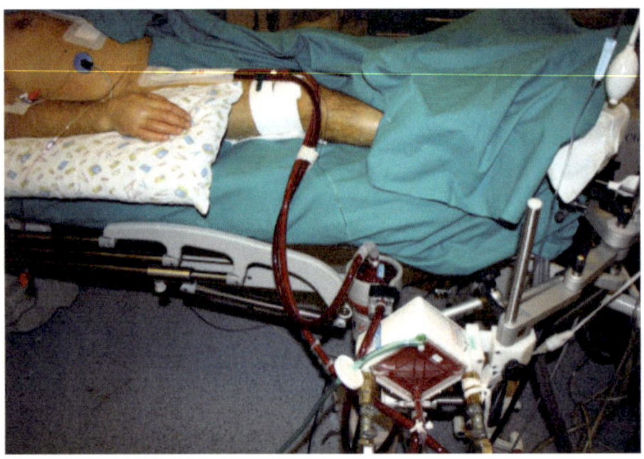

Figure 1. Patient supported with peripheral V-A ECMO

The veno-venous ECMO mode refers to blood, which is drained from the venous system and returned back to the venous system. This mode only provides respiratory support and is obtained by peripheral cannulation, usually of both femoral veins and jugular vein. This ECMO configuration will be not discussed in this chapter.

2.1. Definition of cardiogenic shock

Cardiogenic shock is a state of impaired and non-physiologic end-organ perfusion owing to a low cardiac output. Being characterized by hypotension cardiogenic shock is defined mainly by haemodynamic parameters as follows [9,10]:

a. a systolic blood pressure of less than 90 mmHg for more than 30 min with normovolemia;

b. the need of inotropic drugs to obtain a systolic blood pressure more than 90 mmHg with;

c. a cardiac index less than 1.8 L/min/m2 without inotropic support and 2.0–2.2 L/min/m2 with inotropic and intra-aortic balloon pump (IABP) support;

d. high left ventricular (LV) filling pressures (pulmonary capillary wedge pressure more than 18 mmHg).

End-organ hypoperfusion may be manifested clinically by:

a. pale, cool, and clammy peripheries;

b. alteration in mental status such delirium, confusion, clouded sensorium, psychomotor agitation;

c. decreased urine output (less than 1 ml/kg/min);

d. pulmonary congestion or edema;

e. tachycardia;

f. hyperlactacidemia (more than 3.mmol/L) as expression of impaired peripheral microcirculation;

g. mixed venous saturation of less than 65%.

3. Definition of in-hospital and out-hospital cardiac arrest

Cardiac arrest is a major cause of unexpected death in developed countries with a low probability of patient survival. Survival is influenced by several variables common to both in-hospital and out-of-hospital arrest, such as time to recognition of the cardiac arrest, time to initiation of CPR, rhythm presentation, first defibrillation [2, 11, 12]. In current resuscitation guidelines for in-hospital cardiac arrest (IHCA) patients [13], CPR using ECMO (E-CPR) has been assigned a low-grade recommendation. It is reported that ECMO for out-of-hospital cardiac arrest (OHCA) has worse outcomes compared with ECMO for IHCA patients [7, 14]. In the United States, more than 166,000 patients experience an OHCA annually [15] and approximately 60% are treated by emergency medical services. OHCA survival to hospital discharge range from 0.3% in Detroit [16] to 20.4% in Slovenia [17].Five clinical criteria to predict survival from OHCA [18] have recently been reported. They are: cardiac arrest witnessed by a bystander, arrest witnessed by emergency medical personnel, provision of bystander CPR, shockable cardiac rhythm, and return of spontaneous circulation (ROSC) in the field. These criteria are applicable on IHCA too.

4. Indication and contraindications for v-a ECMO

Patient selection is a crucial point when the physician needs to take the decision to institute ECMO and several considerations must be focused up. Most importantly, it must be consider the likelihood of heart and end organs recovery. If the organs failure is thought to be reversible with ECMO, in such situation the device application is to be encouraged. If the likelihood of recovery of the heart or other end organs is thought to be very low or even impossible, then other factors must be taken into account. In such clinical scenario, the decision to institute ECMO should be based on an experienced ECMO team approach, which has to evaluate the patient's eligibility for heart transplantation or a definitive mechanical assist device (LVAD) implant as destination therapy.

4.1. Indications for v-a ECMO

The following factors need to be evaluated for the indications [19]:

- Age of patient and body surface area;
- sufficient medical expertise in the field of ECMO;
- possibilities for myocardial revascularization therapy, such as a coronary artery bypass grafting or coronary angioplasty;
- possibilities for heart transplantation or LVAD implant as destination therapy;
- status of central organs such as kidney, liver, and brain.

4.2. Contraindications for v-a ECMO

Contraindications to the institution of v-a ECMO include [20]:

- disseminated malignancy;
- advanced age;
- graft vs. host disease;
- known severe brain injury;
- unwitnessed cardiac arrest or cardiac arrest of prolonged duration;
- aortic dissection aortic incompetence.

5. Equipment of v-a ECMO circuit

5.1. ECMO circuit

The ECMO circuit is made of PVC tubing and the diameter of lines varies from ¼ inch for a neonate to ½ inch for pediatric and adult patients. The length of the circuit is kept not more than 2 meters to avoid increasing of resistance within a tube and twisting, but the length should be suitable to allow the movements of the patient by ECMO staff.

Areas of turbulent flow can predispose to clot formation; therefore loop and connectors should be avoided or kept at minimum.

http://dx.doi.org/10.5772/54719

5.2. ECMO cannulas and cannulation techniques

Cannulation is one of the most challenging aspects of ECMO. Peripheral percutaneous approach [6, 21 is the most used in cardiogenic shock and cardiac arrest [7, 22] because is quicker with less bleeding complications and easier decannulation. (Figure 2).

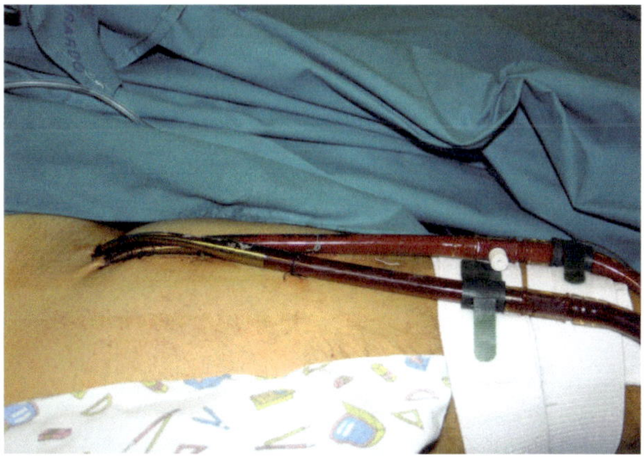

Figure 2. Peripheral cannulation for V-A ECMO.

The open surgical approach is considered for patients with severe peripheral vascular disease or for patients with postcardiotomy syndrome or failure of weaning from cardiopulmonary bypass [23, 24] (Figure 3). The open or central cannulation has more complications such as bleeding, infections, and mediastinitis.

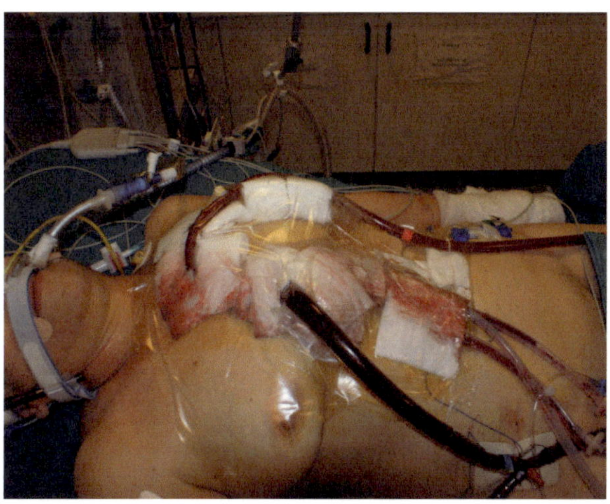

Figure 3. Central cannulation for V-A ECMO

Percutaneous cannulas are usually made of polyurethane (Figure 4) and they are inserted using the Seldinger technique (Figure 5).

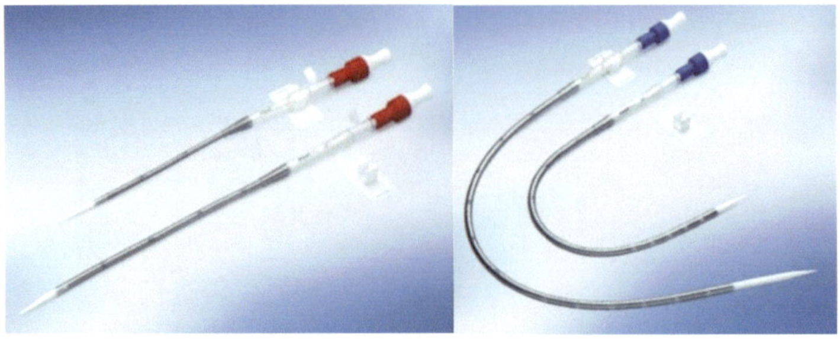

Figure 4. Percutaneous arterial cannulas (right) and percutaneous venous cannulas (left).

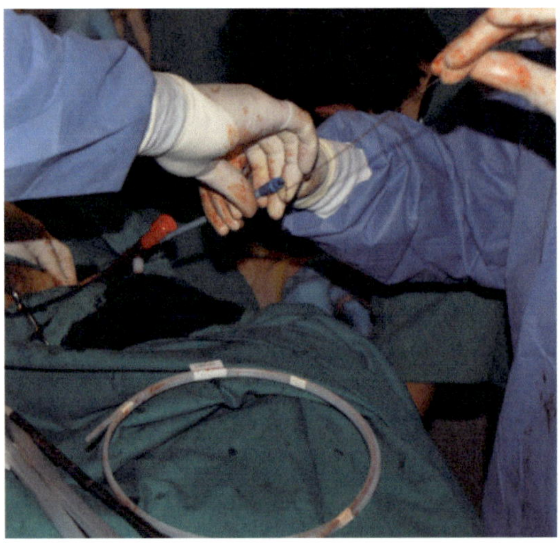

Figure 5. Percutaneous cannula insertion by Seldinger technique.

The size of the cannulas depends on the size of the patient; usually the arterial cannula ranges between 17 Fr to 21 Fr and the venous cannula ranges between 21 Fr and 25 Fr. Cannulas of sufficient size are required to support high blood flow with low resistance. Local complications, particularly at the site of peripheral insertion of VA-ECMO can occur, of which the most concerning is leg ischemia. For this reason all attempts the limb perfusion is restored, after noted the absence of anterior and posterior tibial artery flow, by inserting a 9-Fr catheter distally to the arterial cannula by means of vascular ultrasound scan as soon as possible after ECMO implantation (Figure 6).

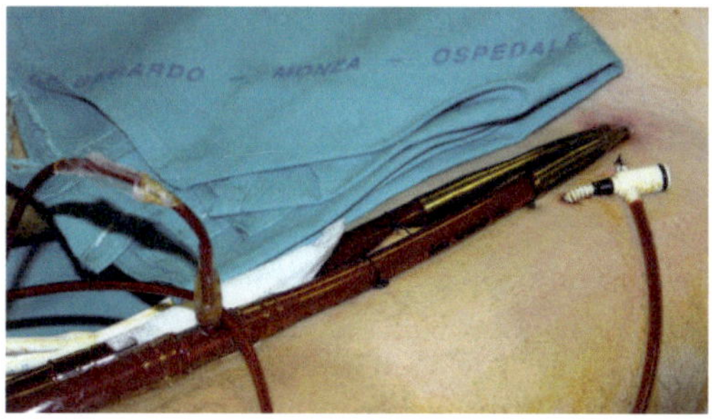

Figure 6. Distal leg perfusion to restore the blood flow.

Some Authors [25] suggested to insert a catheter for a distal perfusion if the mean pressure of the superficial femoral artery is lower than 50 mmHg.

Alternative arterial approach, such as axillary arterial cannulation, has been reported [26] (Figure 7).

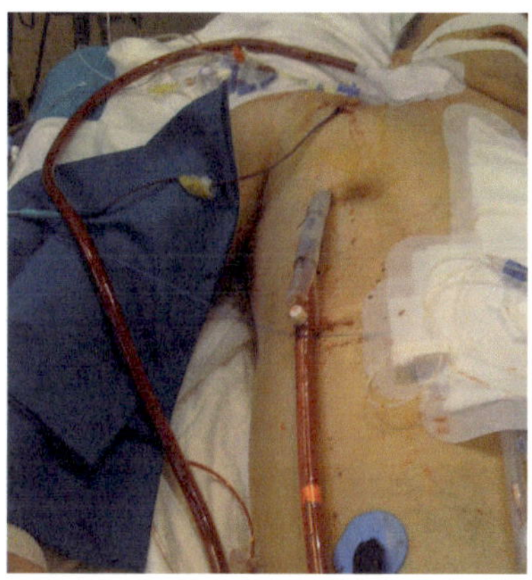

Figure 7. Cannulation of right axillary artery (tube on the right). Cannula is tunneled below the skin to protect by accidental trauma.

Whatever the type of approach cannulation is considered, it requires always a highly skilled medical staff, usually a cardiac or vascular surgeon, who are able to undertake this procedure under often very difficult conditions as the patients are so unstable or even in cardiac arrest.

5.3. Pumps

The pump pushes the blood through the oxygenator and then back to the patient. The most used pump in adult patients is the centrifugal pump. These pumps consist of a polycarbonate housing with a one-point sapphire bearing linked to a magnetic field, which create a vortex flow at an adjustable rate (Figure 8). Vortex creates a negative pressure in the pump head and this negative pressure pulls blood into the pump and then the blood is pushed towards the oxygenator.

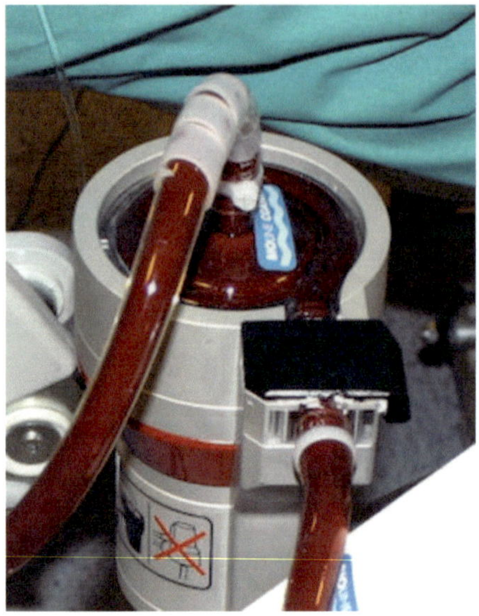

Figure 8. Centrifugal pump.

5.4. Oxygenators

The silicone membrane has been the principal artificial lung used for ECMO for many years and introduced in the clinical practice by Kolobow [27] and Bartlett [28]. The silicone oxygenators were used until the diffusion of microporous hollow fibers oxygenators in the 90s. The silicone surface is homogeneous and does not contain micropores, which can cause plasma leakage. However, the silicone oxygenator has a very large membrane surface to ensure adequate gas exchange and needs both high prime volume and high pressure drop; moreover, the procedure to optimize the efficacy of the oxygenator is cumbersome and lengthy, requiring a $CO2$ gas flush. The hollow-fiber polypropylene membrane oxygenators had advantages over the silicone oxygenators, such as high gas exchange efficiency with a smaller change surface, lower prime volume, and lower pressure gradient. However, this generation of oxygenators has micropores causing plasma leakage for periods more than 6 hours, thus reducing the gas exchange. Recently, a new generation of poly-methylpentene (PMP) membrane oxygenators have been introduced with the aim of allowing longer support without the complications linked to the hollow-fiber oxygenators, such as plasma leakage [29] (Figure 9).

The adjunct equipment that completes the ECMO system includes a heat exchanger for temperature regulation, monitors that measure blood flow, venous and arterial saturation, hematocrit, and other variables. ECMO systems also can measure circuit pressures and changes in circuit resistance. Additional safety features include continuous monitoring of venous drainage and air detection.

http://dx.doi.org/10.5772/54719

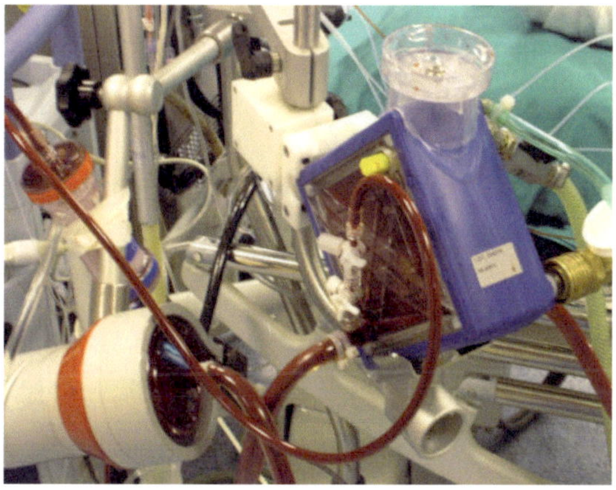

Figure 9. V-A ECMO circuit with polymethilpentene oxygenator (blue case)

Recently a new miniaturized system for V-A ECMO was introduced in the clinical practice. The system has the console directly connected with the oxygenator and the blood pump, which are integrated to each other. The console has a touch screen where is possible to monitor continuously several parameters such has hematocrit, hemoglobin, SVO2, resistance at the inlet and the outlet of oxygenator and the pressure drop (Figure 10).

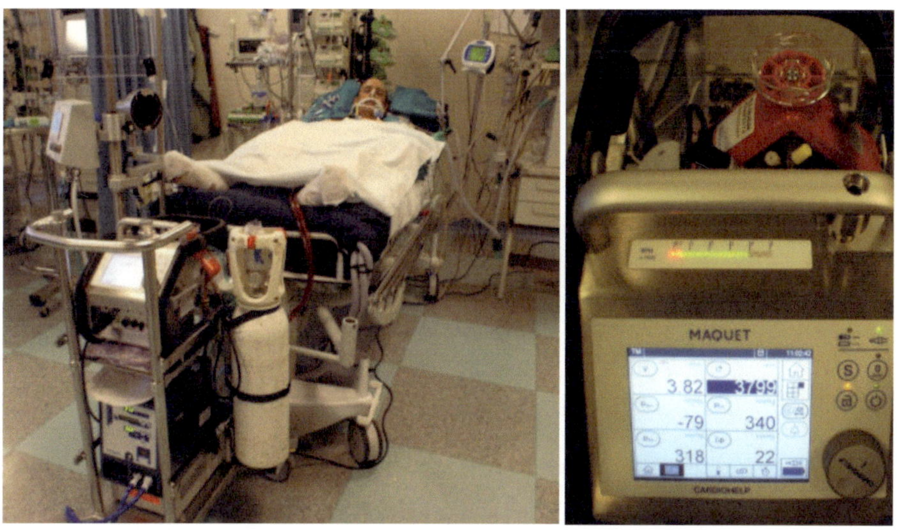

Figure 10. On the left the miniaturized V-A ECMO system (Cardiohelp by Maquet); on the right the particular of console.

This system is very useful because of his reduced dimension and weight (the weight of console is about 10 Kgs); for this reason this system can be used for transportation of V-A ECMO patients within the different sites of the hospital or from hospital to other hospital.

6. Management of v-a ECMO

Systemic heparinization is obtained with an intravenous bolus of 5,000 UI of heparin, 5 minutes prior to vessels cannulation. ECMO blood flow is calculated to maintain a Cardiac Output (CO) index of 2.5 L/min/m^2, an SvO_2 of about 70% and a mean blood arterial pressure of 60-70 mmHg during the first 24-48 hours. Continuous intravenous heparin is administered in order to achieve an activate clotting time (ACT) of 160-180 seconds and a prothrombin time value of 50-60 seconds. Small doses of inotrope (dobutamine, 5 to 7 μg/Kg/min) are given to maintain the ventricular ejection, to allow the opening of aortic valve and to prevent the formation of clots inside the left ventricle (LV). Oxygenator is always connected with a heat exchange to maintain a body temperature of 36 °C. Those patients who had a cardiac arrest before ECMO implantation are gradually cooled to 32-34°C during the first 24-36 hours. The assessment of the neurologic status is initiated by electroencephalography after body rewarming; serial neurologic evaluations and cerebral computed tomography scan are always considered to assess cerebral hemorrhage, stroke or hypoxic encephalopathy. In those patients with criteria of irreversible brain damage, ECMO withdrawn is usually considered.

Multiple heart examinations by transesophageal echo are performed to monitor the LV pulsatility. Left ventricular venting is considered in case of irreversible pulmonary edema, LV distension or pulseless heart with blood stasis. If the heart needs to be decompressed, several techniques can be considered. An 18-20 Fr catheter could be inserted into the apex of LV after surgery when patient cannot be weaned from cardiopulmonary bypass (Figure 11).

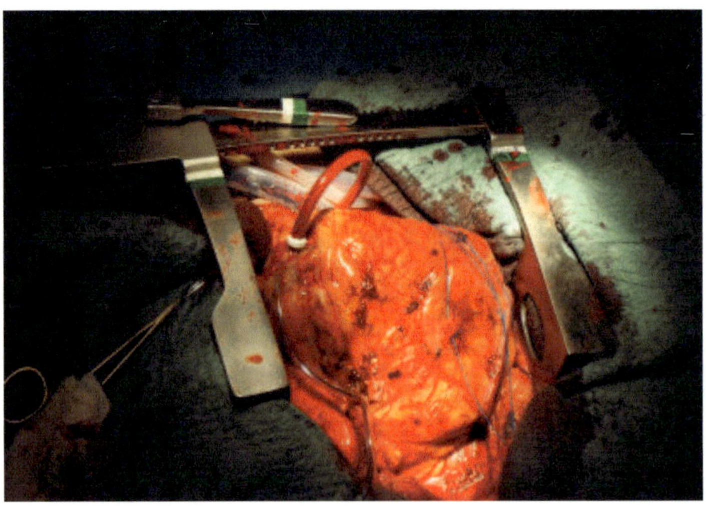

Figure 11. The left ventricle is decompressed by a 20 Fr catheter inserted in the apex of the ventricle.

Alternatively, the LV can be indirectly decompressed with a 16-Fr percutaneous venous cannula inserted in the right internal jugular vein and advanced into the main pulmonary artery; the cannula was connected to the venous arm of the ECMO circuit [30] (Figure 12).

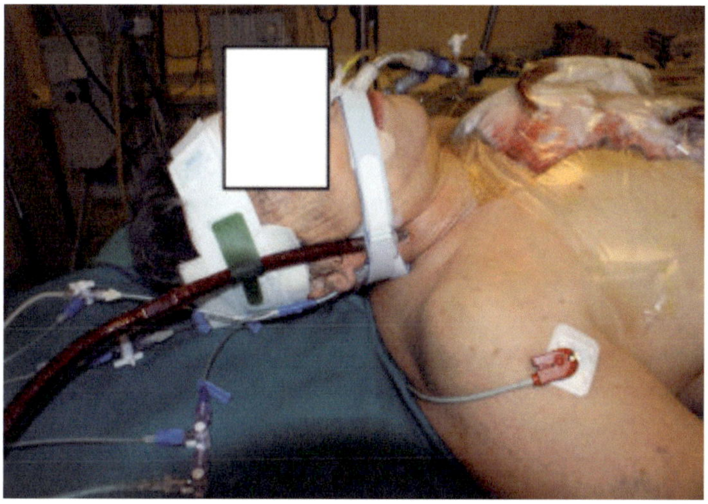

Figure 12. The cannula is inserted in the right jugular vein and advanced up to the main arterial pulmonary trunk.

Other techniques of LV decompression have been described such as the use of Pulse-Cath [31], Insertion of a pigtail inside the LV through the aortic valve [32], use of a transeptal atrial cannula [33].

Red blood cells (RBCs) transfusions are given to achieve a hematocrit of 30-32% and platelets are infused when the platelet count is less than 50,000-60,000/μL. Mechanical ventilation is continued throughout the ECMO support with the same management for each patient. Ventilator setting is commonly set at a tidal volume of 8 ml/Kg, 4 breaths/min, positive end expiratory pressure of 10 cm H_20 and a FiO_2 of 0.40-0.60.

Intraortic balloon pump (IABP) [24, 34] is employed with the aim to reduce the afterload, to increase the coronary and cerebral perfusion [35] and to maintain a pulsatile flow.

No attempts to wean off ECMO are usually considered during the first 48 hours. Step by step is the main strategy for weaning off ECMO using transesophageal echocardiography monitoring. This consists to reduce the pump flow at 1.0 L/min/m^2 for about 40-60 minutes after having obtained an ACT of 180 seconds. In patients who are supported also with IABP, this is set to 1:1 ratio. If systemic pressure, LV contractility, central venous pressure, wedge pressure and SvO_2 had not significant changes without the addition of new inotropes, then heparin is stopped and ECMO is removed at patient's bedside or in operating room within the next few hours.

Transthoracic and transesophageal echocardiography play a very important role in the assessment of LV and RV function and during the delicate phase of weaning from ECMO. Echocardiographic knowledge and facilities are becoming mandatory to start and continue an ECMO program with the aim to improve the outcome. Such echocardiographic parameters, such as transmitral E velocity, E/e' ratio, LV ejection fraction, aortic valve velocity-time integral, tissue Doppler lateral Ea, Sa, and parameters derived from Velocity Vector Imaging, including lateral systolic velocity, strain, and strain rate, are now considered important data [36] to drive a safe weaning from ECMO and they should be frequently collected in each ECMO patient.

7. Results and discussion

Extracorporeal membrane oxygenation is now considered a validate tool to support very ill patients affected by refractory cardiogenic shock to conventional therapy or cardiac arrest [4, 7, 37-39] and it is a well-established technology to provide a rapid and full circulatory support and to reverse the severe hypoperfusion organ injury. The ECMO system has several advantages: a) it can easily be implanted at patient's bedside, b) it can be initiated through a peripheral percutaneous cannulation, c) it is possible to stabilize the patient in the out-center hospital [6,22] d) it provides a full cardiopulmonary support, e) it allows to take time for diagnosis and further decision f) it is a relative *low-cost* support and g) it is a validate system for a "bridge strategy" [40]. However, the use of ECMO for cardiogenic shock has several limitations. All patients need to be anticoagulated during the ECMO support and complications such as neurological damage [41], infections [42], limb ischemia [43], bleeding and transfusion requiring [44] are frequently reported. However, the use of ECMO in patients with acute coronary syndrome complicated by advanced cardiogenic shock or by cardiac arrest is becoming an increasingly accepted procedure [3, 38, 39, 45].

Although the results about the use of IABP before and during ECMO are not univocal, the use of IABP seems to affect positively the early outcome. Some Authors [23, 24, 34, 46] found that the nonuse of IABP was one of the significant predictors of in-hospital death. On the other side, other Authors [39, 40, 47] could not find significant difference about the use of IABP during ECMO support. According to these different results, we cannot confirm whether the use of IABP has a determinant role in the cardiac function improvement. It can be argued that the use of IABP during ECMO, through the increase of coronary blood flow as reported by Madershahian [35], could favorite the cardiac recovery in ischemic patients.

Higher lactate levels are an index of severe acidosis and tissue hypoxia. The trends of blood lactate levels during the first three days of ECMO are considered as independent predictors of early mortality. Hyperlactatemia (level of blood lactate above 3 mmol/l) during cardiopulmonary bypass is associated with an increased mortality and morbidity, and appears to be related primarily to a state of inadequate perfusion [48]. We have already observed [44] that, when blood lactate level is > 3 mmol/l at 48 hours after ECMO initiation, the predicted probability of mortality is 52%. The earlier ECMO initiation should improve the organ perfusion and reduce dramatically the incidence of multi-organ failure. The persistence of hyperlactacidemia during the first days of ECMO support in nonsurvivors patients, even though the flow of the pump during the same period is similar to that of surviving patients, is likely to be referred to the persistent systemic and splanchnic hypoperfusion due to the extent of atherosclerotic disease or other unknown causes.

Bleeding and transfusion requiring can negatively affect the ECMO course and the early outcome and they are considered important complications during ECMO [23, 24, 47]. It is worthy to point out that lower number of RBCs transfused the number of RBCs units transfused was an independent predictor of in-hospital and late mortality. The need for RBCs transfusion depends not only by the fact that some patients on ECMO have undergone surgery; other factors such as systemic heparinization during ECMO and the use of platelet inhibitors after PTCA can cause bleeding and need for transfusions with increased risk of early mortality. Alternative therapy to conventional heparin anticoagulation therapy, such as bivalirudin or fondaparinux, to reduce the risk of bleeding and for the treatment of heparine induced thrombocitopenya have been recently published [49, 50].

High incidences of central nervous system (CNS) injury meeting the criteria of brain death are reported. These patients usually are withdrawn from ECMO sooner than the rest of the other patients. Brain death is frequent in patients who presented with cardiac arrest and received V-A ECMO implantation during cardiopulmonary resuscitation maneuvers. The incidence of brain death is ranging between 10% and 40% [6, 7, 39, 51]. Thiagarajan et al.[5] analyzing data of 297 patients supported by ECPR and extracted from the Extracorporeal Life Support Organization (ELSO) Registry reported an incidence of 33% of CNS damage and 21% had irreversible hypoxic encephalopathy. Other Authors [3, 4] described a very low survival when cardiopulmonary resuscitation (CPR) time is 60 minutes and a survival approaching to 0% when the CPR was more than 90 minutes.

Left ventricular decompression during ECMO support is an important priority in cases in which the contractile activity of the heart is inadequate to allow the opening of the aortic valve. In such scenario, the risk of clotting formation inside the left cavities is very high and the clots may embolize.

Several techniques to unload the left ventricle such as atrial septostomy [4, 33], direct LV apex cannulation [21], insertion of PulseCath iVAC [31], use of Impella [52, 53], percutaneous insertion of a pigtail [32] or percutaneous pulmonary truck drainage [30] have been described. One of the most followed strategies is to use as soon as the IABP associated with low dose of inotrope (dobutamine 5 mcg/min/Kg) with the aim to reduce the systemic resistance, improve the coronary and cerebral flow and increase the cardiac contractility. Whether the use of IABP is a useful tool to dramatically reduce the afterload mainly in such patients with a peripheral retrograde arterial return [21], and whether the IABP simply increases the coronary blood flow [35], is still debated.

Peripheral percutaneous cannulation represents a big challenging for all ECMO teams. Several peripheral complications such as retroperitoneal hemorrhage, cannula dislocation, cannulation failure, leg ischemia and leg amputation are described [43, 54]. According to early or late vascular complication following peripheral cannulation, Huang et al. [25] suggested measuring the mean pressure of the superficial femoral artery and they indicate to insert a catheter for a distal perfusion if the mean pressure is lower than 50 mmHg. It is extremely important to verify the pulsatility of the anterior and posterior tibial artery by an ultrasound vascular Doppler and to restore the limb perfusion signs of hypoperfusion are observed. In such case an 8-9 F catheter is placed distally to the arterial cannula by means of vascular ultrasound scan.

In female patients or in patients with a BSA less than 1.7 m^2 or in patients with a severe peripheral vascular disease, the distal catheter is inserted as soon as possible.

Patients with acute coronary syndrome complicated by advanced cardiogenic shock had a higher survival than patients presented with cardiac arrest. Kim et al. [45] reported an early survival of 59.2% in a group of 27 patients and described a long-term survival of 42.9% at 3 years. Bermudez et al. [39] described an early survival of 64% in a group of 33 patients affected by AMI and advanced CS. The 2-year survival was 48%. Sakamoto et al. [38] reported a cumulative early survival of 32.7% in a group of 98 patients affected by refractory CS following AMI in which 36.7% had CA on arrival. Other early survival rate ranging between 33.3% and 56.8% have been reported [37, 55, 56].

8. Future implications

Recently, some Authors have reported early results about the use of IABP in the setting of cardiogenic shock following acute myocardial infarction and in these articles the IABP seems to have not robust data to be still considered as the tool of first choice in the treatment of cardiogenic shock. Seyfart et al [57], in a randomized study of 25 patients with CS, randomly assigned to IABP (n=13) and percutaneous Impella 2.5 (n=12), reported a superior hemodinamic parameter and a significative increasing of cardiac index in patients treated with Impella; the 30 days mortality (46%) was not different in both groups. In a meta-analisys published by Sjauw et al. [58] about the use of IABP in the setting of ST-elevation myocardial infarction complicated by cardiogenic shock, the Authors could not find robust data in favours of the use of IABP. Different complications such as stroke and bleeding and increasing of 30-days mortality in patients managed with IABP were observed. A very recent article by Thiele and al [59], 600 patients affected by CS following acute myocardial infarction, were randomly assigned to IABP therapy (n = 300) or conventional therapy (n = 298). The Authors could not find significant differences in 30-days mortality and in secondary end points or in process-of-care measures, including the time to hemodynamic stabilization, the length of stay in the intensive care unit. No other significant differences with respect to the rates of major bleeding, peripheral ischemic complications and stroke were reported between the two groups. Howewer all these results have received different criticisms due to small number of patients [57] or a high number of patients with a relatively low mortality risk if treated with conventional therapy [59] and therefore these report could be influenced from some confounding factors.

According to these recent results, in the next close future, it can be argued that the use of ECMO could be more encouraged and anticipated in such patient who are in the setting of "pre-shock", in order to reduce the complications linked to the low cardiac output and to reduce the rate of very late application of ECMO. The current systems are safe and simple to apply, due to the advance in miniaturized centrifugal pumps and circuits, to the increased biocompatibility (heparin-coated system), but they are still associated with major complications in a relatively high percentage. Big efforts are still needed to improve the current techniques and devices.

9. Conclusion

The use of V-A ECMO in patients with acute myocardial infarction complicated by refractory cardiogenic shock and or cardiac arrest is widely increasing due to the improving in the early e mid-term results. The relatively low early survival rate in these very illness patients supported by ECMO should be considered an encouraging data, because in these patients the mortality without the ECMO support is dramatically higher. Bleeding, infections and CNS irreversible damage remain still serious complications and efforts to reduce or prevent them are necessary and strongly recommended to improve the outcome.

Acknowledgements

The Authors wish to thank Dr Giorgia Pavan for her editing and English language support, all the cardiac surgeons and the cardiologist team, the anesthesiologist medical staff, the perfusionist service an the nurse staff of the operating room and the intensive care unit.

Author details

Francesco Formica and Giovanni Paolini

Cardiac Surgery Unit, San Gerardo Hospital, Monza, Department of Surgical Science and Interdisciplinary Medicine, University on Milano-Bicocca, Italy

References

[1] Goldberg RJ, Spencer FA, Gore JM, Lessard D, Yarzebski J. Thirty-year trends (1975 to 2005) in the magnitude of, management of, and hospital death rates associated with cardiogenic shock in patients with acute myocardial infarction: a population-based perspective. Circulation 2009;119:1211-9.

[2] Brady WJ, Gurka KK, Mehring B, Peberdy MA, O'Connor RE, American Heart Association's Get with the Guidelines (formerly NRCPI. In-hospital cardiac arrest: impact of monitoring and witnessed event on patient survival and neurologic status at hospital discharge. Resuscitation 2011;82:845-52.

[3] Chen YS, Chao A, Yu HY, Ko WJ, Wu IH, Chen RJ et al. Analysis and results of prolonged resuscitation in cardiac arrest patients rescued by extracorporeal membrane oxygenation. J Am Coll Cardiol 2003;41:197-203.

[4] Massetti M, Tasle M, Le Page O, Deredec R, Babatasi G, Buklas D et al. Back from irreversibility: extracorporeal life support for prolonged cardiac arrest. Ann Thorac Surg 2005;79:178-83; discussion 83-4.

[5] Thiagarajan RR, Brogan TV, Scheurer MA, Laussen PC, Rycus PT, Bratton SL. Extracorporeal membrane oxygenation to support cardiopulmonary resuscitation in adults. Ann Thorac Surg 2009;87:778-85.

[6] Beurtheret S, Mordant P, Paoletti X, Marijon E, Celermajer DS, Léger P et al. Emergency circulatory support in refractory cardiogenic shock patients in remote institutions: a pilot study (the cardiac-RESCUE program). Eur Heart J 2012.

[7] Avalli L, Maggioni E, Formica F, Redaelli G, Migliari M, Scanziani M et al. Favourable survival of in-hospital compared to out-of-hospital refractory cardiac arrest patients treated with extracorporeal membrane oxygenation: an Italian tertiary care centre experience. Resuscitation 2012;83:579-83.

[8] Sasson C, Forman J, Krass D, Macy M, Kellermann AL, McNally BF. A qualitative study to identify barriers to local implementation of prehospital termination of resuscitation protocols. Circ Cardiovasc Qual Outcomes 2009;2:361-8.

[9] Cove ME, MacLaren G. Clinical review: mechanical circulatory support for cardiogenic shock complicating acute myocardial infarction. Crit Care 2010;14:235.

[10] Thiele H, Allam B, Chatellier G, Schuler G, Lafont A. Shock in acute myocardial infarction: the Cape Horn for trials? Eur Heart J 2010;31:1828-35.

[11] Kayser RG, Ornato JP, Peberdy MA, Resuscitation AHANRoC. Cardiac arrest in the Emergency Department: a report from the National Registry of Cardiopulmonary Resuscitation. Resuscitation 2008;78:151-60.

[12] Peberdy MA, Kaye W, Ornato JP, Larkin GL, Nadkarni V, Mancini ME et al. Cardiopulmonary resuscitation of adults in the hospital: a report of 14720 cardiac arrests from the National Registry of Cardiopulmonary Resuscitation. Resuscitation 2003;58:297-308.

[13] ECC Committee SbaTFotAHA. 2005 American Heart Association Guidelines for Cardiopulmonary Resuscitation and Emergency Cardiovascular Care. Circulation 2005;112:IV1-203.

[14] Le Guen M, Nicolas-Robin A, Carreira S, Raux M, Leprince P, Riou B et al. Extracorporeal life support following out-of-hospital refractory cardiac arrest. Crit Care 2011;15:R29.

[15] Rosamond W, Flegal K, Furie K, Go A, Greenlund K, Haase N et al. Heart disease and stroke statistics--2008 update: a report from the American Heart Association Statistics Committee and Stroke Statistics Subcommittee. Circulation 2008;117:e25-146.

[16] Dunne RB, Compton S, Zalenski RJ, Swor R, Welch R, Bock BF. Outcomes from out-of-hospital cardiac arrest in Detroit. Resuscitation 2007;72:59-65.

[17] Grmec S, Kupnik D. Does the Mainz Emergency Evaluation Scoring (MEES) in combination with capnometry (MEESc) help in the prognosis of outcome from cardiopulmonary resuscitation in a prehospital setting? Resuscitation 2003;58:89-96.

[18] Morrison LJ, Verbeek PR, Vermeulen MJ, Kiss A, Allan KS, Nesbitt L et al. Derivation and evaluation of a termination of resuscitation clinical prediction rule for advanced life support providers. Resuscitation 2007;74:266-75.

[19] Beckmann A, Benk C, Beyersdorf F, Haimerl G, Merkle F, Mestres C et al. Position article for the use of extracorporeal life support in adult patients. Eur J Cardiothorac Surg 2011;40:676-80.

[20] Marasco SF, Lukas G, McDonald M, McMillan J, Ihle B. Review of ECMO (extra corporeal membrane oxygenation) support in critically ill adult patients. Heart Lung Circ 2008;17 Suppl 4:S41-7.

[21] Russo CF, Cannata A, Lanfranconi M, Bruschi G, Milazzo F, Paino R et al. Veno-arterial extracorporeal membrane oxygenation using Levitronix centrifugal pump as bridge to decision for refractory cardiogenic shock. J Thorac Cardiovasc Surg 2010;140:1416-21.

[22] Formica F, Avalli L, Redaelli G, Paolini G. Interhospital stabilization of adult patients with refractory cardiogenic shock by veno-arterial extracorporeal membrane oxygenation. Int J Cardiol 2011;147:164-5.

[23] Bakhtiary F, Keller H, Dogan S, Dzemali O, Oezaslan F, Meininger D et al. Venoarterial extracorporeal membrane oxygenation for treatment of cardiogenic shock: clinical experiences in 45 adult patients. J Thorac Cardiovasc Surg 2008;135:382-8.

[24] Rastan AJ, Dege A, Mohr M, Doll N, Falk V, Walther T et al. Early and late outcomes of 517 consecutive adult patients treated with extracorporeal membrane oxygenation for refractory postcardiotomy cardiogenic shock. J Thorac Cardiovasc Surg 2010;139:302-11, 11.e1.

[25] Huang SC, Yu HY, Ko WJ, Chen YS. Pressure criterion for placement of distal perfusion catheter to prevent limb ischemia during adult extracorporeal life support. J Thorac Cardiovasc Surg 2004;128:776-7.

[26] Javidfar J, Brodie D, Costa J, Miller J, Jurrado J, Lavelle M et al. Subclavian artery cannulation for venoarterial extracorporeal membrane oxygenation. ASAIO J 2012;58:494-8.

[27] Kolobow T, Bowman RL. Construction and evaluation of an alveolar membrane artificial heart-lung. Trans Am Soc Artif Intern Organs 1963;9:238-43.

[28] Bartlett RH, Gazzaniga AB, Jefferies MR, Huxtable RF, Haiduc NJ, Fong SW. Extracorporeal membrane oxygenation (ECMO) cardiopulmonary support in infancy. Trans Am Soc Artif Intern Organs 1976;22:80-93.

[29] Formica F, Avalli L, Martino A, Maggioni E, Muratore M, Ferro O et al. Extracorporeal membrane oxygenation with a poly-methylpentene oxygenator (Quadrox D). The

experience of a single Italian centre in adult patients with refractory cardiogenic shock. ASAIO J 2008;54:89-94.

[30] Avalli L, Maggioni E, Sangalli F, Favini G, Formica F, Fumagalli R. Percutaneous left-heart decompression during extracorporeal membrane oxygenation: an alternative to surgical and transeptal venting in adult patients. ASAIO J 2011;57:38-40.

[31] Anastasiadis K, Chalvatzoulis O, Antonitsis P, Tossios P, Papakonstantinou C. Left ventricular decompression during peripheral extracorporeal membrane oxygenation support with the use of the novel iVAC pulsatile paracorporeal assist device. Ann Thorac Surg 2011;92:2257-9.

[32] Barbone A, Malvindi PG, Ferrara P, Tarelli G. Left ventricle unloading by percutaneous pigtail during extracorporeal membrane oxygenation. Interact Cardiovasc Thorac Surg 2011;13:293-5.

[33] Aiyagari RM, Rocchini AP, Remenapp RT, Graziano JN. Decompression of the left atrium during extracorporeal membrane oxygenation using a transseptal cannula incorporated into the circuit. Crit Care Med 2006;34:2603-6.

[34] Doll N, Kiaii B, Borger M, Bucerius J, Krämer K, Schmitt DV et al. Five-year results of 219 consecutive patients treated with extracorporeal membrane oxygenation for refractory postoperative cardiogenic shock. Ann Thorac Surg 2004;77:151-7; discussion 57.

[35] Madershahian N, Liakopoulos OJ, Wippermann J, Salehi-Gilani S, Wittwer T, Choi YH et al. The impact of intraaortic balloon counterpulsation on bypass graft flow in patients with peripheral ECMO. J Card Surg 2009;24:265-8.

[36] [Firstenberg, 2012, ECMO and ECHO: the evolving role of quantitative echocardiography in the management of patients requiring extracorporeal membrane oxygenation

[37] Chen JS, Ko WJ, Yu HY, Lai LP, Huang SC, Chi NH et al. Analysis of the outcome for patients experiencing myocardial infarction and cardiopulmonary resuscitation refractory to conventional therapies necessitating extracorporeal life support rescue. Crit Care Med 2006;34:950-7.

[38] Sakamoto S, Taniguchi N, Nakajima S, Takahashi A. Extracorporeal life support for cardiogenic shock or cardiac arrest due to acute coronary syndrome. Ann Thorac Surg 2012;94:1-7.

[39] Bermudez CA, Rocha RV, Toyoda Y, Zaldonis D, Sappington PL, Mulukutla S et al. Extracorporeal membrane oxygenation for advanced refractory shock in acute and chronic cardiomyopathy. Ann Thorac Surg 2011;92:2125-31.

[40] Hoefer D, Ruttmann E, Poelzl G, Kilo J, Hoermann C, Margreiter R et al. Outcome evaluation of the bridge-to-bridge concept in patients with cardiogenic shock. Ann Thorac Surg 2006;82:28-33.

[41] Mateen FJ, Muralidharan R, Shinohara RT, Parisi JE, Schears GJ, Wijdicks EF. Neurological injury in adults treated with extracorporeal membrane oxygenation. Arch Neurol 2011;68:1543-9.

[42] Pieri M, Greco T, De Bonis M, Maj G, Fumagalli L, Zangrillo A et al. Diagnosis of infection in patients undergoing extracorporeal membrane oxygenation: a case-control study. J Thorac Cardiovasc Surg 2012;143:1411-6.

[43] Bisdas T, Beutel G, Warnecke G, Hoeper MM, Kuehn C, Haverich A et al. Vascular complications in patients undergoing femoral cannulation for extracorporeal membrane oxygenation support. Ann Thorac Surg 2011;92:626-31.

[44] Formica F, Avalli L, Colagrande L, Ferro O, Greco G, Maggioni E et al. Extracorporeal membrane oxygenation to support adult patients with cardiac failure: predictive factors of 30-day mortality. Interact Cardiovasc Thorac Surg 2010;10:721-6.

[45] Kim H, Lim SH, Hong J, Hong YS, Lee CJ, Jung JH et al. Efficacy of veno-arterial extracorporeal membrane oxygenation in acute myocardial infarction with cardiogenic shock. Resuscitation 2012;83:971-5.

[46] Smedira NG, Moazami N, Golding CM, McCarthy PM, Apperson-Hansen C, Blackstone EH et al. Clinical experience with 202 adults receiving extracorporeal membrane oxygenation for cardiac failure: survival at five years. J Thorac Cardiovasc Surg 2001;122:92-102.

[47] Wang J, Han J, Jia Y, Zeng W, Shi J, Hou X et al. Early and intermediate results of rescue extracorporeal membrane oxygenation in adult cardiogenic shock. Ann Thorac Surg 2009;88:1897-903.

[48] Ranucci M, De Toffol B, Isgrò G, Romitti F, Conti D, Vicentini M. Hyperlactatemia during cardiopulmonary bypass: determinants and impact on postoperative outcome. Crit Care 2006;10:R167.

[49] Pappalardo F, Maj G, Scandroglio A, Sampietro F, Zangrillo A, Koster A. Bioline heparin-coated ECMO with bivalirudin anticoagulation in a patient with acute heparin-induced thrombocytopenia: the immune reaction appeared to continue unabated. Perfusion 2009;24:135-7.

[50] Ranucci M, Ballotta A, Kandil H, Isgrò G, Carlucci C, Baryshnikova E et al. Bivalirudin-based versus conventional heparin anticoagulation for postcardiotomy extracorporeal membrane oxygenation. Crit Care 2011;15:R275.

[51] Jaski BE, Ortiz B, Alla KR, Smith SC, Glaser D, Walsh C et al. A 20-year experience with urgent percutaneous cardiopulmonary bypass for salvage of potential survivors of refractory cardiovascular collapse. J Thorac Cardiovasc Surg 2010;139:753-7.e1-2.

[52] Beurtheret S, Mordant P, Pavie A, Leprince P. Impella and extracorporeal membrane oxygenation: a demanding combination. ASAIO J 2012;58:291-3.

[53] Koeckert MS, Jorde UP, Naka Y, Moses JW, Takayama H. Impella LP 2.5 for left ventricular unloading during venoarterial extracorporeal membrane oxygenation support. J Card Surg 2011;26:666-8.

[54] Zimpfer D, Heinisch B, Czerny M, Hoelzenbein T, Taghavi S, Wolner E et al. Late vascular complications after extracorporeal membrane oxygenation support. Ann Thorac Surg 2006;81:892-5.

[55] Combes A, Leprince P, Luyt CE, Bonnet N, Trouillet JL, Léger P et al. Outcomes and long-term quality-of-life of patients supported by extracorporeal membrane oxygenation for refractory cardiogenic shock. Crit Care Med 2008;36:1404-11.

[56] Aissaoui N, Luyt CE, Leprince P, Trouillet JL, Léger P, Pavie A et al. Predictors of successful extracorporeal membrane oxygenation (ECMO) weaning after assistance for refractory cardiogenic shock. Intensive Care Med 2011;37:1738-45.

[57] Seyfarth M, Sibbing D, Bauer I, Fröhlich G, Bott-Flu®gel L, Byrne R, et al. A randomized clinical trial to evaluate the safety and efficacy of a percutaneous left ventricular assist device versus intra-aortic balloon pumping for treatment of cardiogenic shock caused by myocardial infarction. J Am Coll Cardiol 2008;52:1584–8

[58] Sjauw KD, Engstrom AM, Vis MM, van der Schaaf RJ, Baan J, Koch, et al. A systematic review and meta-analysis of intra-aortic balloon pump therapy in ST-elevation myocardial infarction: should we change the guidelines? Eu Heart Journal 2009;30:459–468

[59] Thiele H, Zeymer U, Neumann F-J, Ferenc M, Olbrich H-G, M.D., Hausleiter J, et al. Intraaortic Balloon Support for Myocardial Infarction with Cardiogenic Shock. N Engl J Med 2012;367:1287-96.

Chapter 11

Management And Controversies of Post Myocardial Infarction Ventricular Septal Defects

Michael S. Firstenberg, Kevin T. Kissling and
Karen Nelson

Additional information is available at the end of the chapter

http://dx.doi.org/10.5772/53396

1. Introduction

Acute myocardial infarction (AMI), despite advances in health care delivery systems, education, and primary prevention still remains a significant problem. Fortunately, with these advances and early interventions, there has been a decline in the incidence of mechanical complications. Unfortunately, while becoming less common, when mechanical complications occur and despite advances and evolving techniques in the surgical management of these problems, morbidity and mortality remain high. Post-myocardial infarction ventricular septal rupture (PI-VSD) has challenged and intrigued clinicians for years. The timing of presentation can be quite variable, as they tend to occur in patients several days after their initial cardiovascular insult (acute PI-VSD) – and unfortunately, they can occur in patients who appear to otherwise be doing well. In addition, while less common, some patients might not present until weeks, if not longer, after their AMI with symptoms prompting a work-up that might reveal a chronic PI-VSD. Early PI-VSDs tend to be catastrophic and can result in death. The pathology is also variable and complex, but common themes include:

1. acute right ventricular (RV) failure from a sudden increase in pressure, volume, and flow from left to right shunts,
2. pulmonary hypertension also from the acute increase in RV work and flow and
3. worsening cardiac output, often with manifestations of shock and end-organ damage, from acute left ventricular (LV) dysfunction and left-right shunting.

Definitive management remains surgical, however, controversies continue to exist regarding the timing of surgery, the role of concomitant coronary revascularization, and the evolving role of percutaneous closure devices. Unfortunately, despite early repair and improvement in techniques and peri-operative management, the short and long-term outcomes remain less than ideal.

2. History

Post-myocardial infarction ventricular septal defects (PI-VSD) were described first at autopsy [30]. It was not until 1923 that the pre-mortem pathophysiology was understood [7]. [40], described the association with coronary artery disease and acute myocardial infarction [40]. The first report of a surgical repair came in 1956 when Denton Cooley described a patient 9 weeks after the initial diagnosis who underwent operative intervention [12]. With advances in the peri-operative and intra-operative management of the cardiovascular surgery patients there were reports of survival in what was previously felt to be an inherently fatal problem. Most of the successful operative cases occurred in patients who presented in congestive heart failure weeks after their initial acute event. Based upon these experiences, for many years it was the belief that operative management should be delayed as long as possible to allow for scaring of the necrotic myocardium to provide for a more stable repair. As experiences grew early repair was advocated, particularly in stable patients before hemodynamic deterioration and associated multi-organ failure.

3. Clinical Presentation

The incidence of PI-VSD has decreased dramatically over the years with advances in myocardial reperfusion and early revascularization strategies. Historically, up to 5% of AMI were associated with mechanical complications such free-wall ruptures, papillary muscle rupture, and PI-VSD [1]. With advanced in therapies that advocate early and aggressive attempts at reperfusion of the acute ischemic myocardial – such as thrombolytic therapy, early percutaneous interventions with coronary stenting (PCI), and, rarely, emergent coronary artery bypass surgery (CABG) – the overall presentation of mechanical complications, such as PI-VSD, has decreased significantly. Large multi-center studies evaluating the pathophysiologies of acute myocardial infarctions have shown a current incidence of approximately 0.2% of all AMI. In patients who present late or in whom there is a delay in therapy and there is a resulting increase in myocardial damage, this incidence increases up to 2%. Despite the low risk of developing a PI-VSD, it accounts for a disproportionally high mortality rate. Five percent of all early deaths after AMI are attributed directly to the complications of PI-VSD [36].

The timing of the development of a PI-VSD can be quite variable. The average time to clinical presentation is between 2 and 4 days. However, some patients can present as early as a few hours after AMI or as long as several weeks.

http://dx.doi.org/10.5772/53396

Risk factors include gender, with men at a greater risk than women (3:2 ratio), increasing age, and current smoking history. In the GUSTO trial, the mean age of presentation with a PI-VSD was 62.5 years and ranged from 44 to 81 years [13].

4. Diagnosis

The diagnosis of a PI-VSD must be considered in any patient presenting with hypotension, cardiogenic shock, or respiratory failure, particularly in the setting of a patient who otherwise had been doing well, either during or after an AMI. A PI-VSD presents in a similar manner as other mechanical complications of AMI, such a papillary muscle rupture with acute mitral regurgitation, free wall rupture with tamponade, or severe LV failure and pulmonary edema. The initial diagnosis must be suspected during initial investigations during a comprehensive work-up.

Patients often complain of recurrent chest pain. The characteristics of the pain are often different than their initial presentation and are typically related to the onset or recurrence of myocardial necrosis. Often a new systolic murmur will develop and it can be harsh, pansystolic, and often-best auscultated at the left lower sternal border. Patients can often have a bundle branch block from disruption of the septal conduction system. Hemodynamic deterioration can be quick and there can be a rapid progression to cardiogenic shock.

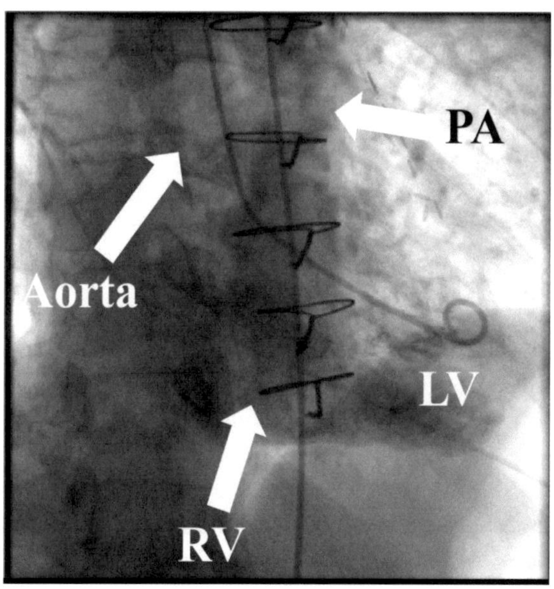

Figure 1. Representative cardiac catheterization in which contrast is injected during left ventriculography crosses the defect into the right ventricle. Contrast flowing into the pulmonary artery is then diagnostic for a ventricular septal defect.

With the acute clinical decompensation, a rapid evaluation of potential causes is critical. Unlike other mechanical complications, such as papillary muscle rupture, PI-VSDs will have imaging confirming a left to right shunt – such as contrast injected into the left ventricle during catheterization crossing the defect into the RV and entering into the pulmonary arteries (Figure 1). Likewise, oxymetric assessment with right heart catheterization will demonstrate a "step-off" from the mixing of de-oxygenated RV blood with the oxygenated LV blood. Quantitative assessment of Qp:Qs can correlate with the size, and more importantly – the physiologic consequences, of the defect.

4.1. Cardiac Catheterization:

Without a doubt, the value of early cardiac catheterization and coronary angiography in the setting of acute myocardial ischemia is well established and standard of care. In patients whom the diagnosis of a PI-VSD is suspected this test can also be diagnostic. Because a septal defect is often with extensive and acute ischemia of a large territory of myocardium, it is not uncommon that the catheterization findings are different from patients with a history of chronic coronary artery disease in which compensatory development of septal collaterals have had time to develop. During the acute presentation, the findings often suggest a complete occlusion of a large coronary artery in the setting of relatively minimal disease. Single vessel disease is found in 64% of patients. The left anterior descending (LAD) artery is often the culprit vessel and this explains why anterior or apical septal defects are found in 60% of cases. Conversely, acute occlusions of a dominant right coronary or circumflex artery accounts for the remaining cases involving the posterior septum. Seven percent have concomitant double vessel disease, and 29% have triple vessel disease.

As mentioned above, quantitative assessment of oxygen step-offs, when performed, will demonstrate an increase in the partial pressure of oxygen (PaO_2) between the right atrium and ventricle – diagnostic of left to right shunting. Left ventricular contrast injections, although less likely to be performed in a deteriorating patient secondary to the concern that additional contrast might further injure already compromised renal function, can be diagnostic of a PI-VSD. Contrast injected into the LV will cross the defect (left-right shunt) and flow into the pulmonary arterial tree. This "pulmonary arteriogram" is characteristic for a VSD (Figure 1, see above)

Arguments against mandatory catheterization suggest that in a clinically deteriorating patient in whom the diagnosis is clear it only delays surgical management, the dye load may worsen already impaired renal function, and some reports suggest that considering the patterns of coronary disease typically encountered that coronary revascularization is a risk factor for a poor outcome [33]. Despite these theoretical arguments, from a practical standpoint it is hard to argue the clear benefits of defining the coronary anatomy prior to a surgical intervention aimed at treating a complication of impaired coronary blood flow – particularly given the importance of optimal and complete revascularization. Since these patients have already undergone catheterization as part of the initial management of their initial ischemic event, the question whether to proceed with catheterization (or repeat catheterization) is rarely encountered. However, as many of the patients develop septal defect several days (or weeks)

http://dx.doi.org/10.5772/53396

after their initial acute coronary insult, it is hard to argue the need for repeat cardiac catheterization if the diagnosis is clear and the coronary anatomy is defined. Conversely, repeat catheterization might suggest an alternative, and potentially more likely, diagnosis such as acute stent thrombosis, coronary dissection, or disruption of an already unstable plaque.

4.2. Echocardiography:

Transthoracic echocardiography (TTE) remains the cornerstone of the non-invasive assessment of PI-VSD [28]. TTE is indicated in any patient who presents with acutely impaired ventricular function or in unexplained hemodynamic deterioration [9]. Echocardiography has the benefit of being able to assess both left and right ventricular function, the presence of co-existing and confounding valvular diseases – typically mitral and/or tricuspid regurgitation, and with color flow imaging it can be 100% specific and sensitive in diagnosing a PI-VSD. Despite the utility of transesophageal echocardiography in the acute assessment of an unstable patient, a high index of suspicion is needed when looking for a PI-VSD as traditional echo windows might miss a small or apical defect. Large pericardial effusions might suggest an associated free wall rupture.

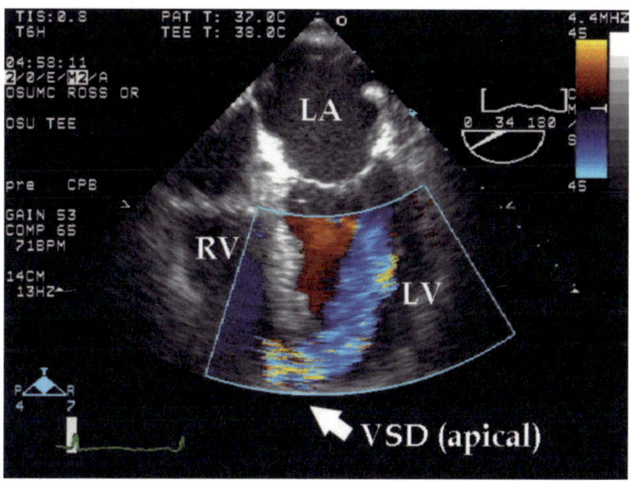

Figure 2. Transesophageal echo, 4-chamber view, demonstration an apical VSD with shunt from the left ventricle (LV) to the right ventricle (RV). The left atrium (LA) is also shown to illustrate the typical relationship of the defect to the mitral valve.

4.3. Cardiac Magnetic Resonance Imaging:

While the diagnosis is often made at the time of initial cardiac catheterization or echocardiography, occasionally a PI-VSD may be encountered as an incidental finding during other diagnostic imaging. While patients might be too hemodynamically unstable or the presence of an intra-aortic balloon pump might contraindicate cardiac MRI, with the growing indications and utilization of MRI for operative planning, PI-VSD might be encountered. Patients with low ejection fractions, cardiomyopathies, or suspicion for unusual cardiac anatomy, might have cardiac MRI performed to assess for myocardial viability, fibrosis, or valvular pathology. In these patients, a PI-VSD may be an unsuspected finding (Figure 3). Although there is little experience describing the role of cardiac MRI in PI-VSDs, using concepts derived from the literature on congenital shunts and defects, cardiac MRI might be of value in assisting in defining the extent of the defect, the shunt fraction, right ventricular function, and other associated pathophysiology [17]. Cardiac MRI might be of additional value in situations of questionable catheterization or echocardiographic results or in the assessment of the post-operative patient when a residual shunt is suspected. Nevertheless, MRI is, in general, not considered a first-line diagnostic imaging tool.

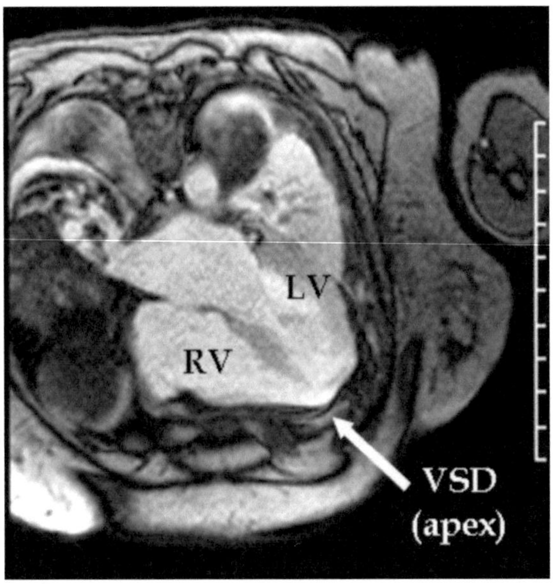

Figure 3. Cardiac MRI demonstrating an apical defect. Gated cine images indicated a left to right shunt in which quantitative assessment can be used to calculate the shunt fraction and size of the defect.

5. Pathophysiology

The pathophysiology reflects two different types of defects. The first, a simple rupture, is a direct through-and-through defect that is typically located anteriorly when associated with a LAD territory infarct. Alternatively, complex defects are believed to result from tracking of blood as it dissects thru the septum with left ventricular entry sites remote from right ventricular exit sites – these tracks then enlarge over time due to the pressure gradient between the left and right ventricle. Obviously, with unpredictable injury to the septum, there can be a combination of the 2 different pathologies. Multiple defects are found in 5-11% of cases and emphasized the need for a complex pre-operative and intra-operative assessment of all pathways to insure a complete repair [18] and the observation that most defects are probably larger than they initially appear. Incomplete closure of residual or secondary defects can account for post-operative recurrences. Transmural infarcts can be quite extensive with defects developing to several centimeters in diameter and can often involve extensive areas of the left ventricular free wall and potentially the annular structures of the mitral valve. For complex defects, as blood dissects through the necrotic myocardium there can be further expansion and damage with loss of cellular integrity. With local cellular destruction there is fragmentation with degeneration of myocytes with enzymatic digestion and destruction. In patients who survive the acute presentation, up to 66% develop chronic ventricular aneurysms and a third will have significant functional mitral regurgitation from the secondary effects on the ventricular free wall.

Interestingly, and clearly an area of further study, the pathologic consequences and outcomes of surgery of anterior and posterior defects are different in ways beyond what can be explained by the varying degree of shunting. Autopsy studies have shown that anterior PI-VSDs were associated with 33% of the LV and only 10% of the RV being infarcted, while posterior defects were associated with only 20% of the LV and 33% of the RV being infarcted [15]. Particularly considering the acute pressure/volume overload and associated RV failure, it becomes understandable why posterior based defects are associated with a worse prognosis.

6. Natural History

The natural history of untreated PI-VSD is also poorly understood. As advances in the acute and chronic management of coronary artery disease continues to evolve, so does complications of CAD such as AMI. In general, 25% of patients with PI-VSDs die within the first 24 hours [6]. Death is most commonly related to pre-existing comorbidities and the potentially irreversible and severe heart failure that comes from not only the acute pump failure from the inciting infarct but also the significant acute left to right heart shunting that only compromises systemic perfusion further. The sudden increase in pulmonary overcirculation also contributes to the development of significant right heart failure. For those patients who survive the acute event, 1, 2, and 4-week survival is 50%, 35%, and 20% respectively [31]. It is easy to appreciate that those patients who survive the first month may have inherently favorable variables that might further self-select for a good post-operative outcome. Prolonged untreated survival has been reported with up to 7% of patient surviving to 1 year – obviously the physiologic insult and over-circulation is minimal in these rare cases.

7. Timing/Indications for surgery

The mere presence of a PI-VSD is considered an indication for surgery with the majority of patients undergoing urgent or emergent operative intervention [38]. The primary goal of VSD closure is to reduce the end-organ damage from the combined insults of acute right ventricular overload/failure and systemic cardiogenic shock.

As soon as the diagnosis is made an intra-aortic balloon pump (IABP) should be placed. Coronary augmentation will assist the ischemic and injured myocardium. More importantly, an IABP will unload the left ventricle and improve cardiac output, and end-organ perfusion. By decreasing afterload, there will also be an improvement in pulmonary shunting and over-circulation. However, the physiologic improvements with IABP and other inotropic or vasoactive medications should only be viewed as transient and allow finishing the pre-operative assessment.

While some advocate a strategy of delayed repair, this approach is rarely successful. The hypothesis of this management plan is to give the friable necrotic myocardium time (3-6 weeks) to fibrosis thereby allowing for an easier and more secure repair. The scarred tissue will better hold suture and less likely to tear apart and result in an early post-operative failure. This approach appears reasonable, in theory, but it is rare that patients remain stable or can be supported during this time period. While guidelines for delayed surgical management are lacking, this might be an option in those who are hemodynamically or physiologically stable with a delayed presentation, have no or minimal signs of pulmonary hypertension or over-circulation, and have a stable fluid balance with good renal function. Unfortunately, such patients are rare and less than 5-10% of all PI-VSD patients will survive to allow for delayed repair. Such an approach may represent a "survival of the fittest" approach in those with minimal shunting and with strict attention to medical comorbidities and nutrition a period of close careful waiting may be clinically successful. This approach may also be used to justify waiting in patients who have other severe comorbidities precluding intervention and would, in theory, require optimization prior to surgery. Nevertheless, it is hard to argue that any other comorbidities would improve enough to the point of making surgery safer in the setting of worsening right ventricular heart failure – a problem that by itself is very difficult to treat both pre and post-operatively. Although, one can also suggest that in these patients, unless early surgical repair is clearly contraindicated, that their physiologic reserve combined with a minimal pathophysiologic insult might predispose them to a good outcome regardless of whether an early or late repair is performed.

Of growing concern regarding the timing of surgery and the implications of peri-operative management is the use of potent, and often irreversible, anti-platelet inhibitors and/or anticoagulants. The data and experience on operating on patients with some of these newer agents, the impact on the ability – or lack thereof – to achieve surgical hemostasis with such drugs is both limited and evolving. As many of these patients might have already been pretreated with P2Y12 inhibitors such as clopidogrel, or the more potent agents such as prasugrel or ticagrelor, the impact on bleeding and the timing of surgery can be worrisome. Furthermore, other agents used to facilitate coronary interventions, such as Gp IIb/IIIa inhibitors such as eptifibatide, or direct thrombin inhibitors such as bivalirudin might require an appropriate 'wash-out' period. The risk for a massive transfusion (particularly with platelets) at the time of surgery with these agents still active cannot be understated. In fact, at patient who already might be considered physiologically high-risk might be considered inoperable in the setting of recent Dabigatran (Pradaxa) exposure due to the risk of catastrophic, irreversible, surgical hemorrhage. In the post-operative period, the decision to restart a P2Y12 inhibitor, if indicated (i.e. for recent coronary stents), clearly needs to be a balance between the risk of bleeding and the risk of a stent thrombosis or recurrent ischemia. Hopefully, newer agents, such as cangrelor, which is an IV, short-acting, reversible, anti-platelet agent might lead to protocols that can assist in bridging patients to such high-risk surgical interventions – such as an acute PI-VSD [2].

8. Operative Management

The initial surgical techniques for PI-VSDs followed a surgical approach similar to that for congenital ventricular septal defects. The approach was through a ventriculotomy in the right ventricular outflow track (RVOT) [12]. It was quickly realized that this approach had significant drawbacks. Firstly, in an already dysfunctional and acutely injured right ventricle, the outflow tract incision only further reduced residual, crucial RV function. As importantly, while suited for many common types congenital septal defects near the aortic valve, the RVOT incisions offered poor exposure of defects that tended to be much further down the septum towards the apex. Most importantly, since the patch and suture line was on the RV side, the defect was still exposed to LV pressures and consequently was at increased risk for patch dehiscence, early recurrence, extension of the defect, and clinical failure. Pioneering animal studies by [22] advocated an approach to the VSD thru the left ventricle in the region of the culprit vessel through infracted myocardium – specifically, anterior defects approached through the anterior wall while posterior defects through the inferior wall. These techniques addressed many of the deficiencies of a RVOT approach [22]. The benefits of these animal studies were subsequently validated clinically within several years [26][8]

8.1. Basic Principles and Considerations

After the patient arrives in the operative room, routine anesthesia is induced. If not already in place, all patients should have arterial monitoring lines and a pulmonary artery (Swan-Ganz) catheter inserted. Pressures and oxygen saturations should be obtained to determine shunt fractions and to assist in determining the completeness of repair. Since these patients have left-to-right shunting, it is of critical importance to avoid pharmacologic agents that cause pulmonary vasodilation. Such agents would worsen the shunt, increase pulmonary over-circulation, and potentially worsening right heart dysfunction. Preoperative antibiotics including a first generation cephalosporin, such as cefazolin, and vancomycin are administered. In cases of antibiotic allergies, appropriate alternatives should be chosen.

Median sternotomy is performed and the patient is prepared for cardiopulmonary bypass. Minimally invasive techniques are typically not advocated for this type of extensive and complex procedure in which complete exposure of heart is helpful. However, in situations of re-operative surgery, depending on surgeon preferences, consideration should be given to peripheral cannulation (i.e. femoral or axillary) prior to sternotomy as a re-entry injury to an already compromised and dilated RV can be fatal. The patient is heparinized prior to standard aortic – right atrial cannulation. Some advocate routine bicaval venous drainage, but typically, as procedures on the tricuspid or mitral valves are not performed unless clearly indicated by pre-operative studies, this is not necessary. Cold-blood antegrade and retrograde cardioplegia is delivered via conventional root and coronary sinus catheters. Topically cooling to further reduce the metabolic demands of the already compromised heart is also liberally used. This author routinely uses ice-slush wrapped in gauze to further cool the right ventricle to assist in reducing the temperature and assists further in myocardial protection – a key component in minimizing post-operative biventricular dysfunction. Active or passive systemic cooling is performed with an ideal temperature of 25º-28ºC to further assist end-organ protection. Regardless, the key concept is an appropriate and well thought out approach to myocardial protection.

In general, once the defect is identified, a piece of either glutaraldehyde-fixed bovine pericardium or Dacron is cut to not only cover the defect but a generous rim of surrounding, and potentially non-viable, myocardium. Continuous suture or interrupted pledgeted sutures are used to suture the patch to the residual septum. Tension on the repair must be avoided to minimize the risk of the sutures tearing through once the ventricle is pressurized and begins to contract. The "Sandwich Technique" approach has been described to minimize the tension and risk for leakage of the final repair. In this technique, a patch is positioned on the RV side and re-enforced with pledgets. The defect, much like a "pot-hole" in the road, is then filled a gelatin-resorcin-formalin (GRF) glue and then covered on the left ventricular side with a similar patch and pledgets. The proposed advantage of this technique is that the glue serves as a cement to re-enforce the repair, minimize tension on the sutures lines, attempts to preserve ventricular geometry, and most importantly, reduces the risk of leaking. Early [24] and midterm results [25], although in limited studies, support this adjuvant to traditional patch repair techniques as described below. Although the "sandwich technique" advocated a repair via a right ventricular incision, such an approach, for reasons already outlined, may not be desirable – nevertheless, experience with this technique is growing and this might be a reasonable approach in selected patients [4]. For posterior defects the patch might require anchoring to the annulus of the mitral valve. For cases in which the annulus of the mitral valve and/or peri-valvular tissues is involved, mitral valve replacement may be required. The choice of prosthesis is up to the surgeon, but given the 5-year limited survival of these patients in general and the post-operative challenges that might come from the need for anticoagulation with a mechanical valve, a tissue valve in these cases is a reasonable option regardless of the patient's age and co-morbidities.

The intra-operative approach and management of the defect is based upon the location of the VSD and the need for concomitant procedures. The pre-operative assessment of the location of the defect is critical in determining the optimal approach to closing it.

8.2. Apical Defects

Apical septal defects involve the apical portion of the right ventricle, septum, and the left ventricle. As mentioned, such defects are typically the result of acute occlusion of the distal left anterior descending artery. Daggett and colleagues first described the technique of apical amputation and repair of the PI-VSD in 1970. The initial incision is created through the infracted tissue of the cardiac apex. The necrotic myocardium is then excised until healthy muscle is exposed and deemed adequate for repair. The healthy tissues of the right and left ventricle are then approximated to the septum using interrupted, felt pledgeted, heavy Tycron suture in a mattress fashion (Figure 4). Felt strips are placed along the right and left septal walls during this process to create a 'felt sandwich'. The apical repair can be reinforced with a second layer of suture. While meticulous hemostasis is critical, too much tension on the suture repair can tear through the muscle and result in uncontrolled post-operative hemorrhage.

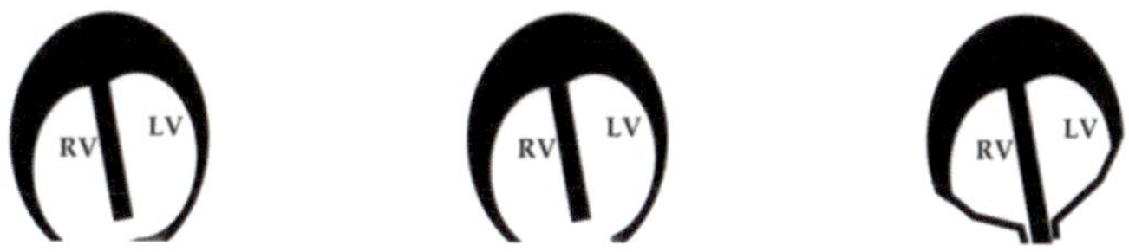

Figure 4. Apical repair involves excising the apical defect and bringing together the residual edges of the left and right ventricular walls using a primary repair reinforced with pledgets.

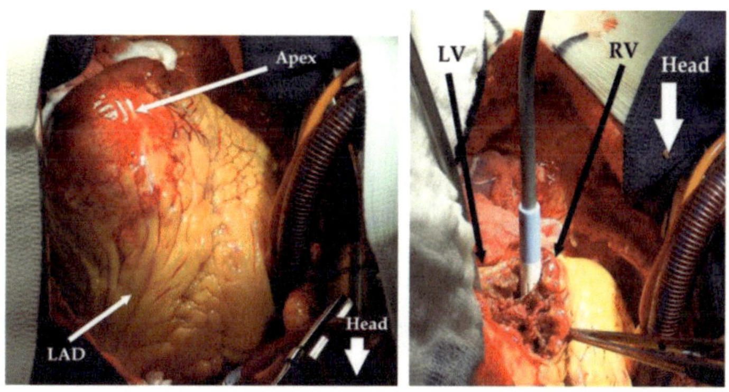

Figure 5. Left: Intra-operative view of the extensive apical infarction that has resulted in the echocardiographic findings demonstrated in Figure 2. The left anterior descending artery (LAD) is shown. Right: The same patient after opening and debridement of the infracted apex. The necrotic septum is visualized with a probe in the left ventricle (LV) and the bypass "pump sucker" is in the right ventricle (RV).

8.3. Anterior Defects

The anterior septal defect involves the anterior septum as well as the anterior left ventricular free wall. This, as discussed earlier, is typically a result of acute infarct of the LAD territory. The initial approach is via an incision in the left ventricular myocardium parallel to the LAD and through the non-viable or ischemic tissue. The infracted area is then excised and debrided back to healthy, viable myocardium. The septum is then inspected and necrotic tissue is excised in the same fashion. This is can be straightforward in a single, obvious defect. However, great care must be taken if the defect is noted to be tracking through the myocardium – a finding that might not be obvious. In general, the larger the patch the better - as a too small of a patch is more likely to pull through and dehisce.

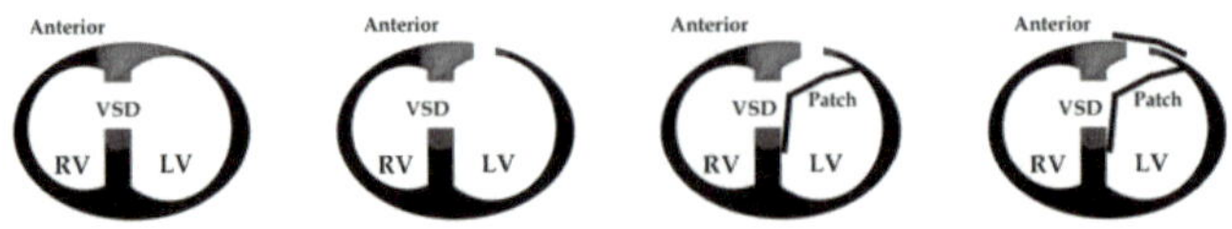

Figure 6. Picture representation of the various steps used to repair an anterior defect with the patch excluding the necrotic septum from the higher pressure left ventricular cavity. The incision is through the infracted muscle on the anterior wall, parallel to the left anterior descending artery.

Small defects can be plicated with a primary repair to the right ventricular free wall using interrupted, pledgeted suture as first suggested by Shumacker [42]. For anything other than very small (<1.0 cm) defects, most anterior septal infarcts will require repair with a patch. This is fashioned in a manner that will allow for a tension-free repair. Excess tension in the repair can lead to devastating consequences either with acutely life threatening bleeding or a delayed dehiscence and residual shunt.

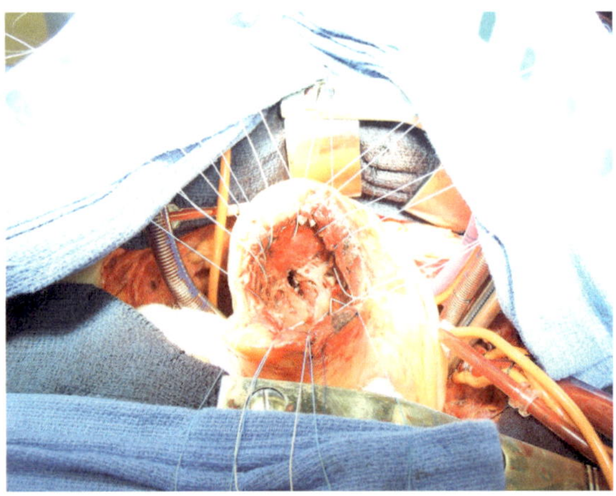

Figure 7. Intra-operative picture with the apex of the heart elevated (head and aortic cannula to the right). The incision is through the infarcted anterior wall. The septal defect is shown in the middle of the cavity with circumferential sutures around a wide margin. The sutured will then be placed through a pericardial patch to exclude the infracted septal muscle and defect from the left ventricular cavity.

Larger defects require the use of a prosthetic patch that is anchored to the posterior wall of the septum using interrupted, pledgeted Tycron or Proline suture to distribute the tension. The suture is passed from the RV through the LV so that the patch-septum interface lies in the left ventricle, as opposed to the RV. The anterior sutures are placed through the right ventricular free wall and tagged with hemostats (Figure 7). All sutures are placed prior to placing them through the patch. They can now be placed through the designated anterior region of the prosthetic patch and then through a second pledget if desired prior to tying the suture knots. The left ventricular free wall is then re-approximated using interrupted, mattress suture similar to apical repairs. A second layer of running suture, often with a strip of felt to distribute the tension of the closure, is placed for reinforcement.

8.4. Posterior Defects

The posterior or inferior septal defect involves a transmural infarction of the myocardium in the posterior descending artery distribution. The inferior wall is often thin and after infarction, is quite friable. For this reason, primary repair is not a durable option and is rarely successful. Attempt at primary repair, in which the myocardium is placed under tension, can have disastrous immediate, and potentially fatal, consequences. Hence, posterior/inferior septal defects are the most technically demanding of the PI-VSDs.

After the heart is arrested, the inferior wall is lifted out of the pericardial well and exposed. The transmural infarct may involve both ventricles, or the septum and left ventricle alone. The transinfarct incision is created in a longitudinal fashion in the left ventricle. The nonviable myocardium is excised, which will create adequate exposure of the septal defect which is critical for a durable repair. The papillary muscles are inspected. If the base is involved in the infarct resulting in ruptured papillary muscle, then mitral valve replacement is indicated. If a small posterior defect (<1.0 cm) is identified, primary repair to the ventricular free wall using pledgetted suture as described earlier is satisfactory – but this situation is very rare and placement of a small patch may result in a more durable outcome than risking a primary repair involving ischemic myocardial tissue.

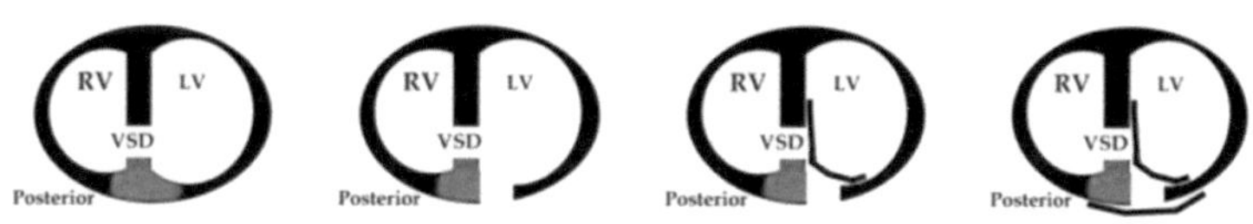

Figure 8. Similar to anterior repairs, the high pressure left ventricular cavity is isolated from the necrotic septum with a patch repair. The incision is along the distal right coronary along and parallel to the posterior descending artery through the infracted basal muscle.

As with anterior defects, most posterior defects will require a tension free repair by utilizing a patch closure. This technique often necessitates the use of two separate patches, one dedicated to the septal repair and the other to the wall of the ventricle. Principles as described previously apply. The pledgetted mattress sutures are placed from the right ventricle to the left along the circumference of the defect. The sutures are passed through the contoured patch and tied down. Great care should be taken to avoid lacerating the myocardium. Some authors suggest placing a second pledget on the patch side of the repair to minimize this risk. The posterior ventricular wall is repaired with the second patch using mattress sutures. Occasionally, depending on the size and quality of free wall myocardium, the free-edges can be approximated and closed primarily (and re-enforced with a pericardial or felt strip) rather than using a second patch.

8.5. General Principles

Closure of the ventriculotomy is performed by folding the free edge of the patch to the edge of the ventricle to exclude it from the circulation. The ventriculotomy repair is then closed with a primary closure re-enforced with strips of either Teflon felt or pericardium. Exclusion of the necrotic myocardium from the left ventricular is also important in minimizing the risk of small debris breaking off at any point and causing a systemic embolism. Biologic glues can be liberally used for small suture leaks, but it should be avoided in more significant bleeding as this might suggest a less than stable closure.

Regardless of the location of the ventriculotomy, it cannot be emphasized enough the importance of a tension free closure. Any unnecessary tension through injured or friable myocardium may predispose to catastrophic and potentially fatal post-operative bleeding once the ventricle becomes pressurized. In extreme cases involving extensive myocardial (free wall and septal) damage, temporary mechanical support with either extra-corporeal membrane oxygenation (ECMO) or a left ventricular assist device may help unload the ventricle to assist in recovery. The hypothesis behind this approach is by reducing the LV pressure, it will encourage recovery, reduce the pressure on the repair, and allow for further decision making in patients in whom there is extensive ventricular destruction and residual ventricular function may not be adequate to support physiologic needs [19].

Although the benefits of concomitant revascularization on long-term outcomes are debatable, complete coronary revascularization, if possible, is typically advocated [23]. As with other risk models for outcomes after surgery (e.g. EuroScore and STS models), it is the need for revascularization and the extent of underlying CAD that defines the long-term outcome rather than the actual performing of the procedure. Overall, the paradigm of complete and/or optimal revascularization should apply in cases of PI-VSD management. It is hard to refute the benefits of revascularization in the setting of an already acutely and chronically ischemic myocardium.

9. Post-operation Management

The post-operative management of patients following successful repair should be similar to that of other high-risk cardiac surgery patients. However, there are several key principles that must be remembered. As these patients often present and are taken to the operating room in acute decompensated heart failure, strict attention to optimizing biventricular function is critical. Post-operative left ventricular dysfunction is common and there should be a low threshold for placement of an intra-aortic balloon pump (IABP), particularly if one was not placed pre-operatively. While, as discussed below, the use of an IABP is often associated with worse outcomes, the relationship to a poor outcome is the need for its use and the potential delay in initiating therapy rather than the therapy itself that influences the adverse outcome. Right heart failure is common and often these patients require considerable therapies directed specifically at assisting in right heart management. Conventional intravenous agents such as epinephrine, milrinone, and dobutamine are often required – and sometimes at high doses. Inhaled agents that selectively reduce pulmonary vascular resistance and assist in reducing RV afterload such as inhaled nitric oxide (20-80 ppm) or epoprostenol (2,500 – 20,000 ng/min) may be required [37]. Ventricular arrhythmias are also common from the residual ischemic/necrotic myocardium (as well as secondary to the ventriculotomy) and anti-arrhythmic medications, such as amiodarone, should be used liberally. In addition, as the repaired septal defect and free wall are often quite friable, strict attention to avoid hypertension is important as even transient elevations in blood pressure can result in disruptions in either the patch repair or the ventriculotomy closure suture line that might precipitate uncontrolled and fatal cardiac bleeding. Any acute increase in chest tube drainage should raise the concern for ventricular suture line dehiscence and there should be a low threshold for returning the patient to the operating room for re-exploration – however, excess manipulation of the heart in the search for bleeding should be avoided at the risk of catastrophic suture-line tearing in a beating and pressurized ventricle. Any post-operative coagulopathy must be aggressively corrected. Although recovery in these patients is unpredictable, it may be prolonged. A slow wean of inotropes may be required and there should be a low threshold for repeat and/or frequent echocardiographic evaluations in a patient who is not improving as anticipated. Repeat echocardiography might show a residual shunt or valvular dysfunction, more importantly may identify easy to correct problems, such as tamponade.

10. Outcomes: Predictors of Survival

The increasing rarity of PI-VSD implies that few centers are able to report an extensive series. Even though several large single center experiences and outcomes have been reported, most summarize years of experience and may not take into consideration the improvements in peri-operative management, surgical skills, and – probably most importantly – the clinical judgment necessary for the management of these critically ill patients.

In the GUSTO trial in which 41,021 patients were randomized to different strategies of reperfusion during AMI, 84 developed a PI-VSD. 34 of these were managed surgically, with 31 (90%) undergoing early treatment and 3 (10%) undergoing delayed surgery. Survival in the surgical group was 53% at 30 days and 47% at 1 year. Conversely, for those treated medically, as an indicator of the lethality of this problem, survival at 30 days and 1 year was 6% and 3%, respectively [13]. All patients who presented in Class III or IV heart failure died.

Deja and colleagues reported their experience with 117 patients from the Glenfield General Hospital in England. In their series, there were 76 anterior defects and 34 posterior defects. The mean age was 65 ± 8 years and 43 of the 117 were females. One third of patients were in cardiogenic shock at the time of presentation. The average time from AMI to the development (or diagnosis) of a PI-VSD was 6 days. The time interval from the point of diagnosis to surgical intervention was 9 days. The overall mortality was 37% and this does not include the 6.4% intra-operative mortality. Forty percent had evidence of a residual left-right shunt with 13 patients undergoing early re-operation. In patients undergoing re-operative surgery, mortality was 30%. Table 1 summarizes their overall results. The predictors of post-operative mortality included:

1. shock at time of surgery,
2. clinical deterioration while awaiting surgery,
3. need for concomitant CABG, and
4. pre-operative renal failure (as a marker for shock and organ failure).

The obvious criticism of this report is the long interval from the time of diagnosis to the time of surgery as earlier intervention, as advocated, might have resulted in less end-organ damage in an already compromised patient (Deja MA, 2002).

Overall surgical mortality (%)	37%
Intra-operative mortality (%)	6.4 %
Need for extra-corporeal membrane oxygenation (ECMO)	2 %
Re-exploration/bleeding	5 %
Average ICU Stay	4.8 days
Average Ventilator Time	40 hours
Major inotropic support	90 %
Use of Intra-aortic balloon pump	75 %
Tracheostomy	5%
Continuous renal replacement	16 %
Stroke	5 %
Residual shunt	40%

Table 1. Post-Operative Complications Following Surgical Repair (From Deja MA, 2002)

National registry data has proven useful to define the real-world experiences with this uncommon problem. In a report from Sweden, outlining the national experience with 189 patients, several factors were found to be predictive of favorable vs. unfavorable short (< 30 days) and long-term (> 30 days) outcomes (Tables 2 and 3) [27].

Favorable Predictors
Short time from MI to Diagnosis
Short time from Diagnosis to Operating Room
Short time from MI to Operating Room
Pre-Op catheterization
Anterior rupture
Unfavorable Predictors
IABP
Stroke/Coma
Renal failure
Re-Op for bleeding
No effect on outcome
Age
Gender
Pre-Op IABP
Pre-Op Lytic therapy
Concomitant CABG
Residual shunt

Table 2. Predictors of short-term (< 30-day) survival based on National Swedish Experience (Adapted from Jeppsson et al. Euro J Cardiothor Surg 2005;27:216-221). CABG: Coronary artery bypass surgery, IABP: Intra-aortic balloon pump, MI: Myocardial infarction.

Favorable Predictors
Younger age
Unfavorable Predictors
Pre-Op IABP
Pre-Op catheterization
Need for CABG
Renal Failure requiring dialysis
Residual shunt
No effect on outcome
Anterior rupture
Time from MI to Operating Room
Post-Op stroke
Pre-Op Lytic therapy
Post-Op IABP
Re-Op for bleeding

Table 3. Predictors of Long-Term (> 30 day) Survival. See above for legend.

The Italians also presented their experience with the outcomes of 58 patients treated between 1992 and 2000 [10]. The mean age was 73 years. Thirty-six percent presented in acute renal failure, 33% were in atrial fibrillation, and 22% were insulin dependent diabetics. Most (57%) were in NYHA Class IV heart failure and 41% were in cardiogenic shock. Intra-aortic balloon pumps were used in only 20% of patients. Sixty percent had associated significant mitral regurgitation. The timing of surgery was 14 ± 12 days from the acute event with 76% undergoing surgery within the first 3 weeks and 31% within the first 24 hours. A key point is again emphasizing the importance of early diagnosis and surgery before the onset of shock and organ failure (Table 4).

	Non-Survivors (n=30)	Survivors (n=28)
Time to OR (days)	11 ± 8	21 ± 13
% to OR < 24hrs	43 %	18 %
Pre-operative Shock	57 %	28 %
Pre-operative sPAP (mmHg)	56 ± 14	42 ± 11
CPB time (time)	126 ± 35	95 ± 28
Post-operative IABP	90 %	39 %
Post-operative LVEF (%)	29 ± 2	45 ± 2
Post-operative Renal Failure	66 %	25 %

Table 4. Italian Registry Data. Legend: CPB: Cardiopulmonary bypass, IABP: Intra-aortic balloon pump, LVEF: Left ventricular ejection fraction, sPAP: Systolic pulmonary artery pressure. Table adapted from Cerin et al. Inter Soc Cardiovasc Surg 2003;11:149-154

In a series of 50 patients, operated on over 19 years (1983-2002), Mantovani et al reported their single center experience. The mean age of 66 ± 9 years (range: 45-81) who presented with either anterior (n=30, 60%) or posterior (n=20, 40%) PI-VSDs. Most patients developed their defects within the first week (76%) with an average of 4 days post-AMI. Only 2 patients presented after 2 days. Cardiac catheterization was performed in 98% of patients. Coronary angiography revealed single vessel disease in 51% of patients, double vessel disease in 35%, and 14% had triple vessel disease. Pre-operative IABP was used in 56% of patients and 74% underwent surgery within 2 days of diagnosis of a PI-VSD. Operative mortality (within 30 days) was 36% with 6 operative deaths. Posterior defects were associated with 50% mortality versus 25% for anterior. Other univariate risk factors for early death included:

cross-clamp time >100 minutes (p=0.035);

emergent surgery (p=0.02); and delayed surgical intervention (>3 days post diagnosis, p=0.0055).

Interestingly, in their experience factors not associated with operative/post-operative mortality included: gender, extent of CAD (single vs. triple vessel disease), need for CABG, age (>65 years), or the year of operation (before/after 1992). In a logistic regression analysis, only emergent surgery (odds ration: 10.23) and a delayed treatment (OR: 4.03) were the only predictors of early post-operative or operative mortality. Long-term survival was 76.5 ± 7.8 and 56.1 ± 11.5% at 5 and 10 years suggesting a reasonable outcome for this catastrophic problem. No significant predictors of long-term survival were found in their analysis.

However, patients with residual myocardium at risk from incomplete revascularization tended to have a worse long-term prognosis [32].

A review of the Society of Thoracic Surgeons National Database has also provided some valuable insight into the management and outcomes of the problem of PI-VSD. Arnaoutakis retrospectively reviewed all adult patients who underwent surgical repair of a PI-VSD between 1999 and 2010 [3]. In this review, there were 2,876 patients – reflecting probably the largest series reviewed. In this cohort, 56.5% were males, almost half (49.7%) underwent emergent surgical intervention, and 65% had a pre-operative IABP. One third (33%) had undergone a previous percutaneous coronary intervention and 7.5% had undergone a previous CABG. The annual incidence of PI-VSD was relatively constant and ranged from 232-297 cases/year and implies that few reporting centers have a significant experience with this complex problem - of the 666 centers reporting data to the database the experience ranged from 0.09 to 3.7 cases/center/year. Consistent with previous reports, the overall operatively mortality was 42.9%. They found an inverse relationship between the timing of surgery and survival. Patients operated on within 6 hours of presentation had a 54% mortality. Survival was ~50% for the patients operated on between 1 and 7 days. However, of the 513 patients operated on >21 days after presentation had a <20% mortality – again, suggesting that those who present late and remain hemodynamically stable have a better long-term prognosis. Furthermore, when classified as elective, survival was 87% versus 20% for salvage operations. Refractory cardiac failure was the most common cause of death post-operatively. Clearly, maintaining hemodynamic and physiologic stability is key to a good outcome. Table 5 lists the predictors of a good outcome.

Favorable	Unfavorable
FAVORABLE FACTORS	**UNFAVORABLE FACTORS**
Male gender	Older age
Hypertension	Chronic kidney disease
Smoking	Need for pre-operative IABP
Chronic lung disease	Pre-operative shock
Pre-operative NYHA Class IV	Previous CABG
Pre-operative beta-blocker	Triple vessel CAD
Pre-operative lipid agent	Lower Ejection Fraction
Elective repair	Salvage surgery
Short bypass time	Longer aortic cross-clamp time

Table 5. Adopted from Society for Thoracic Surgeons National Registry Database on favorable vs. unfavorable predictors of survival after repair of PI-VSD in 2,876 patients.

In a multi-variate analysis of the clinical characteristics, the following variables were found to be predictors of post-operative death:

1. Advancing age (>65 years/old)
2. Lower Ejection Fraction
3. Female (vs. male)
4. Pre-operative cardiogenic shock
5. Pre-operative need for intra-aortic balloon pump
6. Peripheral vascular disease
7. Percutaneous coronary intervention within 6 hours of surgery
8. Re-do cardiac surgery
9. Emergent/Salvage surgery
10. Pre-operative dialysis
11. Pre-operative mitral regurgitation

Of all of the variables, the strongest predictor of a poor outcome was pre-operative renal failure requiring dialysis. Interestingly, favorable variables included a history of hypertension, congestive heart failure, and need for concomitant CABG. The authors emphasized patients, due to their physiologic status, who required earlier intervention tended to have worse outcome. Obviously, the controversies regarding the balance between the timing of intervention and clinical optimization continue.

Unfortunately, there is little data reporting long-term survival. In their report of 68 patients undergoing surgery for PI-VSD between 1988 and 2007, Fukushima and colleagues from Brisbane, Australia provide some valuable insight and predictors of long-term outcomes [21]. In their report, 85% of patients underwent urgent surgery within 48 hours of diagnosis, 71% had concomitant CABG, and 30-day mortality was 35%. The mean follow-up was 9.2 years. Overall short-time outcomes and predictors of survival were similar to previous reports (as discussed above). The actuarial survival at 1 year was 67%, 63% at five years, 51% at 10 years, and 36% at 15 years. However, freedom from main adverse coronary events of the survivors was 91%, 61%, 40%, and 19% at 30 days, 1 year, 5 years, and 15 years respectively. At 5 years, freedom from congestive heart failure was 70% and 85% for ventricular arrhythmias – while at 10 years, 54% were free of heart failure and 71% from arrhythmias. For the cumulative survival analysis, there were 43 patients alive a 1 year, 34 at 5 years, 22 at 10 years, and 6 at 15 years.

11. Controversial Topics

11.1. Percutaneous Closure devices

Successful application of less invasive non-surgical options and closure devices in children with congenital VSDs has prompted enthusiasm for the use of similar closure devices in patients with PI-VSDs. The role of such devices has been proposed for both the primary closure of acute defects and to assist in the closure of recurrent or residual shunts [41].

However, because of the appeal of a less-invasive, non-surgical, option for these critically ill patients, investigators continue to try and define the role of septal occluder devices in patients with PI-VSDs. Attia recently reviewed the literature of such devices [5]. Thirty manuscripts were reviewed, but only 5 studies, consisting of approximately 100 patients, were felt to provide some insight into a "best practice" recommendation – despite numerous case reports. The general recommendations were that 1) surgical management still should be considered the 'gold standard' for patients with PI-VSDs but occluder devices might have a role in small defects (< 15 mm diameter) and in patients who present late (> 3.5 weeks after the index event). Attia also suggested a potential role in attempting to minimize a significant shunt in patients who are too ill to survive surgery as temporizing and potential means of stabilizing a patient prior to urgent surgical intervention.

While conceptually promising, the complex nature of acute defects as compared to congenital defects has tempered some of the early enthusiasm as early experiences were discouraging and improvements in outcomes were not observed [35]. Difficulties in covering not only the actual defect, but also the residual necrotic myocardium predisposed to early recurrence. Challenges remain in the technology because of problems positioning the devices and adequately covering potentially complex defects.

11.2. Mechanical Support

Despite advances in surgical and post-operative management, operative mortality is still high and depending on clinical presentation can vary between 10-60%[14]. Even with early intervention, biventricular failure is often a significant factor in early post-operative deaths. Short and long-term mechanical support, beyond intra-aortic balloon counterpulsation, is a reasonable option in patients with post-operative ventricular (left, right, or bi) failure and who are felt to be salvageable. Short-term support may be required as a bridge to recovery, while long-term device therapy may be indicated for those with irreversible ventricular failure. Since early acute co-morbidities and associated cardiogenic shock predict poor outcomes, there is some evidence and support for pre-operative biventricular mechanical support to allow for clinical optimization and stabilization as a bridge to definitive repair [11].

In cases in which there is extensive ventricular infarction and acute heart failure, associated free-wall rupture, or when there is excessive bleeding or tension from the ventriculotomy, temporary left ventricular support should be considered. With LVAD inflow drainage from the left atrium, the LV is unloaded (i.e. 'atrialized') and may allow time as a bridge to recovery before exposing the compromized left ventricle to systemic pressures and contractile function [19].

Right ventricular mechanical support is also difficult following the acute volume/pressure overload of a PI-VSD with recovery unpredictable and potentially prolonged. Unfortunately, there is little data to guide decision making other than clinical judgment and center experience with management of acute post-cardiotomy right heart failure.

Residual shunts after repair pose a unique challenge for patients requiring mechanical support. Careful attention to left and right ventricular flows and pressures are critical to compensate for the residual shunt – and prevent worsening of over-circulation [39]. If residual shunts are significant then biventricular support, either with long-term ventricular assist devices or extra-corporeal membrane oxygenation, may allow for a period of recovery and stabilization prior to an attempted repair in an otherwise very high-risk surgical patient [44]. The decision to intervene surgically on residual shunts, because of the extremely high operative mortality as discussed above, must clearly be made in the context of the overall clinical condition of the patient. Small defects can be managed medically and can be surprisingly well tolerated physiologically for years.

The need for mechanical support, while attractive in unstable post-operative patients, is also not without substantial risks. Often there is need for aggressive anti-coagulation, multiple surgical procedures (i.e. device change-outs, explants, re-operation for bleeding, etc), and overall patient recovery is more difficult when tethered to external VAD controllers. In addition, the risks for infectious complications with long-term support are considerable.

A total artificial heart, by definition, eliminates native cardiac recovery and mandates cardiac transplantation, nevertheless, it may be an option with appropriate resources and experience in highly selected patient with few other comorbidities and in general, is probably a poor idea.

11.3. Residual/Recurrent Defects

Residual shunts are found in up to 25% of patients after definitive repair [43]. The etiology of residual shunts is either a missed defect at the time of initial repair, dehiscence of a patch (sewn to necrotic or friable tissue), or further extension of the initial defect. Fortunately, most residual shunts tend to be physiologically tolerated and spontaneous closure has been reported. Operative re-intervention is associated with a >60% mortality [27] and surgery is reserved for patients in heart failure failing medical management or those with large shunts (Qp:Qs>2.0) [34]. Because of the high operative mortality with repairing residual or recurrent shunts there has been interest, but limited success, with percutaneous closure devices [41]. Nevertheless, the role of percutaneous closure and the ideal devices are undefined [35] and probably best reserved for use in those centers with extensive experience in the closure of congenital VSDs.

12. Conclusions

Ventricular septal defects after acute myocardial infarction are rare events. With modern reperfusion strategies, septal defects occur in up to 0.02% of acute myocardial infarctions. Despite advances and experiences in the management of these complex patients, operative mortality still approaches 50% with major risks including cardiogenic shock, renal failure, right and/or left ventricular failure, size of the defect with degree of shunting, posterior/inferior locations, and residual post-repair shunting. While some patients may present late or benefit from watchful waiting and a delayed repair, typically surgical intervention is indicated prior to irreversible end-organ damage. Repair techniques emphasize closure of the defect and protecting the injured septum from left ventricular pressures while avoiding additional injury to the already compromised left and right ventricles. Post-operative management is typically challenging considering the inherent pre-operative biventricular dysfunction and often encountered end-organ dysfunction. Those who survive their initial event and operation tend to have favorable 5 and 10-year survivals.

13. Conflicts of Interest

The authors have no conflicts of interest or disclosures related to any of the topics or technologies discussed in this manuscript.

Acknowledgements

This chapter, figures, and tables were adopted from a previous version with permission from InTech for use of copyrighted images [20].

Author details

Michael S. Firstenberg[1*], Kevin T. Kissling[2] and Karen Nelson[1]

*Address all correspondence to: Michael.Firstenberg@osumc.edu

1 Division of Cardiac Surgery, U. S. A.

2 Department of Pharmacy, The Ohio State University Medical Center, U. S. A.

References

[1] Agnihotri, A. K., Madsen, J. C., & Daggett, W. M. (2008). Surgical Treatment of Complications of Acute Myocardial Infarction: Postinfarction Ventricular Septal Defect and Free Wall Rupture. *Cohn L, ed. Cardiac Surgery in the Adult. New York: McGraw-Hill*, 753-784.

[2] Angiolillo, D. J., Firstenberg, M. S., Price, M. J., et al. (2012). BRIDGE Investigators. Bridging antiplatelet therapy with cangrelor in patients undergoing cardiac surgery: a randomized controlled trial. JAMA 18 , 307(3), 265-74.

[3] Arnaoutakis, G. J., Zhao, Y., George, T. J., Sciortino, C. M., Mc Carthy, P. M., & Conte, J. V. (2012). Surgical Repair of Ventricular Septal Defect After Myocardial Infarction: Outcomes From The Society of Thoracic Surgeons National Database. *Annals of Thoracic Surgery*, 94(2), 436-444.

[4] Asai, T., Hosoba, S., & Kinoshita, Suzuki T. (2012). Postinfarction Ventricular Septal Defect: Right Ventricular Approach- The Extended "Sandwich" Patch. *Semin Thoracic Surg*, 24, 59-62.

[5] Attia, R., & Blauth, C. (2010). Which patients might be suitable for a septal occluder device closure of postinfarction ventricular septal rupture rather than immediate surgery? *Interactive Cardiovascular and Thoracic Surgery* [11], 626-629.

[6] Berger, T. J., Blackstone, E. H., & Kirklin, J. W. (1993). Postinfarction ventricular septal defect. *in Kirklin JW, Barratt-Boyes BG (eds): Cardiac Surgery. New York, Churchill Livingstone*, 403.

[7] Brunn, F. (1923). Diagnostik der erworbenen ruptur der kammerscheidewand des herzens. *Wien Arch Inn Med*, 6, 533.

[8] Buckley, M. J., Mundth, E. D., Daggett, W. M., De Sanctis, R. W., Sanders, C. A., & Austen, W. G. (1971). Surgical therapy for early complications of myocardial infarction. *Surgery*, 70(6), 814-20.

[9] Buda, A. J. (1991). The role of echocardiography in the evaluation of mechanical complications of acute myocardial infarction. *Circulation*, 84, 3, I109-21.

[10] Cerin, G., Di Donato, M., Dimulescu, D., Montericcio, V., Menicanti, L., Frigiola, A., & De Ambroggi, L. (2003). Surgical treatment of ventricular septal defect complicating acute myocardial infarction. Experience of a north Italian referral hospital. *Cardiovasc Surg*, Apr, 11(2), 149-54.

[11] Conradi, L., Treede, H., Brickwedel, J., & Reichenspurner, H. (2009). Use of initial biventricular mechanical support in a case of postinfarction ventricular septal rupture as a bridge to surgery. *Ann Thorac Surg*, May, 87(5), e37-9.

[12] Cooley, D. A., Belmonte, B. A., Zeis, L. B., & Schnur, S. (1957). Surgical repair of ruptured interventricular septum following acute myocardial infarction. *Surgery*, 41(6), 930-7.

[13] Crenshaw, B. S., Granger, C. B., Birnbaum, Y., et al. (2000). Risk factors, angiographic patterns and outcomes in patients with ventricular septal defect complicating acute myocardial infaction. GUSTO-1 (Global Utilization of Streptokinase and TPA for Occluded Coronary Arteries). Trial Investigators. *Circulation*, 101(1), 27-32.

[14] Cummings, R. G., Califf, R., Jones, R. N., Reimer, K. A., King, Y. H., & Lowe, J. E. (1989). Correlates of survival in patients with postinfarction ventricular septal defect. *Ann Thorac Surg*, 47, 824-30, (update: 1997;63:1508-9).

[15] Cummings, R. G., Reimer, K. A., Califf, R., Hackel, D., Boswick, J., & Lowe, J. E. (1988). Quantitative analysis of right and left ventricular infarction in the presence of postinfarction ventricular septal defect. *Circulation*, 77(1), 33-42.

[16] Deja, M. A., Szostek, J., Widenka, K., et al. (2000). Post infarction ventricular septal defect-can we do better? *Eur J Cardiothorac Surg*, 18, 194.

[17] Didier, D., & Higgins, C. B. (1986). Identification and localization of ventricular septal defect by gated magnetic resonance imaging. *Am J Cardiol*, 57(15), 1363-8.

[18] Edwards, B. S., Edwards, W. D., & Edwards, J. E. (1984). Ventricular septal rupture complicating acute myocardial infarction: identification of simple and complex types in 53 autopsied hearts. *Am J Cardiol*, 54, 1201.

[19] Firstenberg, M. S., Blais, D., Crestanello, J., Sai-Sudhakar, C., Sirak, J., Louis, L. B., Vesco, P., & Sun, B. (2009). Long-term mechanical support for complex left ventricular postinfarct pseudoaneurysms. *Heart Surg Forum*, 12(5), E291-3.

[20] Firstenberg, M. S., & Rousseau, J. (2012). Post Myocardial Infarction Ventricular Septal Defect. *Front Lines of Thoracic Surgery, Stefano Nazari (Ed.)*, 978-9-53307-915-8, InTech, Available from:, http://www.intechopen.com/books/front-lines-of-thoracic-surgery/post-myocardial-infarction-ventricular-septal-defect.

[21] Fukushima, S., Tesar, P. J., Jalali, H., Clarke, A. J., Sharma, H., Choudhary, J., Bartlett, H., & Pohlner, P. G. (2010). Determinants of in-hospital and long-term surgical outcomes after repair of postinfarction ventricular septal rupture. *J Thorac Cardiovasc Surg*, Jul, 140(1), 59-65.

[22] Heimbecker, R. O., Lemire, G., & Chen, C. (1968). Surgery for massive myocardial infarction. An experimental study of emergency infarctectomy with a preliminary report on the clinical application. *Circulation*, 37(4), II3-11.

[23] Heitmiller, R., Jacobs, M. L., & Daggett, W. M. (1986). Surgical Management of Postinfarction Ventricular Septal Rupture. *Ann Thorac Surg*, 41(6), 683-691.

[24] Isoda, S., Imoto, K., Uchida, K., et al. (2004). Sandwich Technique, via Right Ventricular Incision to Repair Postinfarction Ventricular Septal Defect. *J Card Surg*, 19, 149-150.

[25] Isoda, S., Osako, M., Kimura, T., et al. (2012). Midterm Results of the "Sandwich Technique" via a Right Ventricle Incision to Repair Post-Infarction Ventricular Septal Defect. *Ann Thorac Cardiovasc Surg*, 18, 318-321.

[26] Javid, H., Hunter, J. A., Naiafi, H., Dye, W. S., & Julian, O. C. (1972). Left ventricular approach for the repair of ventricular septal perforation and infarctectomy. *J Thorac Cardiovasc Surg*, Jan, 63(1), 14-24.

[27] Jeppsson, A., Liden, H., Johnsson, P., Hartford, M., & Radegran, K. (2005). Surgical repair of post infarction ventricular septal defects: a national experience. *Euro J Cardiothor Surg*, 27, 216-221.

[28] Kishon, Y., Iqbal, A., Oh, J. K., Gersh, B. J., Freeman, W. K., Seward, J. B., & Tajik, A. J. (1993). Evolution of echocardiographic modalities in detection of postmyocardial infarction ventricular septal defect and papillary muscle rupture: study of 62 patients. *Am Heart J*, 126(3 Pt 1), 667-75.

[29] Labrousse, L., Choukroun, E., Chevalier, J. M., et al. (2002). Surgery for post- infarction ventricular septal defect (VSD): risk factors for hospital death and long term results. *Euro J Cardiothor Surg*, 21, 725-732.

[30] Latham, P. M. (1845). Lectures on Subjects Connected with Clinical Medicine Comprising Diseases of the Heart. *London, Longman Rees.*

[31] Lemery, R., Smith, H. C., Giuliani, E. R., & Gersh, B. J. (1992). Prognosis in rupture of the ventricular septum after acute myocardial infarction and role of early surgical intervention. *Am J Cardiol*, 70, 147.

[32] Mantovani, V., Mariscalco, G., Leva, C., Blanzola, C., & Sala, A. (2006). Surgical repair of post-infarction ventricular septal defect: 19 years of experience. *International Journal of Cardiology*, 108, 202-206.

[33] Muehrcke, D. D., Daggett, W. M., Buckley, M. J., et al. (1992). Postinfarct ventricular septal defect repair: effect of coronary artery bypass grafting. *Ann Thorac Surg*, 54, 876.

[34] Murashita, T., Komiya, T., Tamura, N., Sakaguchi, G., Kobayashi, T., & Sunagawa, G. (2010). The clinical challenge to reduce the postoperative residual shunt in surgical repair of postinfarction ventricular septal perforation. *Interact Cardiovasc Thorac Surg*, 11(1), 38-41.

[35] Pienvichit, P., & Piemonte, T. C. (2001). Percutaneous closure of postmyocardial infarction ventricular septal defect with the CardioSEAL septal occluder implant. *Catheterization and Cardiovascular Interventions*, 54, 490-494.

[36] Poulsen, S. H., Praestholm, M., Munk, Wierup. P., Egeblad, H., & Nielsen-Knudsk, J. E. (2008). Ventricular septal rupture complicating acute myocardial infarction: Clinical characteristics and contemporary outcome. *Ann Thorac Surg*, 85, 1591-1596.

[37] Rich, G. F., Murphy, G. D., Jr Roos, C. M., & Johns, R. A. (1993). Inhaled nitric oxide. Selective pulmonary vasodilation in cardiac surgical patients. *Anesthesiology*, 78(6), 1028-35.

[38] Ryan, T. J., Antman, E. M., Brooks, N. H., et al. update: ACC/AHA guidelines for the management of patients with acute myocardial infarction. A report of the American College of Cardiology/American Heart Association Task Force on Practice Guidelines (Committee on Management of Acute Myocardial Infarction). *J Am Coll Cardiol*, 34(3), 890-911.

[39] Sai-Sudhakar, C. B., Firstenberg, M. S., & Sun, B. (2006). Biventricular mechanical assist for complex, acute post-infarction ventricular septal defect. *J Thorac Cardiovasc Surg*, 132(5), 1238-9.

[40] Sager, R. (1934). Coronary thrombosis: perforation of the infarcted interventricular septum. *Arch Intern Med*, 53, 140.

[41] Shah, N. R., Goldstein, J. A., Balzer, D. T., Lasala, J. M., & Moazami, N. (2005). Transcatheter repair of recurrent postinfarct ventricular septal defects. *Ann Thorac Surg*, 80(5), 1907-9.

[42] Shumacker, H. (1972). Suggestions concerning operative management of postinfarction ventricular septal defects. *J Thorac Cardiovasc Surg*, 64, 452.

[43] Skillington, P. D., Davies, R. H., Luff, A. J., et al. (1990). Surgical treatment for infarct-related ventricular septal defects. Improved early results combined with analysis of late functional status. *J Thorac Cardiovasc Surg*, 99(5), 798-808.

[44] Tsai, M. T., Wu, H. Y., Chan, S. H., & Luo, C. Y. (2012). Extracorporeal membrane oxygenation as a bridge to definite surgery in recurrent postinfarction ventricular septal defect. *ASAIO J*, 58(1), 88-9.

Chapter 12

Diagnostics and Surgical Treatment of Left Ventricular Aneurysm with Ventricular Tachycardia

Vladimir Shipulin, Vadim Babokin, Sergey Andreev, Vladimir Usov, Ruslan Aimanov, Anthony Bogunetsky, Roman Batalov and Sergey Popov

Additional information is available at the end of the chapter

http://dx.doi.org/10.5772/54126

1. Introduction

Left ventricular aneurysm (LVA) in postinfarction period makes for worse prognosis of coronary artery disease (CAD) course due to concomitant complications. With the natural course of postinfarction aneurysms 5 year survival varies from 25 to 60%, according to various authors. Ventricular arrhythmias cause death in 50% of the patients with remodelled left ventricle (LV) after myocardial infarction [1].

Contrast-enhanced magnetic resonance imaging (MRI) is the method of choice for the evaluation of myocardial viability in patients with chronic CAD and with LVA in particular [2,3,4].

Meanwhile, data of contrast-enhanced MRI pictures with condition of electrophysiological activity and topical diagnosis of ventricular tachycardia in patients who had experienced myocardial infarction complicated with LVA have not been compared. At the same time, need for surgical treatment of cardiac aneurysm combined with intraoperative ablation of arrhythmogenic areas of myocardium arises no doubts since it allows for better treatment outcomes in the early postoperative period and in the late follow-up [4,5,6].

Thus, the objective of our study was to enhance efficacy of topical diagnostics and of surgical treatment in patients with postinfarction LV aneurysms complicated with ventricular rhythm disorders through application of contrast-enhanced MRI, electrophysiological study (EPhS) of the heart and optimal dissection or ablation of scarred and arrhythmogenic endocardium.

2. Materials and methods

The study included 188 patients operated for postinfarction anterior septal and apical LVA. The disease was diagnosed basing on the data of echocardiography (EchoCG), coronary ventriculography (CVG) and contrast-enhanced MRI.

Prior to the surgery the patients mostly had III-IV CC angina class, their condition corresponded to that of New York Heart Association (NYHA) class II-III for chronic heart failure. All the patients demonstrated evidence of postinfarction LV remodeling according to the results of ventriculography and EchoCG.

Cardiac inversion recovery and T-1 spin-echo weighed MRI study with ECG synchronization was performed with a patient lying flat with no additional functional stress. Axial slices on the level of thorax with the complete coverage of heart area were recorded. The field of view was 350-380 mm wide and 7-8mm thick slices were recorded into the matrix of 256x256 voxels. Synchronization of the recordings of MRI pictures with ECG was performed by standard means of an open PRI scanner Magnetom-Open (0,2 T by Siemens Medical) or high field open MRI scanner Vantage Titan (1,5 T, by Toshiba) by R-wave of ECG; end-diastolic images were acquired in all the cases. Parameters of the acquired T1-weighed images in spin-echo mode were as follows: repetition time (TR) 550 – 1040ms, echo time (TE) – 20 ms. MRI included slices with long axis two-chamber and four-chamber views as well as short axis view covering all the myocardial volume of LV. The study was performed in 12-20 minutes after injection of paramagnetic contrast agents with the concentration of paramagnetic agent itself of 0,5M (Omniscan, Magnevist, Optimark, Cyclomang, Viewgam) in dosage of 2ml/10kg of a body weight. The short-axis and long-axis slices in four-chamber view were divided semi-automatically into 17 segments taking into account generally accepted segmentation of LV myocardium (Fig.1) [7].

In particular, for each segment i (i = 1 – 17) we calculated the depth of damage by the degree of paramagnetic contrast agent uptake as follows: $[\text{Index of Transmurality}]_i$ = (maximum thicknesses of paramagnetic contrast agent uptake$)_i$ / (thickness of myocardium in a particular segment$)_i$ (Figure 2). (original data)

To see the association between MR images with the data of electrophysiological condition of heart muscle, and in particular with the location of the areas with lowered voltage of local electrical activity, the patients underwent electrophysiological study of the heart (EPhS) with electroanatomical CARTO reconstruction of LV [20]. Besides, there were identified the areas of delayed conduction, zones of possible re-entry and inducible VT (Figure 3).

Locations of intracardiac leads and thus of segmental electrical activity corresponded to the locations of left ventricular segments during contrast-enhanced MRI. In accordance with the amplitude of the curve during EPhS for a definite myocardial segment, degree of potential reduction was graded as follows: 0 – for the amplitude of the potential from 1,5 to 8 mV, when the segment was considered to be a zone of normal potential; 1 — for the amplitude of 0,5 — 1,5 mV, a transient zone; 2 — for the amplitude 0,05 — 0,5 mV, low potential zone; 3 — zone of «electrical scar» - lack of electrical activity when the amplitude was 0 — 0,05 mV. This grading was preconditioned by the fact that myocardial areas with the 1st or 2nd grades of lowered potential were, as a rule, sources of life threatening tachycardias, while for grade 3 "electrical scar" this was less possible and in the zones with normal electrical activity of grade 0 VTs did not occur [9,10].

http://dx.doi.org/10.5772/54126

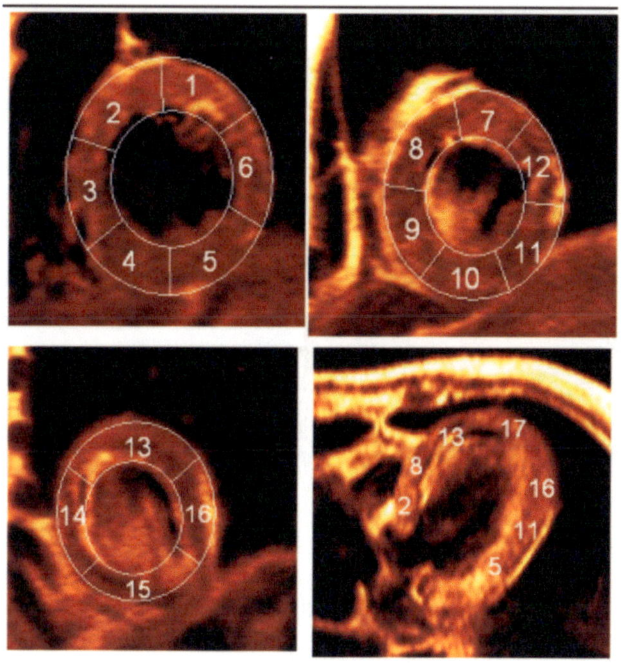

Figure 1. Segmentation of LV myocardium, used in evaluation of a local paramagnetic contrast agent uptake during myocardial MRI

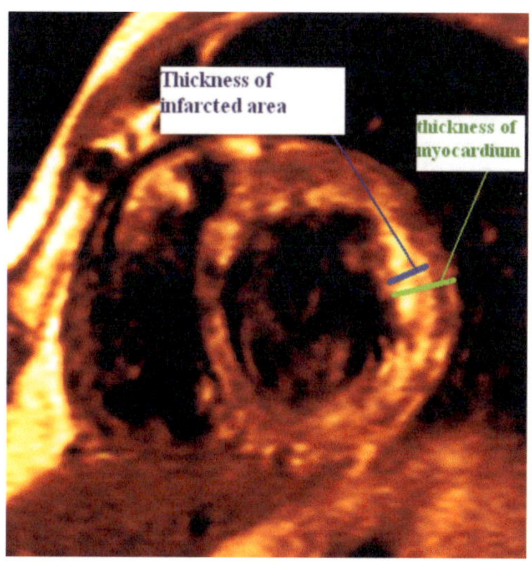

Figure 2. The scheme of TI calculation by the data of delayed contrast-enhanced MRI of myocardium. The values of thickness of the infarction zone (accumulation of paramagnetic) and the value of the total myocardial thickness were identified on the LV slices in short axis. Thickness of the contrast-paramagnetic accumulation in myocardium is thought to be the thickness of lesion resulting from acute myocardial infarction. Thus TI is equal to *{(thickness of an infracted area)/ (thickness of the myocardium)}*. (original data)

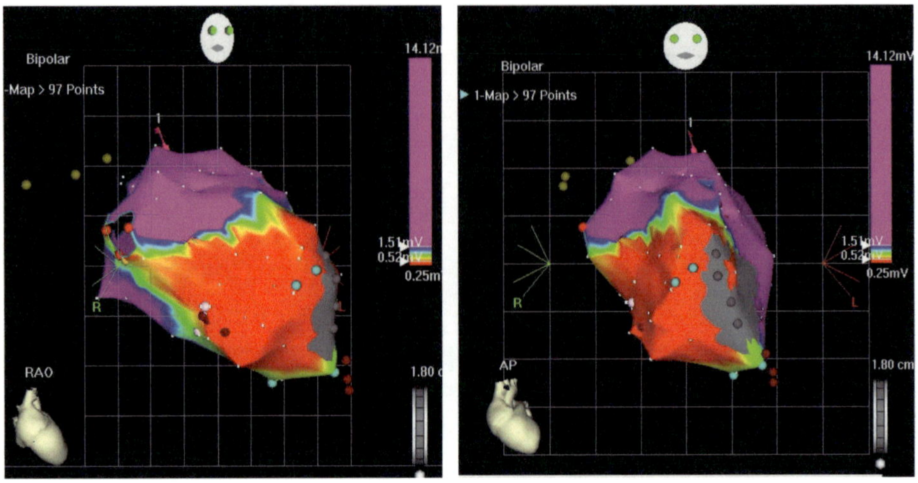

Figure 3. Patient T, 56 year old. Before the surgery. EPhS with LV reconstruction of a patient with LV aneurysm. The area of electrical "silence" (scar) is highlighted with grey color; the low-amplitude ventricular potential area of 0,5 mV – with red; the transient zone of 0,5 - 1,5 mV – with yellow-green; the zone of viable myocardium – with violet; the double potential zone – with blue dots and the zone of delayed potential – with pink dots. Front view, right oblique view. (original data)

Surgical ventricular reconstruction (SVR) was performed by the standard methods by V.Dor and in L.Menicanti modification. [4,6]. After cardiac arrest with a calculated injection of cardioplegia solution (Kustodiol) there was performed grafting of distal coronary anastomoses. Left ventricle was opened with a longitudinal incision in the apical area to be parallel to the anterior descending artery along visually identified scarred tissue. After revision of left ventricular cavity thrombotic mass if any was eliminated. In case of endocardectomy we performed resection of scarred and transient areas of LV. Residual volume of LV cavity was calculated by a physiological norm of 50-60 ml/m^2 of a patient's body surface, and was limited by a special sizer (Chase Medical Richardson, TX, USA). To close LV cavity we used an endocardial synthetic patch (Gore-tex). When L. Menicanti modification was applied, LV neoapex was formed with one or two u-shaped sutures. LV was closed with a double running suture [11,12].

Endocardectomy was performed in 84 patients who were referred to the study group (LVR +EE); on average there was dissected 44cm^2 of LV endocardium (from 17 to 84 cm^2) including ventricular septum. The control group consisted of 104 patients in which endocardial resection was not performed (LVR without EE). The patients were allocated into the groups randomly. All the patients signed the informed consent form. The study was approved by the local ethic committee.

Resection of aneurysm and left ventricular reconstruction (LVR) was performed by V. Dor procedure in 130 patients, by L. Menicanti modification - in 58 patients. In 29 patients from both groups mitral valve fibrous ring repair was done. All the patients underwent coronary artery bypass grafting (CABG). The area of an endocardial synthetic patch varied from 5 to 20 cm^2. Clinical data and the data of instrumental examinations did not show significant differences between the patient groups (Table 1).

Characteristics		LVR with EE n=84	LVR without EE n=104
Age, years old		55	56
Angina class Canadian Cardiovascular Society, (%)	II	10	10
	III	37	40
	IV	34	33
	Unstable angina	19	17
Current NYHA heart failure class, (%)	I	5	6
	II	20	21
	III	70	69
	IV	5	4%
Type of LV aneurysm, (%)	1	56	58
	2	35	34
	3	9	8
Ventricular tachycardia, (%)	Spontaneous	14	13
	Induced	32	30
Ventricular extrasystoly, (%)		44	48
Mitral regurgitation 2+, fibrous ring more than 35 mm, (%)		18	13
Lesions of coronary arteries, (%)	1	30	34
	2	35	36
	3	35	30

Table 1. Clinical characteristics of the patients.

SSPS 11.5 for Windows software was used for the analysis. Shapiro-Wilk test was applied to assess normality of distribution law of quantitative values. The parameters conforming with the normal distribution test were described with the use of a mean value (M) and a standard deviation (SD). Qualitative data were described by the rate of occurrence or its percentage. Student's t-test was used to evaluate significance of the differences of quantitative values in the compared groups when distribution law was normal. To see the significance of differences among quantitative values Z criterion (Fisher's exact test) was used. Evaluation of significance of differences in postoperative mortality was carried out by Kaplan-Meier method. With $p<0.05$ all the statistical parameters were considered significant.

3. Results

3.1. Survival rate

Intraoperative mortality for the patients underwent LVR comprised 5% (9/188). For the patients of the study group (LVR with EE) mortality was 4% (3/84), for the patients of the control group (LVR without EE) – 6% (6/104). One year survival was 92% (77/84) for the patients subjected to LVR with EE and 87% (90/104) for those from the control group. The causes of mortality are shown in Table 2.

Causes of postoperative mortality	LVR with EE (N=7 from 84)	LVR without EE (N = 14 from 104)
Low cardiac output syndrome	1	2
Progressing HF	3	4
Acute myocardial infarction	2	1
Stroke	-	2
Sudden cardiac death	-	4
Non-cardiac reason	1	1

Table 2. Surgical outcomes of the patients in 1 year after the intervention.

4. Cardiac function

Thus, in the study group patients left ventricular end-diastolic volume index (LV EDVI) was increased on average up to 118 ml/m^2, end-systolic volume index (LV ESVI) – up to 74 ml/m^2, LV ejection fraction (EF) was lowered to 38% and in the control group patients these parameters were: LV EDVI - 114 ml/m^2, LV ESVI – 69 ml/m^2, EF - 40%. MRI of diastolic phase in synchronizing mode showed perimeters of affected myocardium; on average they were 52% and 49% of the entire myocardial perimeter in the groups.

EchoCG performed in 2 weeks after the surgical intervention showed statistically significant ($p<0,01$) change of the values in comparison with preoperative data: increased EF up to 49% и 52%, decreased EDVI down to 79 and 77 ml/m^2, ESVI to 49 and 48 ml/m^2 in the patients of the study group and control group correspondingly. There were no statistically significant differences found between the groups as for preoperative and postoperative hemodynamic values.

5. EPhS with LV electroanatomical mapping

Analyzing the results we decided to allocate the patients who underwent EPhS with electro-anatomical LVR before and after the surgery into separate groups. Fourty patients from the study group were included into group 1 and 38 from the control group into group 2. In the early postoperative period in the patients of group 1 the values of EPhS improved: "electrical scar" zones were found on endoventricular patch only, areas of lowered potential disappeared completely, transient zones (from 0,5 to 1,5 mV) took a limited area without possibility of re-entry and VT induction (Figure 2).

In 2nd group patients spontaneous VT spells were registered by Holter monitoring in 6 cases; in 8 cases VT was induced during EPhS which made in total 37% of the patients. In 12 patients cardioverters-defibrillators were implanted for the secondary prevention of a sudden cardiac death.

6. Contrast-enhanced MRI

Analyzing the obtained MRI values characterizing local morphological condition of the myocardium with values of local electrical myocardial potential we found a significant difference as for the thickness of viable myocardium (i.e. myocardium which does not accumulate contrast paramagnetic agent) in comparable segments. Thus in the zones with normal potential (0 decrease) the thickness of viable myocardium was more than 7 mm - on average 9,8mm; in transient zone (lowered potential 1) it was 6,2mm; in low potential zone (lowered potential 2) – 5,3mm and in "electrical scar" zone (lowered potential 3) – 2,8 mm. In the latter case viable myocardium was thinner than 3,5mm in all the segments. Figure 4 shows an example of a typical MR image in a patient with a previous acute myocardial infarction and affected lateral LV wall.

In the segments 10,11, 12 the uptake of contrast with the index of transmurality ranging from 0,20 to 0,55 is obviously seen. Later on during the electrophysiological study the activity of proarrhythmogenic type 2 was revealed. (original data)

Besides, the value of transmural index (TI) of paramagnetic contrast agent accumulation in myocardium differed significantly between unaffected segments with 0 degree potential lowering and segments with the 1st and 2nd degrees of potential lowering –the most arrhythmogenic degrees (Figure 4). In electrically normal myocardial segments, in particular, TI value was 0,072 ± 0,020. In the group of segments in transient zone TI was 0,46 ± 0,046, and in the low potential zone - 0,32 ± 0,052. Finally, the most affected myocardium with TI of 0,32 ± 0,052 was found in the area of an "electrical scar" with no electrical potential.

By the data of ROC analysis and discriminative analysis the most appropriate breaking value allowing to differentiate segments with abnormal electrical activity became TI value of 0,27. In other words, when TI ≥ 0,27 one should consider probable arrhythmogenic activity in such a segment and pay closer attention to such areas during EPhS.

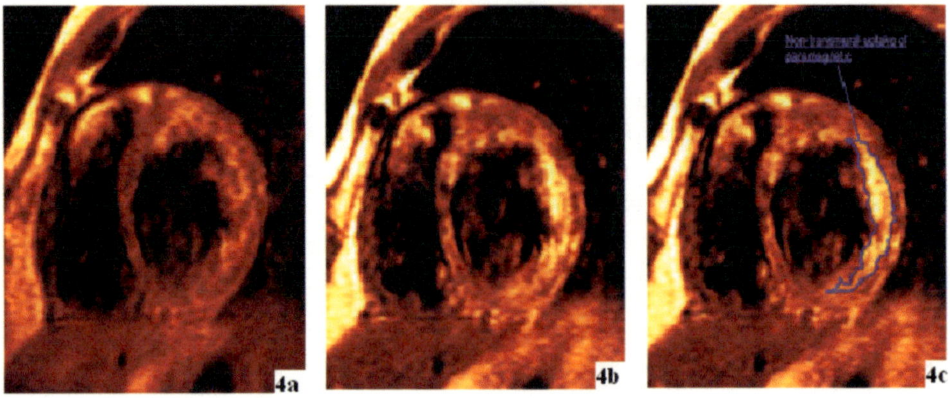

Figure 4. Patient K, has had an acute MI in the circulation of a left circumferential artery with a long area of subendocardial lesion of a lateral wall. Fig.4a – T1- weighed spin-echo ECG-gated MRI study before injection of paramagnetic contrast; Fig. 4b – T1-weighted spin-echo ECG-gated MRI 15 min after injection of paramagnetics, as 2ml of 0,5M solution per 10 kg of BW. Fig. 4c – the same as 4b, after semi-automatic bordering of subendocardial contrast uptake.

7. Clinical case

Patient T, 56 year old was admitted to the department of cardiovascular surgery at Tomsk Institute of Cardiology in 4 months after transmural anterior-septal myocardial infarction with complaints on occasional angina pangs and dyspnea. The patient was examined routinely. Holter monitoring showed ventricular extrasystoly (grade III by Lown). By EchoCG ejection fraction was 25% lower than normal (in B mode), LV was dilated with LV EDVI as high as 154 ml/m2 and LV ESVI of 116 ml/m2; local LV contractility was disturbed, there was found akinesis of apical, medial septal and anterior segments as well as hypokinesis of lateral and posterior-lateral segments. EchoCG also showed the 2nd type aneurysm.

By MRI there were found postinfarction cicatricial changes in all apical and, ventricular septal and anterior segments; perimeter of the affected LV endocardium was 43%. In the apical and septal segments TI varied from 0,35 to 0,56. Data of coronaroventriculography showed LV deformation due to the aneurysm on the plane of anterior-lateral and apical segments and due to atherosclerosis of coronary arteries which included occlusion of the LAD artery in its proximal third and 75% stenosis of the right coronary artery. After mapping and electroanatomical LV reconstruction (Figure 3) there were identified the areas of an "electrical scar" on the apex, ventricular septum and anterior LV wall, zones of delayed conduction (pink dots in the picture) and those of double potential (blue dots) in transient zone, around the scar on ventricular septum and partially on the lateral LV wall. On the border of affected areas and viable myocardium radiofrequent (RF) dotty tags were applied (maroon dots in the picture) by an ablation lead.

After careful examination the decision was made to perform surgical myocardial revascularization and LV endoventriculoplasty with endocardectomy of the affected area. During the

http://dx.doi.org/10.5772/54126

surgery we performed epicardial EPhS with overdriving stimulation of 200 impulses a minute; VT was induced. In conditions of CP bypass and cardioplegia mammary-coronary artery bypass grafting of the LAD artery, LV aneurysm dissection, endocardectomy of the apex, ventricular septum, anterior and lateral LV walls along RF tags were performed as well as SVR including endoventricular circular repair with a synthetic patch by the method of V.Dor. Postoperatively the patient received routine care. Postoperative period was uneventful. By EChoG done in 3 weeks after the surgery one could notice better contractile cardiac function – LV EF grew up to 40% (B-made), LV sizes became smaller – EDVI was 70ml, ESVI – 48ml. The data of 24-hour ECG monitoring did not reveal any signs of ventricular rhythm disturbances. Postoperative mapping (Figure 5) showed significantly smaller transient zone, lack of re-entry and VT.

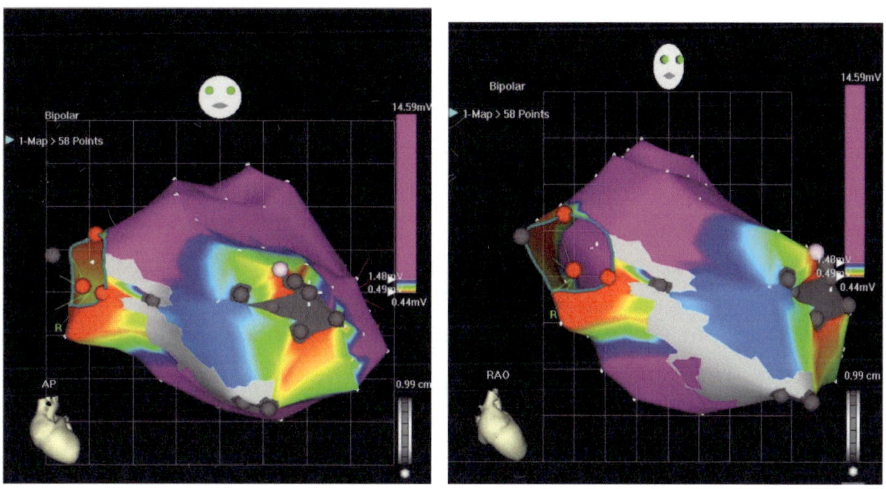

Figure 5. Patient T, 56 year old. EPhS with LV reconstruction of the patient after LV aneurysmectomy (LVR) : electrical scar in the area of the patch. Low-potential areas with the potential from 0,5 mV and transient zones (from 0,5 to1,5 mV) take a limited area with no possibility of re-entry and VT induction. Front view, right oblique view. (original data)

The patient was discharged from the hospital in satisfactory condition.

8. Discussion

In 1956 Couch O.A. performed LV aneurysm resection in a patient with VT thus beginning an era of surgical treatment of ventricular rhythm disorders [13].

It has been more than 50 years since; nevertheless the issue of complications and approaches of surgical treatment associated with the appearance of VT in patients with remodelled LV after previous MI is still quite challenging [14]. It was at that time already when specialists were aware of the fact that LV myocardium affected by infarction was a source of fatal ventricular rhythm disorders. Initially there were offered methods of indirect surgical intervention such as thoracic sympathectomy, CABG, resection of a cardiac wall for the treatment of recurrent ventricular arrhythmias associated with CAD [15,16,17]. Since these methods appeared to be inefficient, over the course of time there were implemented direct endocardial methods performed under control of intraoperative electrophysiological mapping. The first endocardial procedure developed for the treatment of VT combined with CAD was a circular endocardial resection performed by Guiraudon in 1978 [18]. This procedure involves endocardial incision made on the borderline between endocardial fibrosis and viable myocardium and continued around the whole base of aneurysm or infraction area. In 1982 to enhance efficiency of a circular endocardial resection J. Moran modified this procedure by resecting all the fibrous endocardium connected with LV aneurysm or infarction and called it an expanded endocardial resection [19]. Supporting development of the ideas referred to endocardial resection V.Dor offered resection of fibrous endocardium from the side of interventricular septum during surgical LV reconstruction [11].

This kind of intervention appeared to be efficient for the treatment of «refractory» ischemic VTs but did not make any effect on VTs coming from papillary muscles' base or from areas adjacent to a ring of an aortic or mitral valves.

In 1981 Leo Bokeria one of the first in the world began resection of LV aneurysm and cardiodestruction in the areas of early activity after intraoperative epicardial EPhS [20]. Developing cryosurgical methods of intervention in 1985 J.Cox performed endocardial cardiodestruction but the procedure resulted in lethal outcome in 27% of the cases and was ineffective in 17% of the cases [15]. I 1980th M.Mirovsky (the USA) offered an alternative method of VT treatment – implantation of cardioverter-defibrillator [21].

As a result, for the treatment of postinfarction LV aneurysms and associated ventricular tachyarrhythmias there have been used different methods, either alone or in combination. Significant clinical experience have been acquired.

Thus, Bokeria L.A. in his study including 59 patients demonstrated a clear dependence of actuarial survival rate from the type of tachycardia and from the presence of VT relapse in the early postoperative period [20]; the worst prognosis was noticed with the presence of polymorphic ventricular extrasystoly (Figures 6, 7).

Interesting data were presented by the group of authors headed by M. Di Donato [22]; they analyzed data of 382 patients proving that spontaneous VTs after surgical treatment of LV aneurysms and VT significantly worsen prognosis for late postoperative period if compare with induced VTs of cases without arrhythmias (Figure 8).

After careful study of immediate ablation results in 71 patients with LV aneurysm and VT J. Pirk showed that epicardial cryoablation alone was successful in 63,3% of the cases and aneurysmectomy and endocardial cryoablation and/or subendocardial resection were successful in 73,2% of the cases [23].

Sartipy U. studying combination of V. Dor procedure and surgery for VT in 53 patients came to the conclusion that combination of these procedures keeps survival rate high in the postoperative period (Figure 9) and that majority of the patients did not need implantation of an automatic implantable cardioverter-defibrillator (AICD) [24].

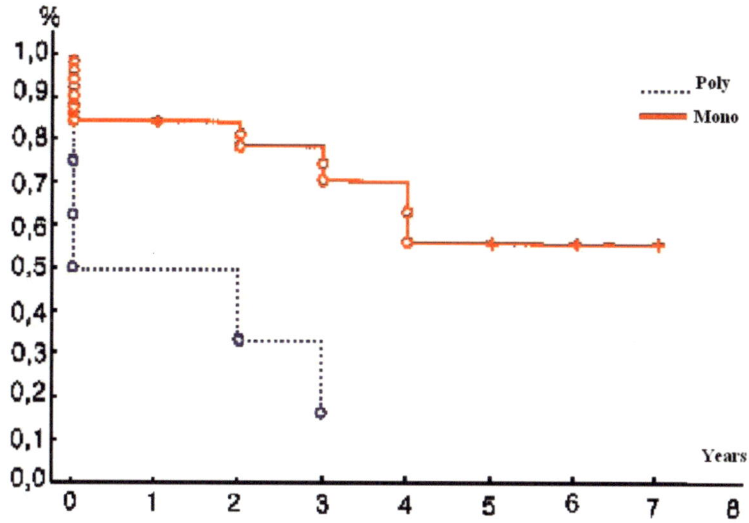

Figure 6. Actuarial survival curve depending on a type of VT (Kaplan-Meier); p=0,00739 (Bokeria L.A et al.// Journal of Thoracic and Cardiovascular Surgery –1999.– №6.).

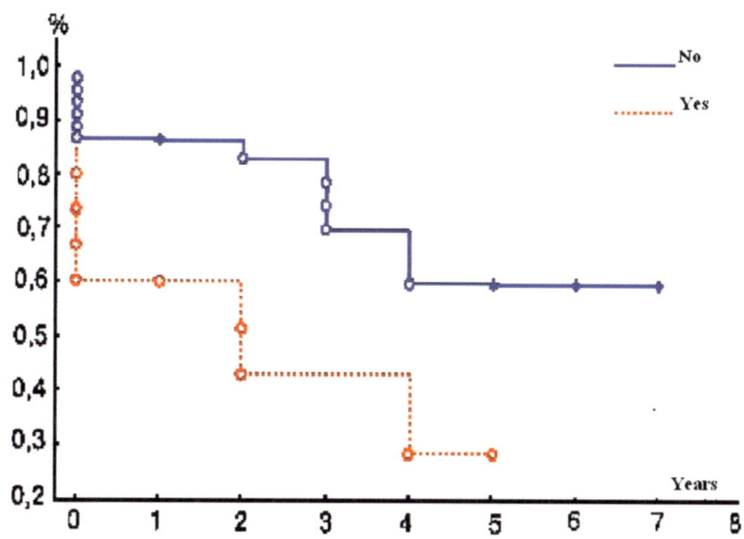

Figure 7. Actuarial survival curve depending on VT relapse (Kaplan-Meier); p=0,012 (Bokeria L.A et al.// Journal of Thoracic and Cardiovascular Surgery –1999.– №6.).

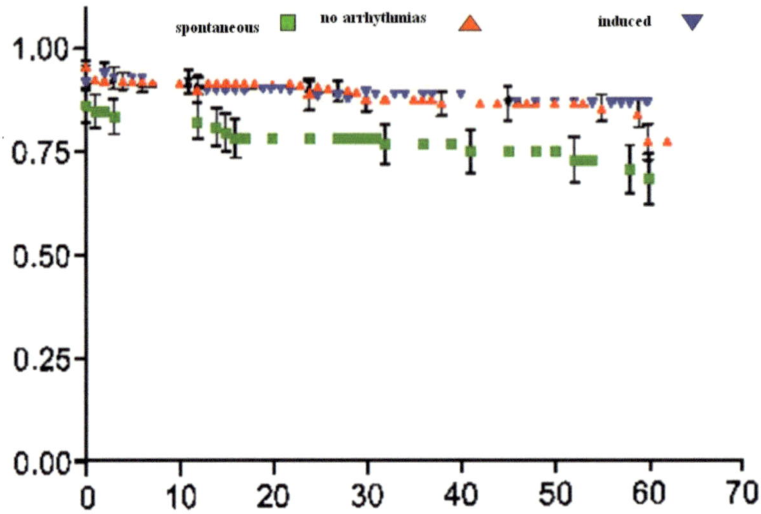

Figure 8. Kaplan-Meier survival curves by the groups with VT in postoperative period (months) after surgical treatment of LV aneurysm and VT. (Di Donato et al. Seminars in Thorac and Cardiovasc Surg.Vol.13;4:480-485).

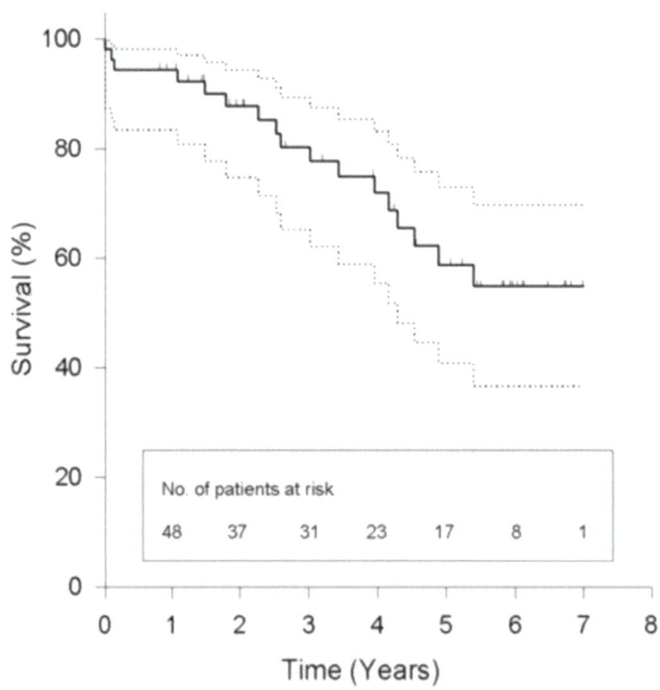

Figure 9. Overall actuarial survival after the Dor procedure including ventricular tachycardia surgery. Dotted curves are upper and lower 95% confidence intervals (Sartipy U. et al.; Ann Thorac Surg 2006;81:65-71).

Contemporary therapeutic methods are not able to solve this problem also. By the data of a multicenter trial MADIT II implantation of AICD in patients with ventricular rhythm disturbances lowers the risk of a sudden cardiac death for 31 % which is more efficient than antiarrhythmic therapy but still is not 100% saving [21]. In a year after endovascular treatment of VT the rate of relapses comprises 20% [25,26]. Nevertheless, antiarrhythmic therapy, implantation of AICD, catheter isolation of ectopic focuses do not touch an issue of coronary arteries lesion.

According to the data of a multicenter STICH trial there were no significant differences found between the patients with ICMP and postinfarction LV aneurysm subjected to CABG only (group 1) and those subjected to CABG with LV reconstruction (group 2) during 5 year follow-up. Nevertheless, postoperatively AICD was implanted into 20% of the patients from group 1 and into 17% from group 2 [27]. The study did not suppose to perform extended endocardectomy during LV reconstruction. Taking into account the aforesaid, one may claim that almost every 5th patient is destined for AICD implantation after surgical remodeling of LV. Although, by the data of multiple authors endocardial resection either with intraoperative mapping or without it prevents VT paroxysms in 90% of the cases and more [19, 24].

Thus, we saw clearly that at that time to treat patients with postinfarction LV aneurysm complicated with ventricular rhythm disorders is was necessary to perform reconstruction of LV cavity with endocardial resection and CABG; to use contemporary antiarrhythmics and AICD implantation in postoperative period if necessary.

Though, at that point there were unclear issues connected with topical diagnostics of potential re-entry zones which was important for adequate resection of affected endocardium. In our study we tried to enhance efficacy of topical diagnostics and surgical treatment of the patients with postinfarction LV aneurysm complicated with VT, due to combined application of contrast-enhanced MRI, EPhS and advanced surgical treatment (SVR and EE). It is well-known that MRI is a golden standard in diagnostics of LV aneurysm [4, 28], but MRI data may provide only indirect evidences about the presence of arrhythmogenic zones.

Prognostic role of contrast-enhanced MRI in evaluation of myocardial viability were reported in literature in as far as 1986 [29]. In particular, it was supposed, that with the presence of irreversible ischemic lesion of myocardium MRI made at rest demonstrated significant decrease of end-diastolic thickness of myocardium (EDTM) and simultaneously – contractility index. At the same time it was assumed that secure thickness of myocardium evaluated by the value EDTM meant also a secure viability of myocardium in that location.

Comparison of myocardial MRI made at rest with the results of PET with 18F-FDG and SPECT with repeated injection of tallim-201 in patients with chronic coronary disease and pronounced LV dysfunction was made in a number of studies [30]. It was found, that as a rule MRI visualized secure thickness of myocardium and the value of EDTM more than 5,5-6,0 mm in the affected areas in LV segments classified as viable by PET and SPECT. Later, Baer et al [31] making a direct comparison of MRI at rest and PET data with 18F-FDG found that with EDTM ≤ 5,5mm there were no signs of viability on myocardial tomography slices during radionuclide study. As for prognosis for restoration of myocardial viability and contractility after CABG in such patients, their criterion { EDTM ≤ 5,5 mm } had high sensitivity up to 92-95%, but low specificity – just about 56-60%.

As a rule, for contrast-enhanced MRI visualization of affected myocardium contrasting agents – paramegnetics are used, usually they are complexes of Gd or Mn with derivatives or analogues of diaethylentriaminpentacetic acid (DTPA). Their intravenous bolus injection makes possible qualitative evaluation of myocardial perfusion by the degree of changing brightness of myocardial image during the first few seconds after injection. Later on, in 12-20 minutes after injection one can evaluate the picture of myocardial lesion by accumulation of contrasting agent in affected areas.

There exist an established and commonly accepted opinion that transmural accumulation of paramagnetics in myocardium during contrast-enhanced MRI means irreversible lesion, and lack of accumulation vice versa evidences viability of myocardium and makes for favourable prognosis [32]. Nevertheless, relationship of contrast-enhanced MRI picture with the possibility of arrhythmogenesis in this or that myocardial area is still of a great interest.

Electrophysiological mechanism of the observed interrelationship between results of cardiac contrast-enhanced MRI and decrease of electrical potential in a definite LV segment is nothing but a particular case of a well-studied pathogenesis of arrhythmias appearance in the area of ischemic myocardial lesion [33].

It is in the area of thickened and partially replaced by subendocardial scarred tissue of myocardium where one can notice lowered electrical potential proportionally to the lowering mass of viable myocardium. This fact, in its turn, is favorable for the functioning of local re-entry circuits which are electrophysiological basis for ventricular tachycardias [33, 34].

That is why during contrast-enhanced MRI it makes sense to calculate TI index value in all the cases keeping in mind further electrophysiological study and evaluation of risks for ventricular tachycardias. Epicardial mapping provides information about the presence of excitement zones in LV and approximate anatomy of their localization for a further surgical treatment [4, 35]. Preoperative endocardial EPhS with electroanatomical LV reconstruction is able to demonstrate vividly disturbances in cardiac conduction system. Examining the results of endocardial EPhS we found consistency of myocardial lesion and its elctrophysiological properties. In patients suffered from extensive myocardial infarction complicated with aneurysm one can identify zones of low-amplitude ventricular potential less than 0,5mV which is a scarred zone more often anatomically involving an apex of LV with a part of anterior wall and ventricular septum. Viable myocardium has potential amplitude higher than 1,5 mV. A subject of a special interest is a transient zone from 0,5 to 1,5 mV situated between the scar and viable myocardium where they register double potential and/or delayed conduction able to cause re-entry and ventricular tachycardia; a surgeon is just to perform dissection of affected endocardium. EPhS and MRI allow to identify borders for endocardial dissection.

Postoperative EPhS worth electroanatomical LV reconstruction performed in patients without endocardectomy showed that re-entry and VT sources revealed preoperatively were still there and made for a high risk for the patients' lives. Contrast-enhanced MRI gives additional prognostic information about arrhythmogenisity of particular areas and segments of LV after myocardial infarction. More often arrhythmogenic areas are located in the areas of a pronounced non-transmural lesion of LV myocardium with TI higher than 0,27.

9. Conclusion

Thus, data of contrast-enhanced MRI not only have diagnostic significance concerning a degree of a cardiac muscle lesion but also identify arrhythmogenisisty of this or that myocardial area. In surgical treatment of postinfarction aneurysm endocardectomy of scarred and transient LV zones' endocardium is an inseparable stage to prevent VT spells. MRI and endocardial EPhS with electroanatomical LV reconstruction allow to find potential areas where re-entry may occur.

Author details

Vladimir Shipulin[1*], Vadim Babokin[1], Sergey Andreev[1], Vladimir Usov[2], Ruslan Aimanov[1], Anthony Bogunetsky[1], Roman Batalov[3] and Sergey Popov[3]

*Address all correspondence to: shipulin@cardio.tsu.ry

1 Cardiovascular Surgery Department, Tomsk Institute of Cardiology, Tomsk, Russia

2 Department of Diagnostic Radiology and Tomography, Tomsk Institute of Cardiology, Tomsk, Russia

3 Department of Heart Rhythm Disorders, Tomsk Institute of Cardiology, Tomsk, Russia

References

[1] Di Donato, M Ventricular arrhythmias after LV remodeling: surgical ventricular restoration or ICD. Heart Fail. Rev. 2005;9(4) 299-306.

[2] Arai A.E. The cardiac magnetic resonance (CMR) approach to assessing myocardial viability. J.Nucl. Cardiol 2011; 18 1095-1102.

[3] Carlsson M., Arheden H., Higgins C.B., Saeed M Magnetic resonance imaging as potential gold standard for infarct quantification. J Electrocardiol 2008; 41 614-620.

[4] Dor, V., Sabatier M., Montiglio F Endoventricular patch reconstruction of Ischemic failing ventricle: A single center with 20 years experience Heart Fail Rev 2004; 9 269-286.

[5] Faxon, D.P., W.O. Myers, C.H. McCabe The influence of surgery on the natural history of angiographically documented left ventricular aneurysm: the Coronary Artery Surgery Study Circulation 1986;74 110-118.

[6] Menicanti, L., Castelvecchio S., Ranucci M Surgical therapy for ischemic heart failure: Single-center experience with surgical anterior ventricular restoration J. Thorac. Cardiovasc. Surg 2007; 134 433 – 441.

[7] Cerqueira MD, Weissman NJ, Dilsizian V et al. Standardized myocardial segmentation and nomenclature for tomographic imaging of the heart: a statement for healthcare professionals from the Cardiac Imaging Committee of the Council on Clinical Cardiology of the American Heart Association. Circulation 2002; 105 539–42.

[8] Kautzner J., Kirstein Pedersen A., Peichl P Electroanatomical mapping of the heart: Remedica Publishing; 2006.

[9] Fernandes V.R., Wu K.C., Rosen B.D. et al. Enhanced infarct border zone function and altered mechanical activation predict inducibility of monomorphic ventricular tachycardia in patients with ischemic cardiomyopathy. Radiology. 2007; 245 712-719.

[10] Suk T., Edwards C., Hart H., Christiansen J.P Myocardial scar detected by contrast-enhanced cardiac magnetic resonance imaging is associated with ventricular tachycardia in hypertrophic cardiomyopathy patients Heart Lung Circ 2008; 17 370-374.

[11] Dor V, Saab M, Coste P, Kornaszewski M, Montiglio F. Left ventricular aneurysm: a new surgical approach. J Thorac Cardiovasc Sug. 1989; 37 11–19

[12] Menicanti L, Di Donato M. The Dor procedure: What has changed after fifteen years of clinical practice? J Thorac Cardiovasc Surg. 2002; 124 886–890

[13] Couch O.A. Cardiac Aneurysm with Ventricular Tachycardia and Subsequent Excision of Aneurysm: Case Report. Circulation. 1959; 20 251-253.

[14] Buxton AE, Lee KL, DiCarlo L, et al Electrophysiologic testing to identify patients with coronary artery disease who are at risk for sudden death. N Engl J Med 2000; 342 1937-45.

[15] Cox J.L. Cardiac surgery for arrhythmias. Pacing Clin Electrophysiol 2004; 27 266—282.

[16] Dor V, Sabatier M, Montiglio F, Rossi P, Toso A, Di Donato M. Results of nonguided subtotal endocardiectomy associated with left ventricular reconstruction in patients with ischemic ventricular arrhythmias. J Thorac Cardiovasc Surg 1994; 107 1301–1308

[17] Josephson ME, Harken AH, Horowitz LN Endocardial excision. A new surgical technique for the treatment of recurrent ventricular tachycardia. Circulation 1979; 60 1430-1439.

[18] Holman W. L., Ikeshita M., Ungerleider R. M. et al. Cryosurgery for cardiac arrhythmias: Acute and chronic effects on coronary arteries Amer. J. Cardiol 1983; 51 149-155.

[19] Moran J.M., Kehoe R.F. et al Extended endocardial resection for treatment of ventricular tachycardia and ventricular fibrillation Ann Thorac Surg 1982; 34 538-552.

[20] Bokeria L.A et al Journal of Thoracic and Cardiovascular Surgery 1999; 6 38-44.

[21] Mirowski M, Reid PR, Mower MM et al. Termination of malignant ventricular arrhythmias with an implanted automatic defibrillator in human beings. N Engl J Med 1980; 303 322—324.

[22] Di Donato M, Sabatier M, Dor V. Surgical ventricular restoration in patients with postinfarction coronary artery disease: effectiveness on spontaneous and inducible ventricular tachycardia. Semin Thorac Cardiovasc Surg 2001;13:480-485.

[23] Pirk J, Bytesnik J, Kautzner J, et al. Surgical ablation of post-infarction ventricular tachycardia guided by mapping in sinus rhythm: long termresults. Eur J Cardiothorac Surg 2004; 26 323-329.

[24] Sartipy U., Albage A. et al. Surgery for Ventricular Tachycardia in Patients Undergoing Left Ventricular Reconstruction by the Dor Procedure. Ann Thorac Surg 2006; 81 65-71.

[25] Buxton A.E., Lee K.L., Fisher J.D. et al. for the Multicenter UnSustained Tachycardia Trial Investigators (MUSTT). A randomized study of the prevention of sudden death in patients with coronary artery diseases. N Engl J Med 1999; 34: 1 1882—1890.

[26] Connoly S.J., Gent M., Roberts R.S. et al. Canadian implantable defibrillator study a randomized trial of the implantable cardioverter defibrillator against amiodarone. Circulation 2000; 101 1297—1302.

[27] Jones R, Velazguez E. et al. Coronary Bypass Surgery with or without Surgical Ventricular Reconstruction. The New England Journal of Medicine 2009; 360 1705-1717.

[28] Marrouch NF, Verna A, Wazni O Mode of initiation end ablation of ventricular fibrillation storms in patients with ischemic cardiomyopathy J. Am. Coll. Cardiol 2004;43 1715 – 1720.

[29] McNamara MT, Higgins CB. Magnetic resonance imaging of chronic myocardial infarcts in man. AJR Am J Roentgenol. 1986; 146(2) 315-20.

[30] Betocchi S, Piscione F, Villari B, Pace L, Ciarmiello A,Perrone-Fillardi P, et al. Effects of induced asynchrony on left ventricular diastolic function in patients with coronary artery disease. J Am Coll Cardiol 1993; 21 1124-31.

[31] Baer FM, Voth E, Theissen P, Schicha H, Sechtem U Gradient-echo magnetic resonance imaging during incremental dobutamine infusion for the localization of coronary artery stenosis. Eur Heart J 1994; 15 97-107

[32] Mahrholdt H, Wagner A, Judd RM, et al . Assessment of myocardial viability by cardiovascular magnetic resonance imaging. Eur Heart J 2002; 23 602–19.

[33] Josephson ME. Electrophysiology of ventricular tachycardia: an hystorical perspective J Cardiovasc Electrophysiol. 2003; 14 1134-1148.

[34] Pokushalov E., Turov A., Shugayev P Successful epicardial catheter ablation of micro-reentrant ventricular tachycardia Pediatr Cardiol 2009; 30 533-535.

[35] Moran J.M Postoperative Ventricular Arrhythmia Ann. Thorac. Surg 1984; 38 312 - 313.

Chapter 13

Cardiac Trauma

Daniel Eiferman,
R. Nathan Cotterman and
Michael Firstenberg

Additional information is available at the end of the chapter

http://dx.doi.org/10.5772/55723

1. Introduction

1.1. History of cardiac trauma

The treatment of trauma to the heart has been written about since 3000 BC and had an inauspicious beginning. Until the late 19th century, the commonly held belief agreed with Boerhaave's sentiments that, "all penetrating cardiac trauma is fatal." Theodore Billroth warned, "The surgeon who should attempt to suture a wound of the heart would lose the respect of his colleagues." Paget believed that "surgery of the heart has probably reached the limits set by nature to all surgery: no new method of discovery can overcome the natural difficulties that attend a wound of the heart." However, reports of successful treatment of cardiac injuries began to surface toward the beginning of the 20th century. Like many surgical advances, times of war brought about new innovations and techniques for treating injuries.

Around the time of World War II, it was recognized that cardiac tamponade could be successfully managed by pericardiocentesis. With the advent of cardiopulmonary bypass by Gibbon in 1953, repair of more complex injuries became possible. This ushered in the modern era of treating injuries to the heart. Diagnosis of cardiac injury and tamponade has also been facilitated by portable ultrasound becoming the standard of care in the evaluation of trauma patients. The focused assessment with sonography for trauma (FAST) scan allows for simple, quick, and non-invasive assessment and recognition of cardiac trauma [1].

Cardiac trauma, especially penetrating injuries to the heart, still carries a very high mortality, but certainly is no longer considered uniformly fatal and attempt at repair is now the standard of care in patients presenting with signs of life upon arrival to the hospital[2, 3].

2. Initial assessment and general assessment

The initial care of the trauma patient with cardiac injuries does not vary from standard Advanced Trauma Life Support (ATLS) protocols. The primary priority is ensuring the patency of the airway and establishing adequate oxygenation and ventilation. This may include tube thoracostomy for drainage of hemothorax from the pleural space to allow re-expansion of the lung. Subsequently, the circulatory system is assessed. Priority is given to establishing intravenous access for the administration of crystalloid and/or blood products. If cardiac tamponade is suspected, this should be confirmed with sonographic confirmation of hemopericardium and/or right ventricular collapse during diastole[4]. If tamponade physiology is present, treatment for immediate drainage of the pericardial space should be initiated. This can be accomplished percutaneously by pericardiocentesis or via open pericardial window.

The treatment algorithm for cardiac injured patients branches at this point depending on the mechanism of injury and hemodynamic status. As is the standard in all trauma care, cardiac injuries are categorized as either blunt or penetrating and we will explore their assessment and treatment separately.

3. Penetrating trauma

Penetrating trauma to the heart most frequently occur with trauma to the anterior chest, but should also be suspected with wounds to the upper abdomen, chest, back, and neck [5]. Of the patients that do present to the hospital, the majority of the injuries are to the low pressure, anteriorly located right side of the heart (Table 1) [6]. Survival following penetrating trauma is often dependent on the state of the pericardial wound.[7] When the pericardial wound is open and blood is able to flow freely into the pleural space, the patient can often be supported with fluid resuscitation and chest tube thoracostomy. Persistent drainage from the thoracostomy tube should warn of possible cardiac injury and surgical exploration is indicated. Conversely, if the blood is retained in the pericardial space, cardiac tamponade and physiology will ensue if not drained immediately.

Right Atrium	14%	Left Atrium	5%
Right Ventricle	43%	Left Ventricle	33%
Coronary Arteries Involved	3.1-4.4%		

Table 1. Anatomic Location of Penetrating Cardiac Injuries

The protocol for treatment of patients with penetrating cardiac trauma can be further subdivided based upon the patient's vital signs upon presentation to the hospital (Figure 1). Management of the stable patient (systolic blood pressure greater than 90 mm Hg) allows for a more complete evaluation including chest x-ray and echocardiography. Unstable patients (systolic blood pressure less than 90 mm Hg) are taken directly to the operating room for exploration while patients with loss of vitals during transport or upon presentation to the hospital are treated with Emergency Department thoracotomy.

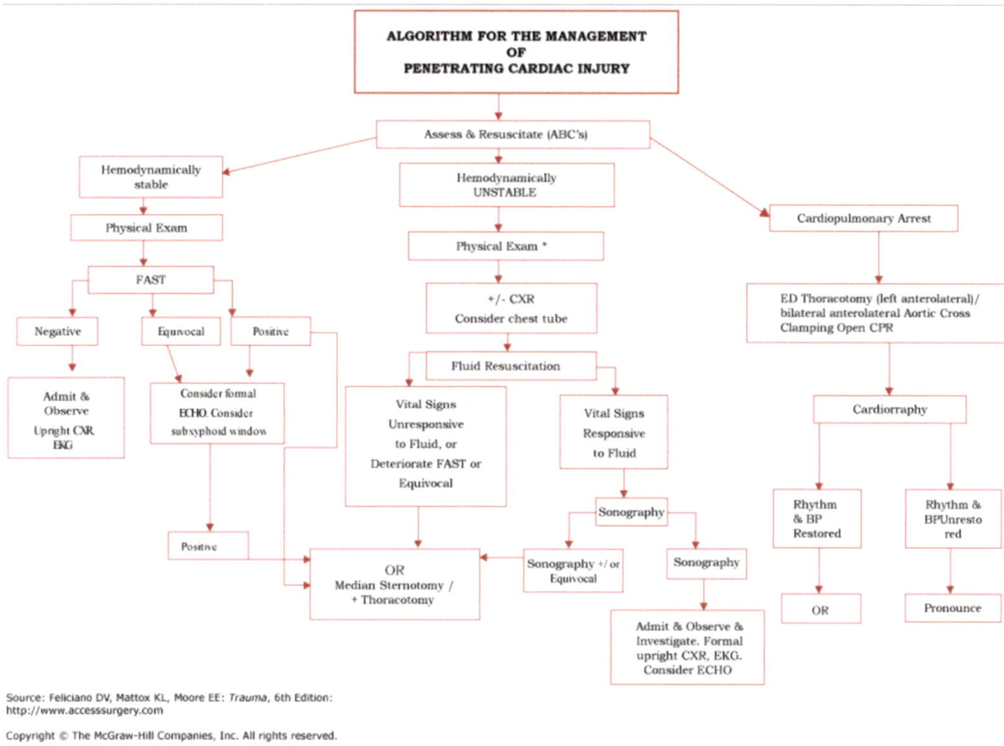

Figure 1. Algorithm for the Management of Penetrating Cardiac Injury

If the diagnosis of penetrating cardiac injury is suspected but not confirmed, a subxiphoid pericardial window should be performed. Surgeons should be prepared to do a median sternotomy if an injury is identified in order to definitely address the wound. Upon opening the pericardial sac, any blood or fluid should be evacuated to allow the heart to properly fill and contract. The surgeon's finger can be used to apply pressure and temporarily control hemorrhage while further exposure is gained. This will also allow for replacement of blood volume and restoration of tissue perfusion.

Repair of the myocardium should be done with interrupted sutures utilizing pledgets and performed in a horizontal mattress fashion [7, 8]. Injuries to small coronary arteries can be treated with simple ligation. Larger coronary arteries require either direct repair or bypass and the operating room should be capable of cardiopulmonary bypass (CPB).[7] Intracardiac injuries require CPB to be definitively addressed.

Whatever injury is encountered and method of repair utilized, the operative principles are universal: relieve tamponade, stop the bleeding, and restore circulating volume. [8]

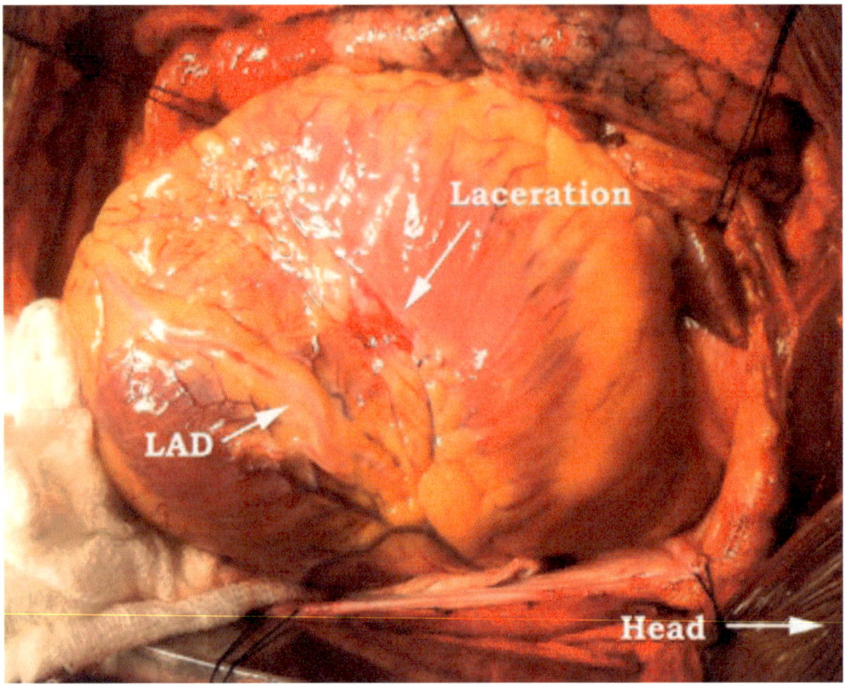

Picture 1. Cardiac Laceration from anterior stab woundPicture

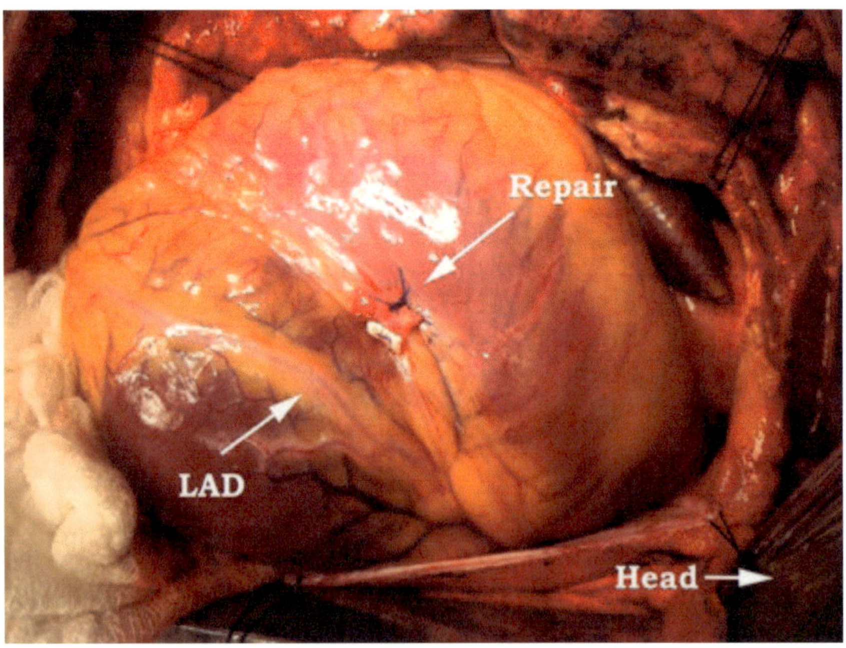

Picture 2. Successful pledgeted repair

http://dx.doi.org/10.5772/55723

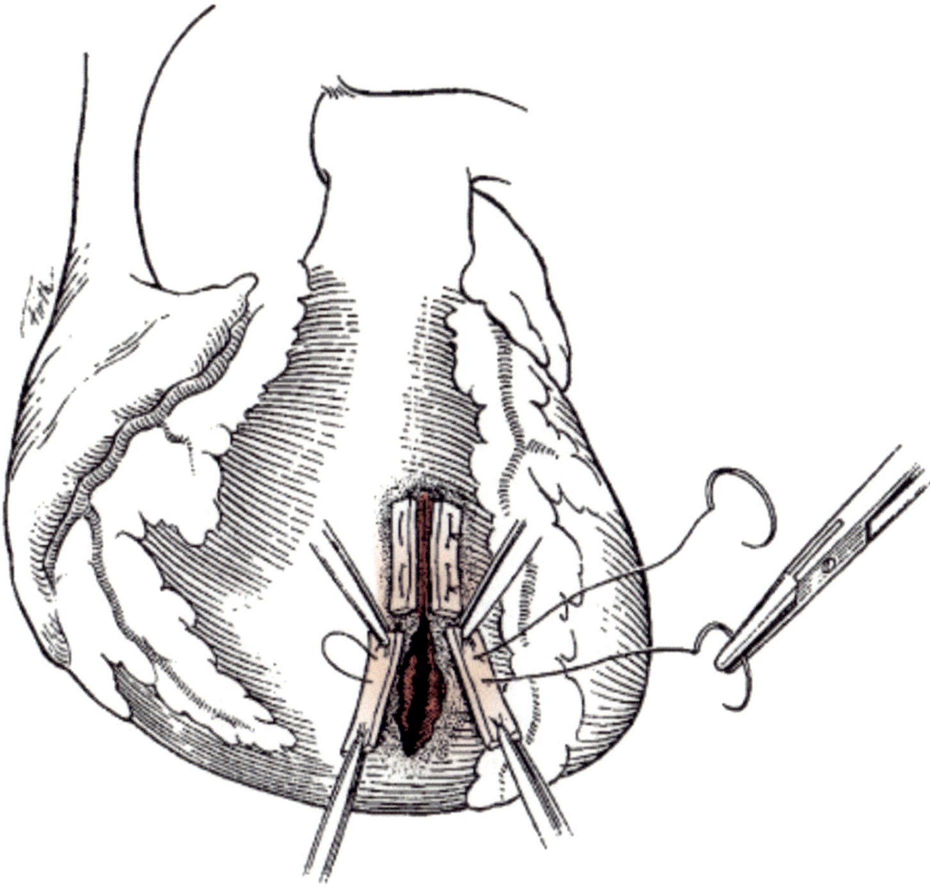

Source: Feliciano DV, Mattox KL, Moore EE: *Trauma*, 6th Edition:
http://www.accesssurgery.com

Figure 2. Schematic Depiction of Right Ventricular Repair

3.1. Iatrogenic injuries

Another form of penetrating cardiac injury that has increased in the modern era is iatrogenic injuries. As the fields of interventional and electrophysiology cardiology continue to increase the number of percutaneous procedures performed, there is a concomitant increase in iatrogenic injuries to the heart. Pacemaker and ICD placement, ASD occlusion devices, coronary catheterization, pericardiocentesis, and even central line placement can cause cardiac trauma. Usually the treatment is observational, but sometimes intervention is necessary. Fortunately these are rare complications but the incidence of iatrogenic injury has been reported as high as 6% for certain radiofrequency ablation procedures.[9] Awareness and prompt recognition of an injury are essential to successful treatment.

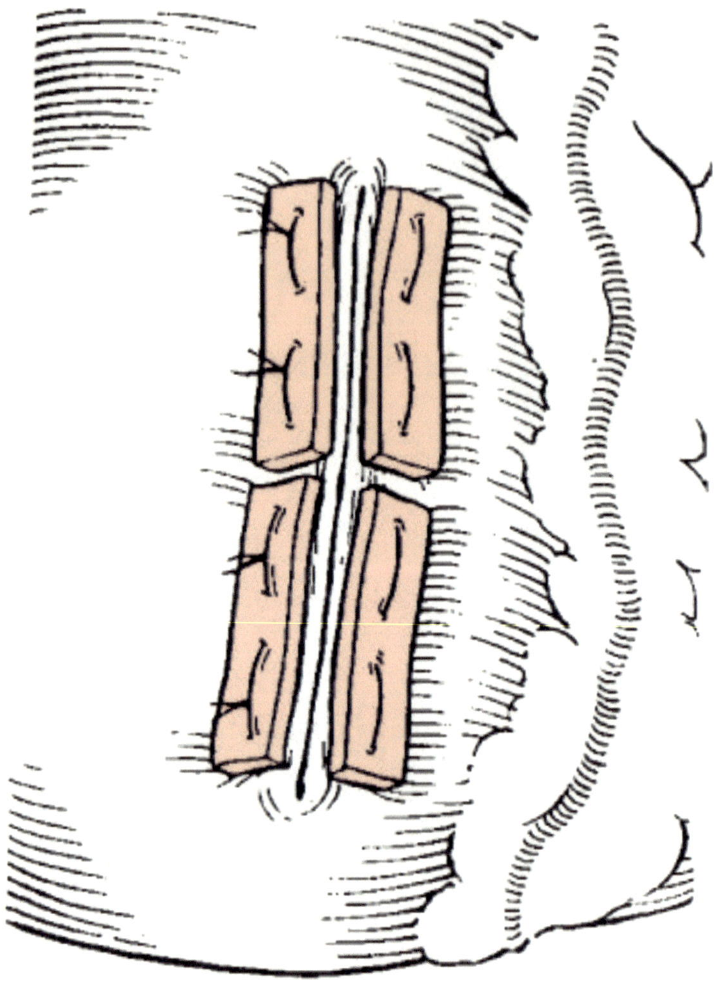

Source: Feliciano DV, Mattox KL, Moore EE: *Trauma*, 6th Edition:
http://www.accesssurgery.com

Figure 3. Pledgets are used to reinforce the suture line

3.2. Cardiac fistulas

Although hemorrhage and tamponade are the most common injuries seen in penetrating cardiac trauma, cardiac fistulas are another uncommon yet dramatic complication from cardiac trauma (including iatrogenic injuries). Fistulous connections can occur between coronary arteries, aorta, and directly with the cardiac chambers. Patients, if symptomatic, usually present with congestive heart failure and surgical repair is usually required.[10, 11]. Presentation is variable from acutely after the injury to decades post-injury. Echocardiography and coronary angiography are the cornerstones of diagnosis and necessary to plan surgical repair.

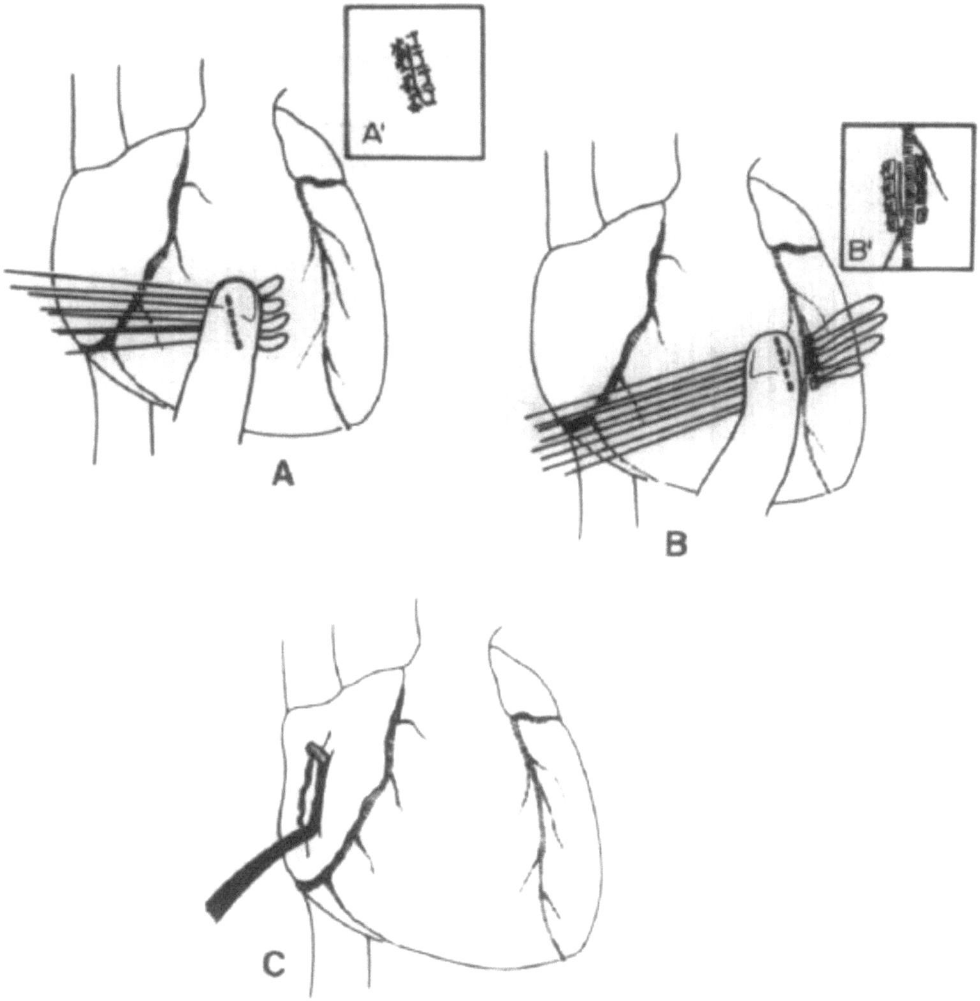

Figure 4. Various maneuvers used to repair penetrating wounds of the heart. Suturing of cardiac wound underneath the wound-occluding finger (A). Wound sutured (A'). Placement of horizontal mattress sutures through the myocardium underneath the cardiac wound-occluding finger and underneath the coronary artery adjacent to the wound (B). Wound sutured (B'). Control of atrial bleeding with a vascular clamp (C). (From Symbas PN: Cardiothoracic Trauma. Philadelphia, WB Saunders Co, 1989, p 42. Used by permission.)

4. Blunt injury

4.1. Background (mechanism, incidence, and pathophysiology)

Blunt cardiac injury (BCI) is a spectrum of traumatic heart diseases with severity that can range from myocardial contusion and EKG changes to septal rupture and death. Earlier in the century, cardiac contusion or concussion were terms used to diagnose cardiac changes from blunt thoracic trauma. More recently, BCI is the term used to better incorporate and classify

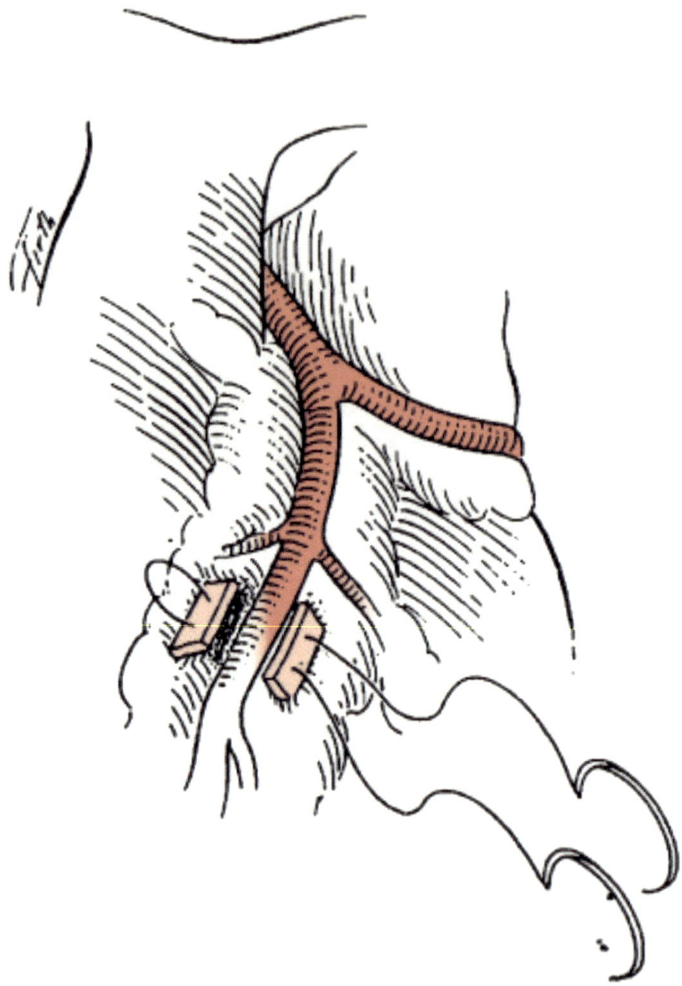

Source: Feliciano DV, Mattox KL, Moore EE: *Trauma*, 6th Edition: http://www.accesssurgery.com

Figure 5.

the myriad of cardiac injuries that result from blunt trauma. BCI is estimated to occur in 20% of motor vehicle collisions and in greater than 75% of thoracic blunt injuries independent of the mechanism. The primary mechanism of injury to the heart is from high-speed motor vehicle collision, but any injury that applies force in the form of kinetic energy to the chest wall and heart can result in a form of BCI. The following mechanisms of injury may result in BCI: direct precordial impact, a crush injury between the sternum and spine, a deceleration injury causing injury from the fixation points of the aorta and vena cava, a hydraulic effect from an intraabdominal injury that sends force to the great vessels and heart, or a crush injury [12].

http://dx.doi.org/10.5772/55723

Since blunt cardiac injury is a spectrum of injuries to the heart, a classification scheme was developed to allow clinicians to categorize the types of injury based on outcomes and treatment options. These categories are as follows: 1) BCI with free wall rupture, 2) BCI with septal rupture, 3) BCI with coronary artery rupture, 4) BCI with cardiac failure, 5) BCI with complex arrhythmias, and 6) BCI with minor ECG or cardiac enzyme abnormalities. The American Association for the Surgery of Trauma (AAST) has also published a cardiac injury scale (Table 2) that may help to codify injury for diagnosis and research. Injuries sustained with blunt cardiac injury (BCI) include contusion, ruptures, septal defects, valvular injuries, and coronary artery injuries. Table 3 lists each of these types and the incidence seen from both autopsy and clinical series. Contusion is the most common type of injury with left atrial chamber rupture being least common. Injuries can often occur concomitantly; approximately 20% of injuries with chamber rupture will have another chamber involved. The right heart is the most commonly injured as it is closest to the sternum which is impacted anteriorly by the steering wheel in motor vehicle collisions. Besides having concomitant cardiac injuries, the force needed to cause a BCI will often cause associated injuries such as chest pain, rib fractures, pulmonary contusions, and solid organ injuries; the most common associated injuries that occur with BCI are listed in Table 5.

4.2. Diagnosis

The best test for diagnosing blunt cardiac injury has been debated for many years. Cardiac enzymes, radionuclide scans, EKG, cardiac ultrasound and continuous monitoring are some of the major methods that have been investigated. Although cardiac enzymes and radionuclide scans have had many supporters these have not shown reliable predictability in diagnosing blunt cardiac injury and have therefore been left out of the Eastern Association for the Surgery of Trauma (EAST) guidelines (figure 6). Cardiac enzymes, specifically serial troponin measurements are mentioned in the suggested BCI algorithm by Schultz and Trunkey 2004 (figure 7) as an adjunct to increase the negative predictive value of the normal EKG when you have a patient who has either a history of cardiac disease or increased age. EKG has emerged as the primary screening tool for blunt cardiac injury. There are no pathognomonic findings; however, the presence of a new arrhythmia is a sign that workup needs to be escalated. If the EKG is negative in a young hemodynamically stable patient without a history of cardiac disease there is no further need for workup [12]. If the EKG is abnormal, and the patient has a history of cardiac disease, increased age or hemodynamic instability then continuous telemetry monitoring for 24-48 hours is recommended. Those with hemodynamic instability require continuous monitoring in a surgical ICU. Any arrhythmia may be detected after BCI including sinus tachycardia, supraventricular arrhythmias, ventricular arrhythmias, any type of heart block, ST-T changes or Q waves [13].

Although, these patients are likely to have had a FAST exam in the emergency room, it is important to figure out who needs a formal echocardiogram. The key indication is hemodynamic instability and a possible diagnosis of blunt cardiac injuiry. Anyone meeting these criteria requires a formal echocardiogram. There has been debate over whether to use transthoracic or transesophageal echocardiography. The recommendations are that the patient receive the first available study method. If transthoracic echocardiography is used and adequate imaging cannot be obtained, then a transesophageal echocardiogram should be initiated immediately.

Grade	Description of injury	ICD-9	AIS-90
I	Blunt cardiac injury with minor ECG abnormality (nonspecific ST or T wave changes, premature arterial or ventricular contraction or persistent sinus tachycardia)	861.01	3
	Blunt or penetrating pericardial wound with out cardiac injury, cardiac tamponade, or cardiac herniation	861.01	3
II	Blunt cardiac injury with heart block (right or left bundle branch, left anterior fascicular, or atrioventricular) or ischemic changes (ST depression or T wave inversion) without cardiac failure	861.12	3
	Penetrating tangential myocardial wound up to, but not extending through endocardium, without tamponade	861.01	3-4
III	Blunt cardiac injury with sustained (≥6 beats/min) or multilocal ventricular contractions	861.01	3-4
	Blunt or penetrating cardiac injury with septal rupture, pulmonary or tricuspid valvular incompetence, papillary muscle dysfunction, or distal coronary arterial occlusion without cardiac failure	861.01	3-4
	Blunt pericardial laceration with cardiac herniation	861.12	3-4
	Blunt cardiac injury with cardiac failure	861.12	3-4
	Penetrating tangential myocardial wound up to, but extending through, endocardium, with tamponade	861.03	3
IV	Blunt or penetrating cardiac injury with septal rupture, pulmonary or tricuspid valvular incompetence, papillary muscle dysfunction, or distal coronary arterial occlusion producing cardiac failure	861.03	3
	Blunt or penetrating cardiac injury with aortic mitral valve incompetence	861.13	3
	Blunt or penetrating cardiac injury of the right ventricle, right atrium, or left atrium	861.03	5
V	Blunt or penetrating cardiac injury with proximal coronary arterial occlusion	861.13	5
	Blunt or penetrating left ventricular perforation		5
	Stellate wound with < 50% tissue loss of the right ventricle, right atrium, or of left atrium		5
VI	Blunt avulsion of the heart		6
	Penetrating wound producing > 50% tissue loss of a chamber		6

*Advance one grade for multiple wounds to a single chamber or multiple chamber involvement.

Table 2. Cardiac Injury Scale

4.3. Management

Since blunt cardiac injury describes a spectrum of disease states, the treatment depends on the actual problem. Arrhythmia can be managed medically with the caveat that anticoagulation needs to be used cautiously in trauma patients. Hemopericardium can be seen with or without

http://dx.doi.org/10.5772/55723

Cardiac Injury	Incidence of injury in autopsy series of patients with BCI	Incidence of injury in clinical series of patients with BCI
Myocardial contusion	60% to 100%	60% to 100%
Chamber Rupture		
Right Ventricle	19% to 32%	17% to 32%
Right Atrium	10% to 15%	8% to 65%
Left Ventricle	5% to 44%	8% to 15%
Left Atrium	1% to 7%	0% to 31%
Atrial Septal Defect	7%	Case reports
Valve Injury in BCI	5%	Case reports
Ventricular Septal Defect	4%	Case reports
Coronary Artery Injury	3%	Case reports

Table 3. BCI Patterns of Injury

Associated Injuries	Incidence of finding in patients with BCI
Chest Pain	18% to 92%
Rib Fracture	18% to 69%
Aortic or great vessel injury	20% to 40%
Hemothorax	7% to 64%
Pulmonary Contusion	6% to 58%
Pneumothorax	7% to 40%
Flail Chest	4% to 38%
Sternal Fracture	0% to 60%
Traumatic Brain Injury	20% to 73%
Extremity Injury	20% to 66%
Abdominal Solid Organ Injury	5% to 43%
Spinal Injury	10% to 20%

Table 4. Injuries Associated with BCI

hypotension or tamponade. If hemopericardium is suspected and the patient is stable a subxiphoid pericardial window can be used to verify the hemopericardium. Once a pericardial window is performed, the surgeon must be prepared to proceed with a median sternotomy. If the patient is hypotensive and tamponade is expected then either a subxiphoid pericardial window or a thoracotomy can be performed. As a rule free wall rupture is more common in the atria than the ventricles and more common on the right than the left. This is thought to be

EAST guidelines

A. Level I

1. An admission EKG should be performed on all patients in who there is suspected BCI.

B. Level II

1. If the admission EKG is abnormal (arrhythmia, ST changes, ischemia, heart block, unexplained ST), the patient should be admitted for continuous EKG monitoring for 24 to 48 hours. Conversely, if the admission EKG is normal, the risk of having a BCI that requires treatment is insignificant, and the pursuit of diagnosis should be terminated.
2. If the patient is hemodynamically unstable, an imaging study (echocardiogram) should be obtained. If an optimal transthoracic echocardiogram cannot be performed, then the patient should have a transesophageal echocardiogram.
3. Nuclear medicine studies add little when compared to echocardiography and, thus, are not useful if an echocardiogram has been performed.

C. Level III

1. Elderly patients with known cardiac disease, unstable patients, and those with an abnormal admission EKG can be safely operated on provided they are appropriately monitored. Consideration should be given to placement of a pulmonary artery catheter in such cases.
2. The presence of a sternal fracture does not predict the presence of BCI and, thus, does not necessarily indicate that monitoring should be performed.
3. Neither creatinine phosphokinase with isoenzyme analysis nor measurement of circulating cardiac troponin T are useful in predicting which patients have or will have complications related to BCI.

Screening of Blunt Cardiac Injury. **Pasquale, N K and Clark, J.** s.l. : The Eastern Association for the Surgry of Trauma, 1998.

Figure 6. EAST guidelines for Blunt Cardiac Injury

due in part to the position of the heart in the chest. The method of repairing the atria is to grasp each side of the atrial wound, place a vascular clamp across the defect, and sew it closed. The method of repair of the ventricle is to place a finger of the non-dominant hand over the injury occluding the wound and stopping the blood loss. Then pledgeted mattress sutures are placed under the finger in order to approximate the wound without tearing through the injured myocardium. Septal rupture requires the patient to be placed on bypass. Coronary artery injury, valve injury and papillary muscle rupture are all very rare. These entities generally

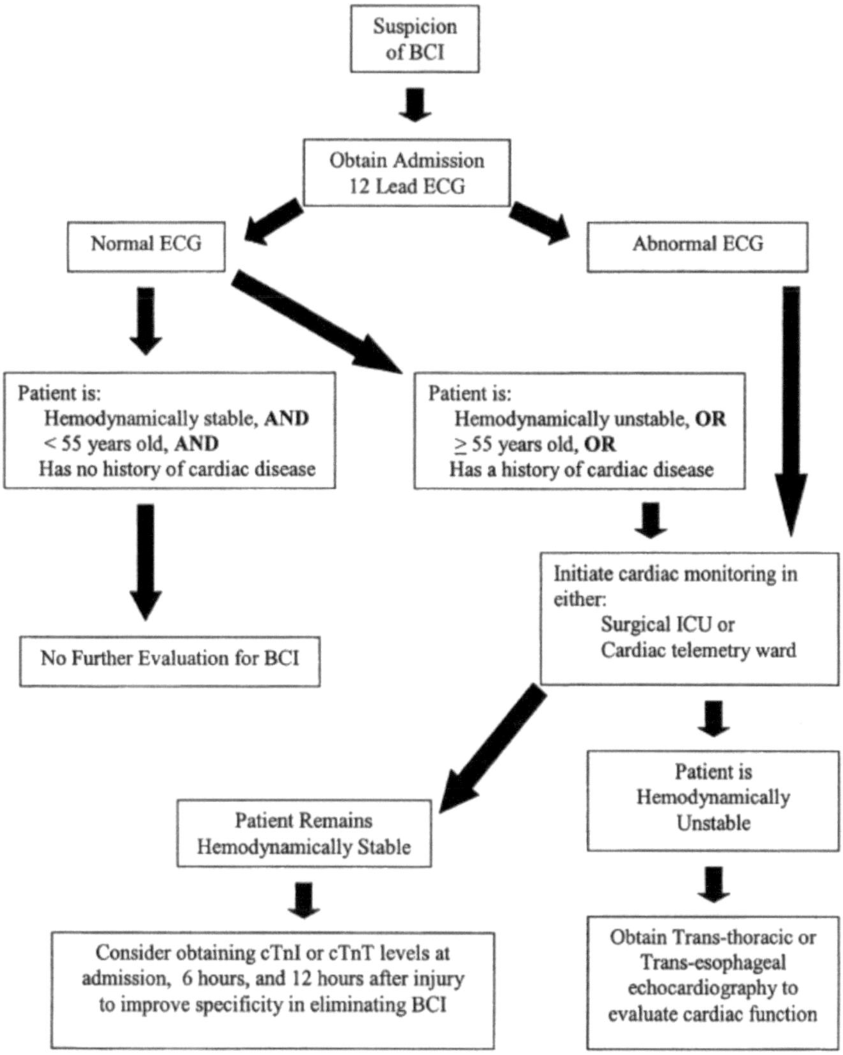

Blunt Cardiac Injury. Schultz JM, Trunkey DD. Critical Care Clin. 20 (2004) 57-70[12]

Figure 7. Algorithm for treatment of suspected BCI

present with clinically significant acute congestive heart failure. Another rare entity is pericardial rupture with cardiac herniation. This requires opening the chest with replacement of the heart in the normal anatomic position and repair of any injured vasculature. Whether you utilize a thoracotomy or sternotomy will depend on the details of the cardiac herniation.

Outcomes of emergency department thoracotomy for blunt trauma are universally poor. The salvage rate of patients with or without vital signs on arrival to the emergency department is 1%-2% [14]. This low survival rate mandates that before an emergency department thoracot-

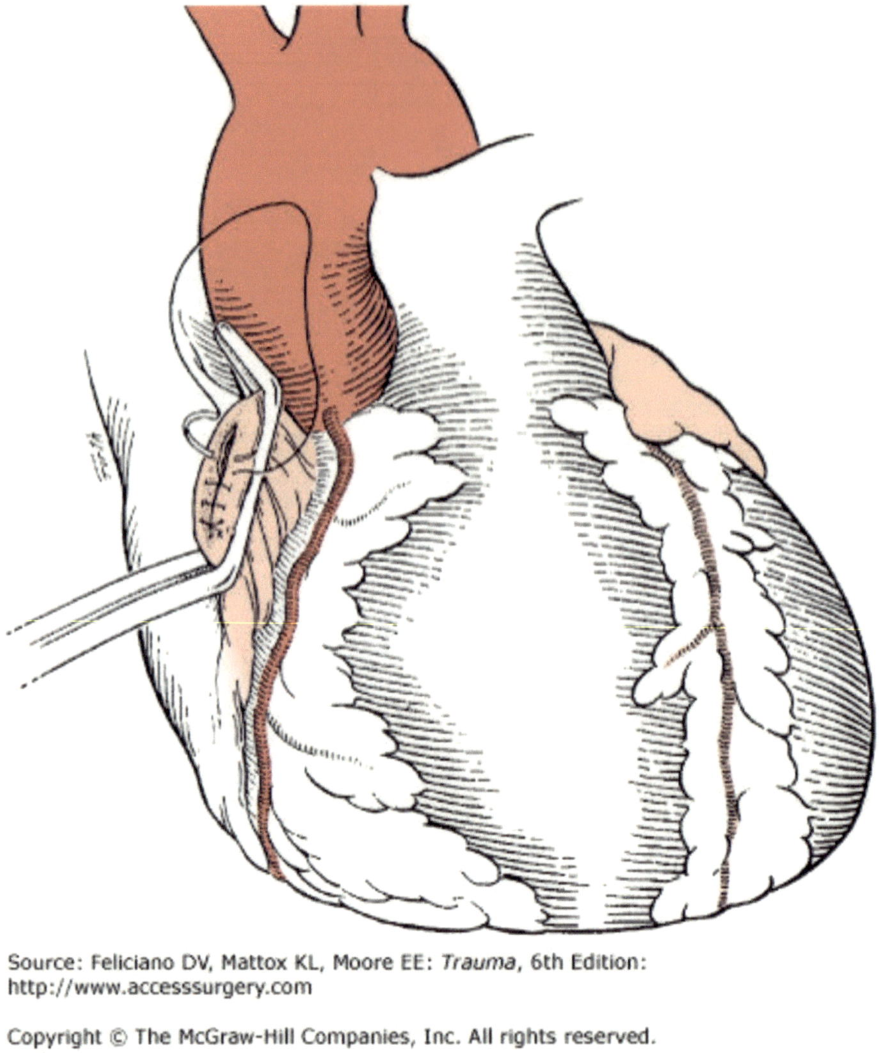

Figure 8. Schematic Representation of right atrial repair

omy is undertaken both the mechanism of injury and the length or presence of CPR be taken into consideration.

Author details

Daniel Eiferman*, R. Nathan Cotterman and Michael Firstenberg

Ohio State University Medical Center, Department of Surgery, Division of Trauma, Critical Care, and Burn, Columbus, OH, USA

References

[1] Rozycki, G.S., et al., The role of ultrasound in patients with possible penetrating cardiac wounds: a prospective multicenter study. J Trauma, 1999. 46(4): p. 543-51; discussion 551-2.

[2] Thourani, V.H., et al., Penetrating cardiac trauma at an urban trauma center: a 22-year perspective. Am Surg, 1999. 65(9): p. 811-6; discussion 817-8.

[3] Velmahos, G.C., et al., Penetrating trauma to the heart: a relatively innocent injury. Surgery, 1994. 115(6): p. 694-7.

[4] Plummer, D., et al., Emergency department echocardiography improves outcome in penetrating cardiac injury. Ann Emerg Med, 1992. 21(6): p. 709-12.

[5] Karrel, R., M.A. Shaffer, and J.B. Franaszek, Emergency diagnosis, resuscitation, and treatment of acute penetrating cardiac trauma. Ann Emerg Med, 1982. 11(9): p. 504-17.

[6] Asensio, J.A., et al., Penetrating cardiac injuries: a prospective study of variables predicting outcomes. J Am Coll Surg, 1998. 186(1): p. 24-34.

[7] Symbas, P.N., Cardiothoracic trauma. Curr Probl Surg, 1991. 28(11): p. 741-97.

[8] Evans, J., et al., Principles for the management of penetrating cardiac wounds. Annals of Surgery, 1979. 189(6): p. 777-84.

[9] Kang, N., et al., Penetrating cardiac injury: overcoming the limits set by Nature. Injury, 2009. 40(9): p. 919-27.

[10] Hancock Friesen, C., J.G. Howlett, and D.B. Ross, Traumatic coronary artery fistula management. Ann Thorac Surg, 2000. 69(6): p. 1973-82.

[11] Lowe, J.E., et al., The natural history and recommended management of patients with traumatic coronary artery fistulas. Ann Thorac Surg, 1983. 36(3): p. 295-305.

[12] Schultz, J.M. and D.D. Trunkey, Blunt cardiac injury. Crit Care Clin, 2004. 20(1): p. 57-70.

[13] Sutherland, G.R., et al., Anatomic and cardiopulmonary responses to trauma with associated blunt chest injury. J Trauma, 1981. 21(1): p. 1-12.

[14] Cothren, C.C. and E.E. Moore, Emergency department thoracotomy for the critically injured patient: Objectives, indications, and outcomes. World J Emerg Surg, 2006. 1: p. 4.

Chapter 14

Gastrointestinal Complications in Cardiothoracic Surgery: A Synopsis

Jennifer Schwartz, David E. Lindsey,
Hooman Khabiri and Stanislaw P. A. Stawicki

Additional information is available at the end of the chapter

http://dx.doi.org/10.5772/54348

1. Introduction

Gastrointestinal complications (GIC) in cardio-thoracic surgery (GIC-CTS) constitute a heterogenous group of non-cardiac/thoracic complications. Although relatively infrequent, these complications are associated with significant mortality and severe clinical sequelae. It is also well recognized that GIC-CTS are often difficult to identify clinically [1], and the presentation of each specific complication may differ from the presentation of said complication in non-CTS patient populations. The incidence of gastrointestinal complications following CTS ranges from <1% to 4.1% patients [2-4], and is associated with mortality rates between 13.9% and 63% [5-7]. Commonly reported GIC-CTS include gastrointestinal hemorrhage, esophagitis/gastritis, perforated ulcer, acute cholecystitis, acute pancreatitis, and mesenteric ischemia [5]. Predominant factors associated with increased mortality following a gastrointestinal complication after cardiac surgery include patient age, COPD, smoking, NYHA class III and IV heart failure, and hepatic insufficiency [8].

2. Risk factors for GIC-CTS

Numerous studies report on specific risk factors for GIC-CTS. Although some of the factors seem to be universally present across different studies, some others are likely unique to specific study populations. A comprehensive list of commonly cited risk factors compiled from the literature includes: (a) decreased left ventricular ejection fraction (<40%) including postoperative low cardiac output; (b) advanced patient age; (c) pre-existing conditions such as diabetes, renal failure, peripheral vascular disease; (d) valvular surgery or combined coronary artery bypass/valve operation; (e) prolonged mechanical ventilation; (f) emergency surgery; (g) prolonged pump time; (h) need for intra-aortic balloon pump (IABP) or vasopressors during or after surgery; (i) need for re-exploration following surgery (re-sternotomy or re-thoracotomy); (j) pre-existing gastric ulcer disease; (k) stroke; and (l) postoperative sepsis/infectious complications including sternal wound infection [3-5, 9-12].

3. Physiologic and bowel motility changes following cardiac surgery

Despite significant hemodynamic implications of cardiac surgery, the effects on gastrointestinal system function are only modest at best. It is important to note that cardiopulmonary bypass impairs small intestinal transport and increases gut permeability, especially when pump times exceed 100 minutes [13]. Intestinal absorption also appears to be affected in cardio-thoracic surgical patients [14].

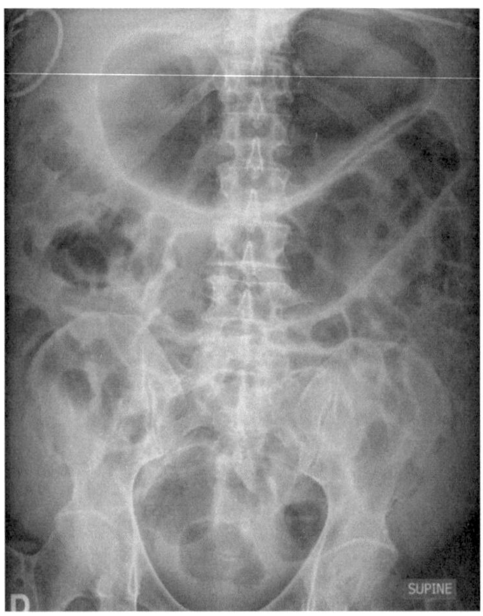

Figure 1. Postoperative ileus following thoracoscopic right upper lobe resection. The patient improved markedly following 5 days of therapy consisting of nasogastric suction, electrolyte correction and bowel rest.

The incidence of ileus (Figure 1) in cardio-thoracic surgical patients is between 1-2% [15]. Ileus is among the more common complications following cardio-thoracic procedures [16]. Various forms of ileus following CTS constitute approximately 10% of GIC [4]. Gastrointestinal motility dysfunction following cardio-thoracic procedures can take a number of clinical manifestations, from isolated gastric distention to prolonged bowel dysfunction [9]. It is important to note that the appearance of clinically significant new ileus, especially when accompanied by severe abdominal pain, may indicate a more serious underlying problem such as mesenteric ischemia or pancreatitis [15]. Mandatory perioperative fasting, the effect of anesthetic agents, and decreased patient mobility during immediate postoperative recovery, all contribute to temporary intestinal dysfunction, which in the vast majority of cases regresses automatically after the initiation of enteral intake. In a small proportion of patients the ileus persists past the fourth postoperative day, requiring the use of suppositories, enemas, and pro-motility agents (i.e., metaclopramide, erythromycin) to facilitate clinical resolution [17, 18]. In addition, the use of opioids has to be minimized due to the inhibitory effect of these analgesic agents on bowel motility [19]. The abovementioned measures, in conjunction with close clinical monitoring and normalization of serum electrolyte concentrations, are usually successful in restoring or improving intestinal function [20]. Cases that remain unresponsive are treated with a course of nasogastric suction, which should be continued until the return of bowel function.

4. Colonic pseudo-obstruction

Colonic pseudo-obstruction is a rare, poorly understood surgical complication with multifactorial origins [21]. Characterized by marked colonic distention in the absence of distal obstruction (Figure 2), this condition seems to be associated with the disturbance of the autonomic innervation of the colon [22]. Untreated, colonic pseudo-obstruction leads to cecal over-distention and subsequent perforation, with reported mortality as high as 15-50% [21, 22]. The critical cecal diameter range at which perforation is more likely to occur is between 9-12 centimeters [23]. The two main management modalities for colonic pseudo-obstruction, used alone or in combination, are neostigmine administration and colonoscopic decompression [22, 24]. Depending on whether indicated by the finding of bowel perforation or repeated episodes of pseudo-obstruction, surgical options vary from cecal decompression (i.e., cecostomy) to colonic resection with entero-enterostomy or ostomy creation [25]. In the presence of sepsis with hemodynamic instability, damage control surgery may be justified [26-28].

5. Dysphagia

Dysphagia is a common complaint following cardio-thoracic operations [29]. Undoubtedly, there is an association between history of endotracheal intubation, median sternotomy or thoracotomy incisions, postoperative inflammatory changes in the chest/mediastinum and dysphagia in the CTS patient population. The etiology of postoperative dysphagia is multifactorial, including contributions from gastroesophageal reflux, local tissue trauma from surgery and endotracheal intubation, intraoperative trans-esophageal echocardiography (TEE), and other potential factors such as recurrent/superior laryngeal nerve dysfunction or injury [30]. One of the more interesting contributors to post-CTS dysphagia is the performance of intraoperative TEE, with nearly 8 times greater odds of developing dysphagia among patients who underwent TEE versus those who did not [31].

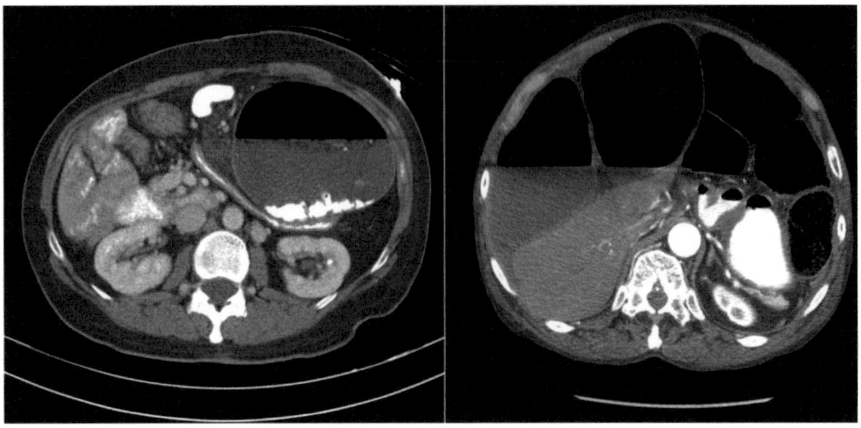

Figure 2. Colonic pseudo-obstruction following cardiac surgery. The first patient (left) presented with increasing abdominal pain/distention, nausea and vomiting following mitral valve replacement. Abdominal CT showed massively dilated left colon with compressive effect on the surrounding small bowel. The pseudo-obstruction resolved with neostigmine therapy. The second patient (right) developed diffuse colonic dilatation following coronary artery bypass grafting. His pseudo-obstruction resolved promptly following emergent colonoscopic decompression.

6. Gastritis and esophagitis

Gastritis and esophagitis are among the more commonly seen gastrointestinal complications in the CTS patient population [32]. In addition to clinical symptoms and history, endoscopy is the most commonly utilized diagnostic modality [33, 34]. Although esophagitis is often associated with gastro-esophageal reflux (GER), the most pressing concern for post-CTS patients with GER is the potential for pulmonary aspiration and associated complications [35]. The etiology of gastritis is multi-factorial, with major contributing elements including mucosal hypoperfusion, previous history of gastric mucosal disorder, and the use of non-steroidal anti-inflammatory drugs [36, 37]. Management includes avoidance of hypotension and hypoperfusion, and aggressive management with H2-receptor blockers or proton pump inhibitors. For postoperative patients with GER and high pulmonary aspiration risk, the maintenance of 45 degree head-of-bed elevation is an important preventive measure [38].

7. Gastrointestinal hemorrhage

Gastrointestinal bleeding is among the most common GIC following cardio-thoracic procedures. In one study, gastrointestinal bleeding constituted nearly 29% of all GIC-CTS [32]. In general, upper gastrointestinal bleeding occurs more frequently than lower gastrointestinal bleeding, with most hemorrhages (>90%) occurring proximal to the ligament of Treitz [5]. Patients with previous history of peptic ulcer disease may be at higher risk for developing an upper gastrointestinal perforation or hemorrhage following cardiac surgery, although other traditional risk factors such as *H. pylori* infection alone do not seem contributory [39]. Prolonged mechanical ventilation significantly elevates the risk of upper gastrointestinal bleeding [39]. The two most common etiologies of upper gastrointestinal bleeding are duodenal ulceration and gastric erosion. The appearance of gastric erosions following CTS is likely secondary to systemic hypoperfusion with subsequent development of mucosal ischemia and erosion [40].

The initial step in diagnosis of gastrointestinal bleeding is the placement of a nasogastric (NG) tube and lavage of gastric contents. This aids in determining if the gastrointestinal hemorrhage is proximal to the ligament of Treitz. Medical therapy is attempted first, and includes the administration of H2-receptor blockers or proton pump inhibitors, red blood cell transfusion, correction of coagulopathy, and temporarily withholding anticoagulation when applicable/possible [41, 42]. If medical management fails, upper endoscopy is the next step in evaluation and treatment of potential bleeding source(s) [43]. Endoscopic attempts aimed at stopping the bleeding by cauterization, vasoconstrictive agent injection, or both are usually effective [42, 43]. In one report, approximately half of the patient with upper gastrointestinal bleeding required upper endoscopy with cauterization to stop the hemorrhage while the other half required surgical intervention to control the bleed [32]. Early surgical intervention if patient fails medical and endoscopic treatment or if significant rebleeding occurs, is recommended. In general, the presence of continued hemodynamic instability, or a pre-determined transfusion threshold (i.e., >4-6 units of packed red blood cells) are utilized as "surgical triggers". Mortality related to gastrointestinal bleeding, even when requiring an operation has decreased over the past two decades.

Lower gastrointestinal bleeding following cardio-thoracic procedures is usually approached according to established clinical algorithms [44]. The first step in management is hemodynamic resuscitation and normalization of coagulation parameters. The bleeding usually stops following these initial maneuvers. If the bleeding does not stop, the next step is the identification of the source of hemorrhage, either endoscopically [45] or by imaging (nuclear scan versus angiography) [46, 47]. In many cases, the bleeding can be controlled endoscopically [48, 49]. Select cases can be treated with endovascular embolization [47]. Surgery should be reserved for refractory cases, with the major determinants for surgery being the failure of non-operative therapies, hemodynamic instability and/or the requirement for transfusion (usually 4-6 units of packed red blood cells) [48, 49].

8. Mesenteric ischemia

Mesenteric ischemia (Figure 3) is a well known complication of CTS that usually occurs within hours to several days after surgery. The gastrointestinal tract is vulnerable to ischemia because it is often unable to acutely compensate for systemic hypotension. Further, due to the potential for persistent vasoconstriction following the initial "low flow" state, gastrointestinal ischemia may continue despite return of hemodynamic stability (i.e., non-occlusive mesenteric ischemia or NOMI). Intestinal ischemia may lead to complications such as mucosal sloughing, gangrenous changes of the bowel wall, and perforation. Mortality may exceed 65% for patients with acute mesenteric ischemia [8]. Early recognition of signs and symptoms of bowel ischemia and early intervention are integral to successful outcomes and lower mortality rates [50]. One of the earliest signs of mesenteric ischemia is abdominal pain out of proportion to physical examination findings [51]. However, this can be quite difficult to elicit in postoperative CTS patients as many are mechanically ventilated and sedated following surgery. In the setting of high clinical suspicion, sigmoidoscopy or colonoscopy can aid in diagnosis of colonic ischemia [52]. The subsequent sections will discuss post-CTS mesenteric ischemia as divided into two major pathophysiologic types: (a) "low flow state" secondary to systemic hypoperfusion; or (b) thrombo-embolic events.

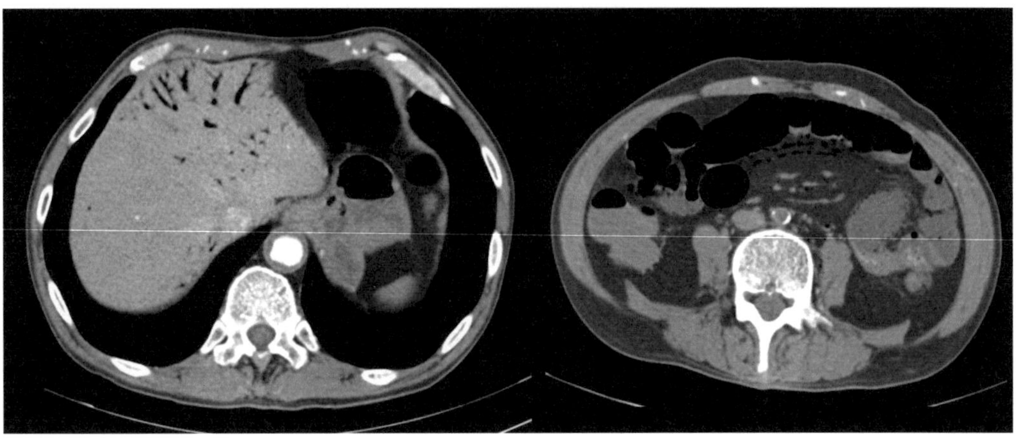

Figure 3. Abdominal CT scan of a patient who developed peritonitis several days after undergoing coronary artery bypass grafting. The study shows diffuse portal venous gas (left) and pneumatosis of the bowel and the mesentery (right). The patient underwent laparotomy with segmental resection of necrotic small bowel. A planned "second-look" laparotomy showed no further bowel necrosis and primary small bowel anastomosis was performed.

9. Ischemia secondary to low flow state

Patients with poor cardiac functional status are at risk for splanchnic hypoperfusion secondary to a number of pre-operative (i.e., pre-existing mesenteric arterial disease), intra-operative (i.e., hypotension/tissue hypoperfusion), and post-operative (i.e., low cardiac output) risk factors. Preoperative presence of conditions such as low left ventricular ejection fraction and peripheral vascular disease have been shown to be significant risks for developing post-operative gastrointestinal ischemia [32].

Intraoperatively, hypovolemia and use of vasoconstrictors can contribute to splanchnic hypoperfusion [53]. Additionally, patients requiring longer cardiopulmonary bypass times may be at greater risk for developing intestinal hypoperfusion [53]. This may be due to the non-pulsatile cardiopulmonary bypass flow characteristics, in conjunction with other factors such as the associated hemolysis, inflammatory cascade activation, the use of anticoagulation, the presence of hypothermia, and the reduced end-organ perfusion. Further, cardiopulmonary bypass may be associated with increased gastrointestinal permeability and enhanced cytokine release, contributing to microcirculatory dysfunction and mucosal injury [32].

In the postoperative setting, inadequate blood flow to the intestines and subsequent intestinal ischemia/infarction can be associated with hypotension and/or cardiogenic shock [10]. In one study, patients with renal failure (Creatinine >1.4), prior myocardial infarction, and those requiring intra-aortic balloon pump support were at higher risk of developing mesenteric ischemia secondary to "low flow" state [8]. Prolonged mechanical ventilation requiring high positive end-expiratory pressure (PEEP) can also result in hypotension and impaired cardiac output, leading to splanchnic vasoconstriction and hypoperfusion. Furthermore, high PEEP is associated with activation of the renin-angiotensin-aldosterone system and increases in catecholamine levels [54]. This, in turn, results in shunting of blood away from the gastrointestinal system, leading to mismatch between oxygen delivery and demand. Persistent deficit in oxygen delivery then leads to mucosal ischemia and damage. Moreover, during the process of tissue re-perfusion after restoration/normalization of adequate oxygen delivery, the persistent vasoconstrictive state of non-occlusive mesenteric ischemia (NOMI) may be seen [32]. Management of NOMI consists of restoration of adequate circulating intravascular volume, maintenance of adequate cardiac output, and selective angiographic approaches utilizing intra-arterial vasodilating agent infusion therapy [55]. Surgery is reserved for cases requiring resection of necrotic bowel, exploration for suspected perforation, and/or revascularization procedure.

10. Embolic phenomena

Mesenteric ischemia following cardiac surgery results from embolic disease secondary to macrovascular embolism or thrombosis, such as SMA embolus, or microvascular emboli, such as embolic cholesterol "showering" secondary to aortic manipulation. Septic embolization with occlusive phenomena has also been reported in cases of endocarditis following open heart surgery [56]. The size of the embolus may be an important prognostic factor. For example, patients with large vessel emboli may have better outcomes when compared to patients with microvascular or "distal" emboli [8]. High index of suspicion is critical to optimal patient outcomes. If recognized promptly, occlusive emboli to the mesenteric circulation can be treated via either endovascular and/or open surgical approaches, with acceptable success rates [51]. Patients with hypotension, cardiogenic shock, and/or pump failure requiring intra-aortic balloon pump not only are at risk of significant intestinal hypoperfusion, but are also at risk secondary to embolization and thrombus formation which may further exacerbate the original insult to the intestinal tract. Surgical therapy is indicated if the patient develops peritonitis, perforation, sepsis, and/or end-organ failure in the setting of elevated clinical suspicion [57]. Planned or "second look" surgery is warranted if ischemic (but non-necrotic) bowel segments are noted at the conclusion of the initial procedure [58, 59]. Open abdominal approaches using temporary abdominal coverage with negative pressure wound therapy have been described in such situations [27].

11. Pancreatitis

Acute pancreatitis is relatively uncommon (incidence 1-3%) following cardiopulmonary bypass [15]. Clinically apparent pancreatitis usually occurs slightly later following cardiac surgery than other gastrointestinal complications, such as bleeding or mesenteric ischemia. Patients typically complain of upper abdominal and left upper quadrant pain, nausea, vomiting, and/or abdominal distension. Laboratory values including elevated amylase and lipase are usually present. However, due to high incidence of hyperamylasemia in cardiac surgery patients (>33%) [15], clinical correlation is required before definitive diagnosis of pancreatitis is made.

The severity of pancreatitis ranges from subclinical (i.e., noted only on laboratory values) to severe hemorrhagic, necrotic pancreatitis (seen in <0.5% of patients) (Figure 4) [60]. In one study, nearly 20% of patients who underwent cardiac surgery were found to have evidence of pancreatitis on autopsy [61]. Although the mechanism explaining the development of pancreatitis after cardiac surgery has not been discovered, it has been hypothesized that low flow state, tissue ischemia, gallstone disease, micro-embolization, and history of pre-existing pancreatic disease all contribute to post-CTS acute pancreatitis.

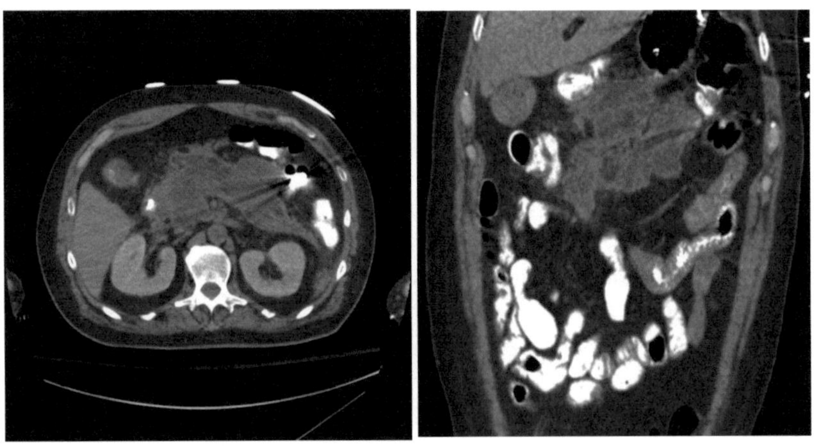

Figure 4. Abdominal CT of a patient who developed acute upper abdominal pain following aortic valve replacement surgery. Representative images of severe necrotizing pancreatitis are shown. Non-operative management resulted in resolution of pancreatitis approximately 2 weeks after the diagnosis was made.

12. Acute cholecystitis

Acute cholecystitis is another commonly seen gastrointestinal complication following CTS (Figure 5). In one study, incidence of acute cholecystitis was approximately 8% among all postoperative gastrointestinal complications [5]. Many cases of acute cholecystitis associated with CTS are termed "acalculous cholecystitis" and are secondary to biliary stasis as a result of multiple factors such as lack of enteral feeding and gallbladder wall ischemia secondary to a "low flow" state. Mortality rates associated with acalculous cholecystitis are significant (>50%) which may reflect the overall poor general health status of patients at risk for this complication [62, 63]. Typical symptoms include right upper quadrant pain and tenderness on examination. However, diagnosis is often delayed secondary to the presence of mechanical ventilation and sedation in significant proportion of patients with acalculous cholecystitis. Patients with acute cholecystitis, diagnosed most often on right upper quadrant ultrasound or cholescintigraphy scan, require surgical intervention or percutaneous cholecystostomy tube placement for treatment of cholecystitis. For poor surgical candidates, percutaneous cholecystostomy can serve as "bridging" therapy that facilitates the patient's recovery until he or she is ready to undergo cholecystectomy [64].

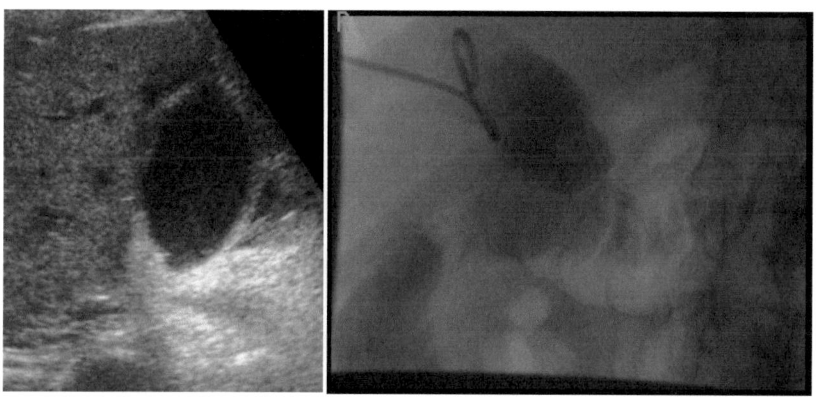

Figure 5. Elderly male patient developed cerebral infarction 2 days after undergoing aortic valve replacement. His recovery was further complicated by acute cholecystitis, as demonstrated by right upper quadrant ultrasound showing distended gallbladder with wall thickening, sludge and pericholecystic fluid (left). His operative risk for cholecystectomy was prohibitive at that time, prompting the placement of percutaneous cholecystostomy (right). Following good functional recovery and hospital discharge, the percutaneous drain was removed and the patient underwent elective laparoscopic cholecystectomy.

13. Gastrointestinal complications unique to transplant recipients and immunosuppression

Immunosuppressive regimens administered to transplant recipients predispose this patient population to elevated risk for bacterial, fungal, parasitic, and viral infections [65]. Within this broad pathophysiologic spectrum, gastrointestinal infection and associated manifestations feature prominently. While a complete discussion of this topic is beyond the scope of this chapter, we thought it would be important to mention some of the more prominent among these post-transplant sequelae. The list of potential gastrointestinal complications seen after solid organ transplantation is diverse, including cytomegalovirus enteritis [65], herpes simplex virus mucocutaneous manifestations [66], candidal esophagitis [67], *Clostridium difficile* and *Yersinia enterocolitica* infections [4], parasitic (protozoan/metazoan) enteritis [67], and *Helicobacter pylori* infection [68]. Among other post-transplant gastrointestinal complications, organ recipients may be more likely to exhibit diarrhea, luminal ulcerations, perforations, biliary tract complaints, pancreatitis, and gastrointestinal malignancy (i.e., post-transplant lymphoproliferative disorder) [65, 69]. For more detail regarding post-transplant and immunosuppresion-related gastrointestinal complications among heart and lung recipients, the reader is referred to more specialized literature on this expansive topic [65, 67, 68].

14. Miscellaneous gastrointestinal and abdominal complications related to cardiac surgery

Among less commonly encountered (and reported) complications of cardiac surgery are those associated with trans-esophageal echocardiography (TEE). Likely under-reported, TEE-related complications in cardiac surgical patients occur in as many as 1.2% of patients [70]. In one series, esophageal and gastric tears were seen within 24 hours of the TEE in 2 patients, with additional gastric ulceration and gastric tear seen within 5 days of the procedure. Moreover, gastric perforations were described presenting between 4-11 days post-TEE. Among the 6 reported cases, 3 required a laparotomy, 2 were treated endoscopically, and 1 patient required transfusion [70].

Epigastric (sub-xiphoid) and chest tube site hernias [71] following cardiac surgery occur in as many as 3-4% of patients following median sternotomy [72]. Another, much less common complications related to the mediastinal tube thoracostomy is superior epigastric artery pseudoaneurysm [73]. Management of these rare conditions is mostly surgical, although minimally symptomatic high-risk surgical patients may be followed with clinical observation.

Due to the growing volume of mechanical cardiac and pulmonary assistive technologies (i.e., ventricular assist devices, intra-aortic balloon pumps, extra-corporeal membrane oxygenation devices), it is important to mention potential gastrointestinal and abdominal complications associated with these devices. Not unexpectedly, the use of cardio-respiratory mechanical assistive devices has been found to be associated with clinically significant abdominal and gastrointestinal complications [32, 74, 75]. For example, extracorporeal membrane oxygenation has been associated with embolic phenomena of the systemic circulation, end-organ ischemia, gastrointestinal hemorrhage, and abdominal compartment syndrome [74, 76-78]. Patients who undergo ventricular assist device placement are also exposed to a number of potential gastrointestinal and abdominal complications, including abdominal infection, bowel injury, acalculous cholecystitis, pancreatitis, various hernias (i.e., incisional,

http://dx.doi.org/10.5772/54348

inguinal, diaphragmatic), peritoneal fluid leaks, and mesenteric ischemia [75, 79-83]. Of note, gastrointestinal hemorrhage has also been reported in patients with ventricular assist devices [84, 85], with higher bleeding rates seen among recipients of non-pulsatile devices as compared to pulsatile devices [86]. There is a trend toward higher mortality among patients receiving ventricular assist devices who experience abdominal complications [75]. Intra-aortic balloon pumps are among known risk factors for gastrointestinal complications following CTS [8, 32]. Some of the reported GIC associated with intra-aortic balloon pump use include gastrointestinal bleeding, bowel ischemia, and pancreatitis [78, 87, 88].

15. Conclusions

Gastrointestinal complications following cardio-thoracic procedures continue to significantly contribute to morbidity and mortality in this patient population. Preventive strategies, coupled with early recognition and aggressive management of GIC-CTS constitute the foundation of the general clinical approach to these complications. Therefore, it is imperative that all practitioners who care for postoperative cardiac and thoracic surgical patients are familiar with the full spectrum of potential gastrointestinal complications in this patient population, as well as with general therapeutic approaches to these complications.

Author details

Jennifer Schwartz[1], David E. Lindsey[1,2], Hooman Khabiri[3] and Stanislaw P. A. Stawicki[1,2]

1 Department of Surgery, The Ohio State University College of Medicine, Columbus Ohio, USA

2 Division of Critical Care Trauma and Burn, The Ohio State University College of Medicine, Columbus Ohio, USA

3 Department of Radiology, Section of Interventional Radiology, The Ohio State University College of Medicine, Columbus Ohio, USA

References

[1] Andersson, B, et al. Gastrointestinal complications after cardiac surgery. Br J Surg, (2005). , 326-333.

[2] Zacharias, A, et al. Predictors of gastrointestinal complications in cardiac surgery. Tex Heart Inst J, (2000). , 93-99.

[3] Negargar, S, et al. Gastrointestinal complications after cardiac surgery. Journal of Iranian Society of Anesthesiology and Intensive Care, (2003). , 66-74.

[4] Geissler, H. J, et al. Incidence and outcome of gastrointestinal complications after cardiopulmonary bypass. Interact Cardiovasc Thorac Surg, (2006). , 239-242.

[5] Yilmaz, A. T, et al. Gastrointestinal complications after cardiac surgery. Eur J Cardiothorac Surg, (1996). , 763-767.

[6] Huddy, S. P, Joyce, W. P, & Pepper, J. R. Gastrointestinal complications in 4473 patients who underwent cardiopulmonary bypass surgery. Br J Surg, (1991). , 293-296.

[7] Lazar, H. L, et al. Gastrointestinal complications following cardiac surgery. Cardiovasc Surg, (1995). , 341-344.

[8] Mangi, A. A, et al. Gastrointestinal complications in patients undergoing heart operation: an analysis of 8709 consecutive cardiac surgical patients. Ann Surg, (2005). discussion 901-4., 895-901.

[9] Halm, M. A. Acute gastrointestinal complications after cardiac surgery. Am J Crit Care, (1996). quiz 119-20., 109-118.

[10] Christenson, J. T, et al. Postoperative visceral hypotension the common cause for gastrointestinal complications after cardiac surgery. Thorac Cardiovasc Surg, (1994). , 152-157.

[11] Franz, W. D. Postoperative abdominal complications after thoracic surgery (author's transl)]. Zentralbl Chir, (1977). , 621-623.

[12] Mlekodaj, S, & Musialek, W. Acute abdominal complications following thoracic surgery]. Gruzlica, (1971). , 541-546.

[13] Ohri, S. K, et al. Cardiopulmonary bypass impairs small intestinal transport and increases gut permeability. Ann Thorac Surg, (1993). , 1080-1086.

[14] Berger, M. M, et al. Intestinal absorption in patients after cardiac surgery. Crit Care Med, (2000). , 2217-2223.

[15] Akpinar, B, et al. Acute gastrointestinal complications after open heart surgery. Asian Cardiovasc Thorac Ann, (2000). , 109-113.

[16] Simic, O, et al. Abdominal complications after heart surgery interventions]. Zentralbl Chir, (1997). , 893-897.

[17] Miller, F, & Fenzl, T. C. Prolonged ileus with acute spinal cord injury responding to metaclopramide. Paraplegia, (1981). , 43-45.

[18] Korolkiewicz, R. P, & Kuziemski, K. Use of erythromycin in prevention or treatment of postoperative ileus. Urology, (2008). , 231.

[19] Kraft, M. D. Methylnaltrexone, a new peripherally acting mu-opioid receptor antagonist being evaluated for the treatment of postoperative ileus. Expert Opin Investig Drugs, (2008). , 1365-1377.

[20] Karangelis, D, et al. Gastrointestinal Complications Following Heart Surgery: An Updated Review. European Journal of Cardiovascular Medicine, (2011). , 34-37.

[21] Apostolakis, E. R, & Thiel, W. Bircks, Acute pseudo-obstruction of the colon (Ogilvie's syndrome) following open heart surgery. Thorac Cardiovasc Surg, (1990). , 371-373.

[22] Vanek, V. W, & Al-salti, M. Acute pseudo-obstruction of the colon (Ogilvie's syndrome). An analysis of 400 cases. Dis Colon Rectum, (1986). , 203-210.

[23] Nanni, G, et al. Ogilvie's syndrome (acute colonic pseudo-obstruction): review of the literature ((October 1948 to March 1980). and report of four additional cases. Dis Colon Rectum, 1982. 25(2): , 157-166.

[24] Connor, F. L. and C. Di Lorenzo, Chronic intestinal pseudo-obstruction: assessment and management. Gastroenterology, (2006). Suppl 1): , S29-S36.

[25] Simic, O, et al. Incidence and prognosis of abdominal complications after cardiopulmonary bypass. Cardiovasc Surg, (1999). , 419-424.

[26] Stawicki, S. P, et al. The concept of damage control: extending the paradigm to emergency general surgery. Injury, (2008). , 93-101.

[27] Smith, B. P, et al. Review of abdominal damage control and open abdomens: focus on gastrointestinal complications. J Gastrointestin Liver Dis, (2010). , 425-435.

[28] Stawicki, S. P, Cipolla, J, & Bria, C. Comparison of open abdomens in non-trauma and trauma patients: a retrospective study. OPUS 12 Scientist, (2007). , 1-8.

[29] Gundry, S. R, et al. Candida esophagitis following cardiac operation and short-term antibiotic prophylaxis. J Thorac Cardiovasc Surg, (1980). , 661-668.

[30] Andersson, B, et al. Gastrointestinal complications after cardiac surgery- improved risk stratification using a new scoring model. Interact Cardiovasc Thorac Surg, (2010). , 366-370.

[31] Ziegelin, M, et al. Does clopidogrel rather than aspirin plus a proton-pump inhibitor reduce the frequency of gastrointestinal complications after cardiac surgery? Interact Cardiovasc Thorac Surg, (2007). , 534-537.

[32] Ancona, D, et al. Determinants of gastrointestinal complications in cardiac surgery. Tex Heart Inst J, (2003). , 280-285.

[33] The role of endoscopy in the management of esophagitis. Guidelines for clinical application. Gastrointest Endosc, (1988). Suppl): , 9S.

[34] Sartori, S, et al. Role of endoscopy in the diagnosis of gastritis. Medicina (Firenze), (1988). , 309-310.

[35] Russell, G. N, et al. Gastroesophageal reflux and tracheobronchial contamination after cardiac surgery: should a nasogastric tube be routine? Anesth Analg, (1996). , 228-232.

[36] Bennett, J. S, et al. The use of nonsteroidal anti-inflammatory drugs (NSAIDs): a science advisory from the American Heart Association. Circulation, (2005). , 1713-1716.

[37] Yapici, N, & Ince, C. Gastrointestinal complications and its predictors after cardiac surgery. Turk J Gastroenterol, (2010). , 3-6.

[38] Keeley, L. Reducing the risk of ventilator-acquired pneumonia through head of bed elevation. Nurs Crit Care, (2007). , 287-294.

[39] Halm, U, et al. Helicobacter pylori infection: a risk factor for upper gastrointestinal bleeding after cardiac surgery? Crit Care Med, (2000). , 110-113.

[40] Egleston, C. V, et al. Gastrointestinal complications after cardiac surgery. Ann R Coll Surg Engl, (1993). , 52-56.

[41] Lau, J. Y, et al. Effect of intravenous omeprazole on recurrent bleeding after endoscopic treatment of bleeding peptic ulcers. N Engl J Med, (2000). , 310-316.

[42] Sung, J. J, et al. Endoscopic clipping versus injection and thermo-coagulation in the treatment of non-variceal upper gastrointestinal bleeding: a meta-analysis. Gut, (2007). , 1364-1373.

[43] Soehendra, N, Grimm, H, & Stenzel, M. Injection of nonvariceal bleeding lesions of the upper gastrointestinal tract. Endoscopy, (1985). , 129-132.

[44] Barnert, J, & Messmann, H. Diagnosis and management of lower gastrointestinal bleeding. Nat Rev Gastroenterol Hepatol, (2009). , 637-646.

[45] Green, B. T, et al. Urgent colonoscopy for evaluation and management of acute lower gastrointestinal hemorrhage: a randomized controlled trial. Am J Gastroenterol, (2005). , 2395-2402.

[46] Winzelberg, G. G, et al. Radionuclide localization of lower gastrointestinal hemorrhage. Radiology, (1981). , 465-469.

[47] Gordon, R. L, et al. Selective arterial embolization for the control of lower gastrointestinal bleeding. Am J Surg, (1997). , 24-28.

[48] Zuckerman, G. R, & Prakash, C. Acute lower intestinal bleeding. Part II: etiology, therapy, and outcomes. Gastrointest Endosc, (1999). , 228-238.

[49] Zuckerman, G. R, & Prakash, C. Acute lower intestinal bleeding: part I: clinical presentation and diagnosis. Gastrointest Endosc, (1998). , 606-617.

[50] Chang, R. W, Chang, J. B, & Longo, W. E. Update in management of mesenteric ischemia. World J Gastroenterol, (2006). , 3243-3247.

[51] Park, W. M, et al. Contemporary management of acute mesenteric ischemia: Factors associated with survival. J Vasc Surg, (2002)., 445-452.

[52] Brandt, C. P, Piotrowski, J. J, & Alexander, J. J. Flexible sigmoidoscopy. A reliable determinant of colonic ischemia following ruptured abdominal aortic aneurysm. Surg Endosc, (1997)., 113-115.

[53] Moneta, G. L, Misbach, G. A, & Ivey, T. D. Hypoperfusion as a possible factor in the development of gastrointestinal complications after cardiac surgery. Am J Surg, (1985)., 648-650.

[54] Aneman, A, et al. Hemodynamic, sympathetic and angiotensin II responses to PEEP ventilation before and during administration of isoflurane. Acta Anaesthesiol Scand, (1997). Pt 1):, 41-48.

[55] Trompeter, M, et al. Non-occlusive mesenteric ischemia: etiology, diagnosis, and interventional therapy. Eur Radiol, (2002)., 1179-1187.

[56] Misawa, S, et al. Septic embolic occlusion of the superior mesenteric artery induced by mitral valve endocarditis. Ann Thorac Cardiovasc Surg, (2011)., 415-417.

[57] Caleb, M. G. Acute bowel ischemia after coronary bypass surgery--a catastrophic event. Singapore Med J, (2001)., 33-37.

[58] Wang, Y. Z. Staged second-look laparoscopy to evaluate ischemic bowel. JSLS, (2009)., 560-563.

[59] Slutzki, S, et al. The laparoscopic second look for ischemic bowel disease. Surg Endosc, (1996)., 729-731.

[60] Haas, G. S, et al. Acute pancreatitis after cardiopulmonary bypass. Am J Surg, (1985)., 508-515.

[61] Feiner, H. Pancreatitis after cardiac surgery; a morphologic study. Am J Surg, (1976)., 684-688.

[62] Leitman, I. M, et al. Intra-abdominal complications of cardiopulmonary bypass operations. Surg Gynecol Obstet, (1987)., 251-254.

[63] Krasna, M. J, et al. Gastrointestinal complications after cardiac surgery. Surgery, (1988)., 773-780.

[64] Elmunzer, B. J, et al. Percutaneous cholecystostomy as a bridge to definitive endoscopic gallbladder stent placement. Clin Gastroenterol Hepatol, (2011)., 18-20.

[65] Bennett, S. M, et al. The scope and impact of perinatal loss: Current status and future directions. Professional Psychology-Research and Practice, (2005)., 180-187.

[66] Brajtman, S, et al. Providing direction for change: assessing Canadian nursing students learning needs. Int J Palliat Nurs, (2007)., 213-221.

[67] Prendergast, T. J, & Puntillo, K. A. Withdrawal of life support: intensive caring at the end of life. JAMA, (2002). , 2732-2740.

[68] Dimitrakakis, G, Keefe, P. A. O, & Von Oppell, U. O. eComment. Gastrointestinal complications in cardiac surgery. Interact Cardiovasc Thorac Surg, (2012). , 627-628.

[69] Rodriguez, R, et al. Gastrointestinal complications following cardiac surgery: a comprehensive review. J Card Surg, (2010). , 188-197.

[70] Lennon, M. J, et al. Transesophageal echocardiography-related gastrointestinal complications in cardiac surgical patients. J Cardiothorac Vasc Anesth, (2005). , 141-145.

[71] Kesieme, E. B, et al. Tube thoracostomy: complications and its management. Pulm Med, (2012). , 256878.

[72] Davidson, B. R, & Bailey, J. S. Repair of incisional hernia after median sternotomy. Thorax, (1987). , 549-550.

[73] Sadat, U, et al. Superior epigastric artery pseudoaneurysm--a rare complication of chest drain insertion in coronary artery bypass grafting. J Cardiothorac Surg, (2007). , 21.

[74] Augustin, P, et al. Abdominal compartment syndrome due to extracorporeal membrane oxygenation in adults. Ann Thorac Surg, (2010). , e40-e41.

[75] Costantini, T. W, Taylor, J. H, & Beilman, G. J. Abdominal complications of ventricular assist device placement. Surg Infect (Larchmt), (2005). , 409-418.

[76] Park, P. K, et al. Extracorporeal membrane oxygenation (ECMO) in patients with ARDS. (2012 [cited 2012 September 9). Available from: http://www.thoracic.org/clinical/critical-care/salvage-therapies-h1n1/pages/ecmo.php.

[77] Sarosiek, K, et al. Adult extracorporeal membrane oxygenation and gastrointestinal bleeding from small bowel arteriovenous malformations: a novel treatment using spiral enteroscopy. J Thorac Cardiovasc Surg, (2012). , 1221-1222.

[78] Muthiah, K, et al. Gastrointestinal (GI) hemorrhage in patients undergoing extracorporeal membrane oxygenation (ECMO). (2012 [cited 2012 September 9). Available from: http://www.pulsus.com/cddw2012/abs/082.htm.

[79] Chatterjee, S, et al. Diaphragmatic hernias associated with ventricular assist devices and heart transplantation. Ann Thorac Surg, (2004). , 2111-2114.

[80] Herman, S. C, et al. Colonic perforation from left ventricular assist device: a rare complication. Interact Cardiovasc Thorac Surg, (2010). , 369-370.

[81] Cipolla, J, et al. Negative pressure wound therapy: Unusual and innovative applications. OPUS 12 Scientist, (2008). , 15-29.

[82] Baradarian, S, et al. Case series: clinical management of persistent mechanical assist device driveline drainage using vacuum-assisted closure therapy. ASAIO J, (2006). , 354-356.

[83] Scherer, M, et al. Extracorporeal membrane oxygenation as perioperative right ventricular support in patients with biventricular failure undergoing left ventricular assist device implantation. Eur J Cardiothorac Surg, (2011). discussion 944., 939-944.

[84] Meyer, M. M, et al. Endoscopic evaluation and management of gastrointestinal bleeding in patients with ventricular assist devices. Gastroenterol Res Pract, (2012). , 630483.

[85] Smith, V, et al. Surgical management of unusual gastrointestinal bleeding and a left ventricular assist device. Interact Cardiovasc Thorac Surg, (2010). , 612-613.

[86] Crow, S, et al. Gastrointestinal bleeding rates in recipients of nonpulsatile and pulsatile left ventricular assist devices. J Thorac Cardiovasc Surg, (2009). , 208-215.

[87] Rivard, J, Vergis, A, & Kassum, D. Case report of visceral ischemia: the "tail" of an intra-aortic balloon pump. J Thorac Cardiovasc Surg, (2008). , 1167-1168.

[88] Rizk, A. B, & Rashkow, A. M. Acute pancreatitis associated with intra-aortic balloon pump placement. Cathet Cardiovasc Diagn, (1996). , 363-364.

Section 3

Great-Vessel Surgery

Chapter 15

Penetrating Aortic Ulcers

Arman Kilic and Ahmet Kilic

Additional information is available at the end of the chapter

http://dx.doi.org/10.5772/54107

1. Introduction

Penetrating aortic ulcers were initially described by Shennan in 1934 [1]. Shumacker and King reported the first operative repair of a ruptured descending aorta secondary to a penetrating aortic ulcer in 1959 [2]. The clinical and pathologic entity of penetrating aortic ulcers was not established, however, until 1986 by Stanson [3]. Since that time, the body of literature on this disease has increased significantly. This chapter provides a broad overview of penetrating aortic ulcers.

2. Pathophysiology

Acute aortic syndromes are a group of disease entities that include penetrating aortic ulcers in addition to aortic dissections and intramural hematomas. Aortic dissections are defined by a tear of the intima that results in passage of blood and separation of the intimal and medial or adventitial layers of the vessel wall (Figure 1) [4]. This typically occurs in patients with cystic medial necrosis or medial degeneration. This creates a false lumen, and propagation of the tear either antegrade or retrograde can result in aortic valve insufficiency, cardiac tamponade, and/or organ malperfusion [5]. Intramural hematomas are caused by rupture of the vaso vasorum. This leads to hemorrhage within the aortic media, and can subsequently lead to rupture of the aortic wall or inward disruption of the intima with resultant secondary aortic dissection [6,7].

As the name suggests, penetrating aortic ulcers arise from atheromatous plaques that ulcerate, causing disruption of the internal elastic lamina [6]. Erosion into the medial layer can lead to development of an intramural hematoma or dissection, complications that can eventually lead to pseudoaneurysm formation or aortic rupture. Penetrating aortic ulcers tend to occur in patients with advanced atherosclerosis. Furthermore, they can occur in isolation or in multiples

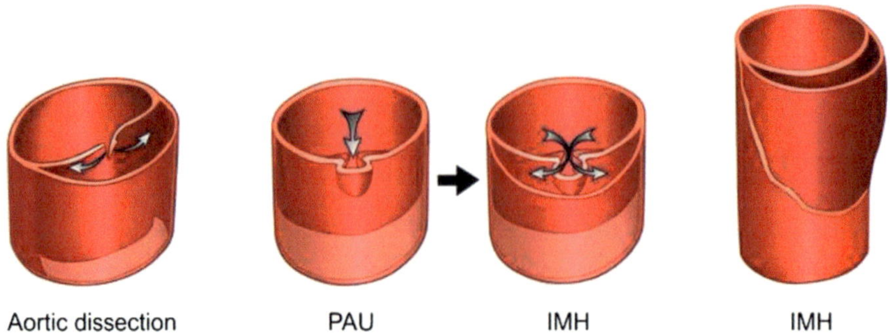

Figure 1. Acute aortic syndromes include aortic dissections, penetrating aortic ulcers (PAU), and intramural hematomas (IMH), each with different pathophysiologies. Aortic dissections are defined by a tear in the intima and separation of the intimal and medial or adventitial layers. Penetrating aortic ulcers result from lesions that ulcerate and disrupt the internal elastic lamina. Intramural hematomas can arise from penetrating aortic ulcers, or can occur in isolation after disruption of the vaso vasorum (from Reference 4 – permission granted).

[8]. Most commonly, penetrating aortic ulcers affect the descending thoracic aorta and less commonly the aortic arch, abdominal aorta, or ascending aorta [9].

3. Epidemiology

Penetrating aortic ulcers comprise 2% to 11% of acute aortic syndromes [10]. In a classic autopsy study, only 4.6% of aortic dissections were found to originate from penetrating aortic ulcers [11]. In one study of incidental findings during cardiac computed tomography for acute chest pain in an emergency department setting, only 1 (0.3%) of 395 consecutive patients was found to have a penetrating aortic ulcer [12]. Another study of incidental findings during cardiac computed tomography similarly found a low prevalence of penetrating aortic ulcers, with only 2 (0.2%) detected in a sample of 966 patients [13].

4. Clinical presentation

The risk factors and clinical presentation of penetrating aortic ulcers are similar yet different in some ways from intramural hematomas and aortic dissections. Similar to patients with intramural hematomas, patients with penetrating aortic ulcers tend to be elderly and are typically older than patients with aortic dissection. As with the other acute aortic syndromes, symptoms include severe chest pain or midscapular pain. An important difference between penetrating aortic ulcers and aortic dissections is that the former tends to be focal disease with absent signs of malperfusion or branch vessel occlusion, whereas the latter can be extensive and present with aortic insufficiency or organ malperfusion. The atherosclerotic burden also tends to be the greatest in patients with penetrating aortic ulcers as compared to those with intramural hematomas or aortic dissections in whom the degree of atherosclerosis is variable.

http://dx.doi.org/10.5772/54107

In a study of 19 patients with penetrating aortic ulcers, common comorbidities included hypertension (95%), chronic obstructive pulmonary disease (63%), cardiac disease (42%), chronic renal insufficiency (26%), and diabetes mellitus (16%) [14]. This comorbidity profile was similar to that seen in patients with intramural hematomas. Patients with penetrating aortic ulcers were found to have the highest rate of concomitant abdominal aortic aneurysms (42%).

A large series of 105 patients with penetrating aortic ulcers demonstrated similar results [15]. Moreover, patients tended to be elderly with an average age of 72 years, and most patients were males (70%) and symptomatic (75%). Common comorbidities included hypertension (92%), smoking (77%), coronary artery disease (46%), chronic obstructive pulmonary disease (24%), and chronic renal insufficiency (21%). Concomitant abdominal aortic aneurysms were found in 61% of patients, and 30% had a pleural effusion on presentation.

5. Diagnosis

5.1. History and physical examination

The diagnosis of penetrating aortic ulcers relies first upon a thorough history and physical examination. The typical patient is elderly with a history of hypertension. As mentioned previously, these patients can also have a history of coronary artery disease, chronic obstructive pulmonary disease, renal disease, and tobacco use. They typically present with anterior chest or midscapular pain. Similar to aortic dissections, those with anterior chest pain usually have ascending aortic involvement and those with back pain typically have descending aortic involvement. The differential diagnosis with this typical presentation includes acute coronary syndrome, aortic aneurysm, aortic dissection, intramural hematoma, and pulmonary embolism.

Physical examination should initially include a review of airway, breathing, and circulation to ensure that the patient is stable. Murmurs indicative of aortic insufficiency typically reflect aortic dissection as opposed to isolated penetrating ulcers, which are focal in nature. Similarly, signs of malperfusion such as neurologic deficits, acute renal insufficiency, visceral vessel compromise, or limb pain with pulse deficit usually occur with dissection as opposed to isolated penetrating aortic ulcers. It is important to note, however, that penetrating aortic ulcers and aortic dissections can occur concomitantly, and therefore, the presence of these signs on physical examination does not exclude a diagnosis of penetrating aortic ulcer. Penetrating aortic ulcers may also be discovered incidentally in asymptomatic patients with imaging performed for other indications.

5.2. Diagnostic modalities

Radiological imaging is essential to the diagnosis of penetrating aortic ulcers given its similarities to other acute aortic syndromes with respect to clinical presentation. A plain chest roentgenogram is frequently obtained in patients presenting with these symptoms and may demonstrate findings that support a diagnosis of penetrating aortic ulcer, although these findings are often nonspecific. Such findings including enlargement of the thoracic aorta, pleural effusion, widened mediastinum, and deviated trachea.

Although once considered the gold standard in diagnosis, angiography has fallen out of favor as the preferred diagnostic modality for acute aortic syndromes. Indeed, contrast-enhanced computed tomography and magnetic resonance imaging are currently the modalities most frequently employed for diagnosis of penetrating aortic ulcers. The typical radiological features of penetrating aortic ulcers appreciated by these modalities includes severe aortic atherosclerosis, aortic calcification, thickening or enhancement of the aortic wall, and a crater-like focal outpouching of the aortic wall (Figure 2) [16]. If associated with an intramural hematoma, inward displacement of the intima may be appreciated. Transesophageal echocardiography can also be used for diagnosis with a reported high sensitivity and specificity, although its invasive nature and need for a skilled operator are relative disadvantages.

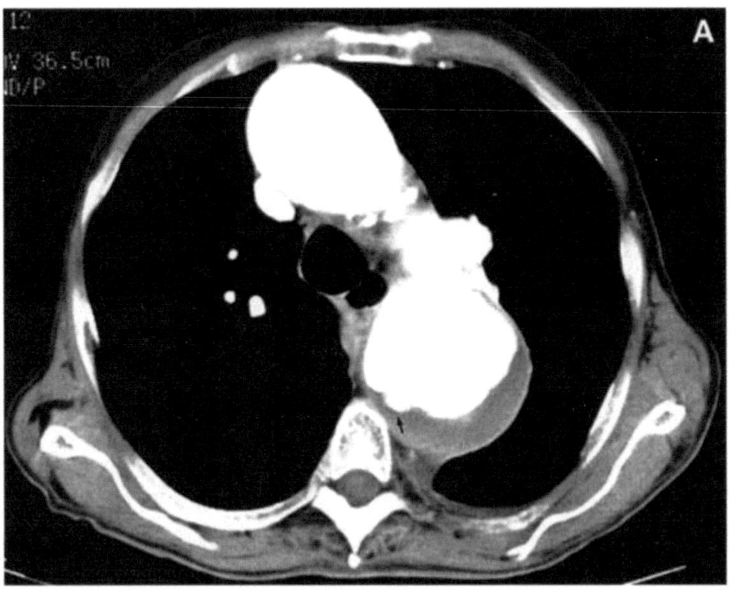

Figure 2. Computed tomography demonstrating a penetrating aortic ulcer as indicated by the black arrow (from Reference 18 – permission granted).

6. Treatment

6.1. Medical management

Patients diagnosed with a penetrating aortic ulcer without rupture or impending rupture, and without involvement of the ascending aorta, can initially be treated medically. Medical management includes afterload reduction and beta-blockade to reduce shear stress on the aortic wall. Intravenous analgesia should also be used to control pain in symptomatic patients. In symptomatic patients whose pain resolves and no evidence of hemodynamic instability, recurrent symptoms, expanding hematoma, or pseudoaneurysm formation occurs, transitioning to oral antihypertensives and re-imaging in 6 to 12 weeks is a reasonable approach. Asymptomatic patients should also be monitored for disease progression and be placed on an antihypertensive regimen.

6.2. Indications for operative repair

Although there is general agreement to treat ulcers with involvement of the ascending aorta surgically, indications for operative management of penetrating aortic ulcers particularly in the descending aorta remain controversial. A single institution series spanning 25 years and including 105 patients with penetrating aortic ulcers employed nonoperative management in the majority of cases (n=76) [14]. In this nonoperative cohort, 89% of those with an associated intramural hematoma had a decrease in the mean thickness of the hematoma at 1-month, and 85% had a completely resolved hematoma at 1-year. The 30-day mortality rate was significantly lower in the nonoperative (4%) versus operative (21%) group. The only predictors of nonoperative management failure were aortic rupture and earlier era (prior to 1990).

Another study provided a longitudinal analysis of computed tomography scans in patients with aortic ulcers [17]. Of 33 lesions with available follow-up scans, 21 (64%) were found to be stable at a mean follow-up of 18.4 months. In 10 (30%) cases, there was progression of the lesion at a mean follow-up of 19.8 months, with the most common changes consisting of an increase in aortic diameter along with increase in size of lesion (n=7), increase in aortic diameter with incorporation of the ulcer into the aortic wall contour (n=2), and increase in aortic diameter without changes in the ulcer itself (n=1). In the remaining 2 (6%) patients, an associated intramural hematoma decreased in thickness over 1 to 2 months with no changes in the ulcer itself.

Based on these reports, many groups have recommended a conservative approach to penetrating aortic ulcers, with surgical repair indicated only in cases of rupture, impending rupture, persistent pain, or enlarging ulcer or aortic diameter. Other reports, however, have indicated that penetrating aortic ulcers should be treated more aggressively. In a single institution series, the risk of aortic rupture with penetrating aortic ulcers was found to be significantly greater than with type A or type B aortic dissection (40% versus 7% versus 4%; $p<0.0001$) [18]. An updated series by the same group similarly advocated operative management in all patients with penetrating aortic ulcers as long as comorbidities do not preclude surgery given the high early rupture rate, risk of late rupture, and frequency of radiographic progression [19]. Another group advocated aggressive management in patients with penetrating aortic ulcers associated with intramural hematoma given a 48% rate of disease progression [20]. Predictors of disease progression in this latter series included increasing pleural effusion, increasing ulcer diameter, increasing ulcer depth, and persistent or recurrent pain.

6.3. Operative approach

Open repair of the descending thoracic aorta in patients with penetrating aortic ulcers is a significant operation with mortality rates as high as 15-20% [20, 21]. This is in part a reflection of the advanced age and comorbidity burden of the typical patient with this disease. Given the frequently segmental nature of aortic ulcers and the higher risk patient profile, an endovascular approach to treatment appears particularly well suited. However, it is important to mention that patients with penetrating ulcers typically have extensive atherosclerotic disease, and therefore, access for endovascular delivery of grafts is challenging if not unfeasible in many patients.

A single-center experience with endovascular treatment of penetrating aortic ulcers in 21 patients demonstrated successful deployment in all patients, with no endoleaks or mortalities at 30-days (Table 1) [22]. Another single institution study compared open repair in 37 patients with endovascular repair in 58 patients [23]. The endovascular cohort was significantly older and had a higher frequency of prior cerebrovascular disease. As expected, the open group involved repair of the aortic arch more frequently. The operative mortality rate was 5.1% in the endovascular group, which was one-third of that observed in the open cohort (16.2%; $p=0.07$). Furthermore, rates of perioperative stroke and prolonged ventilation were higher in those treated with an open approach.

In a European study of 72 patients undergoing endovascular repair of penetrating aortic ulcers, there was an in-hospital mortality rate of 4%, with an early endoleak rate of 7% and late endoleak rate of 4% [24]. Long-term survival was also favorable, with 1-, 5-, and 10-year survival being 93%, 72%, and 60%. Age greater than 75 years was an independent predictor of survival in their analysis. Another European study of 22 patients undergoing endovascular treatment of aortic ulcers similarly demonstrated excellent outcomes, with no in-hospital mortalities and no complications aside from stroke in 1 (5%) patient [25].

Although outcomes of an endovascular approach to penetrating aortic ulcers appear favorable, it is unclear if lower volume institutions or surgeons can attain comparable results to those reported in the literature. Referral to centers with significant experience in endovascular surgery is therefore advisable. Furthermore, open surgical repair will always remain an important component of the treatment armamentarium, as certain ulcers are not anatomically amenable to an endovascular approach due to their location, due to unfavorable aortic dimensions or anatomy, or due to an inability to gain access given the frequently extensive atherosclerotic burden of these patients.

7. Conclusions

Understanding the defining characteristics of the various acute aortic syndromes is essential as their pathophysiology and potential therapeutic implications are different. Penetrating aortic ulcers are defined by their focal nature and a patient population that tends to be elderly with significant comorbidities. Given these characteristics, endovascular approaches to

Study	No. of Patients	Patient Characteristics	In-hospital or 30-day Mortality	Complications
Brinster et al [22]	21	Mean age = 73 years 33% male 76% acute symptoms 76% smoking history 73% hypertension 18% COPD 18% diabetes mellitus 18% coronary artery disease 9% renal failure	0%	Reoperation 5% Endoleak 0% Stroke 0% PE 0% Wound infection 0%
Patel et al [23]	58	Mean age = 73 years 47% male 43% aortic rupture 50% smoking history 81% hypertension 89% COPD 12% diabetes mellitus 52% coronary artery disease Mean creatinine = 1.4 mg/dL	5.1%	Stroke 3.4% Dialysis 3.4% Prolonged ventilation 1.7% Endoleak 13.8%
Czerny et al [24]	72	Median age = 67 years 70% male 58% emergency cases 36% aortic rupture 93% hypertension 27% COPD 12% diabetes mellitus 32% coronary artery disease 14% renal insufficiency 8% cerebrovascular accident	4%	Overall complications 29% Early endoleak 7% Late endoleak 4% Open conversion 1% Secondary intervention 21%
Eggebrecht et al [25]	22	Mean age = 69 years 73% male 64% acute presentation 14% aortic rupture 100% hypertension 5% COPD 55% coronary artery disease 41% renal insufficiency	0%	Early endoleak 5% Open conversion 0% Paraplegia 0% Stroke 5%

Table 1. Operative Outcomes following Endovascular Repair of Penetrating Aortic Ulcers.

treatment in those with suitable anatomy appear particularly attractive, and indeed, initial reports from experienced centers have demonstrated favorable outcomes. A growing cumulative experience with penetrating aortic ulcers will hopefully be met with continuing advances and improvements in therapy. This will be particularly important as the population ages and imaging techniques improve, changes that will likely result in increases in the prevalence of this disease.

Author details

Arman Kilic[1*] and Ahmet Kilic[2*]

*Address all correspondence to: akilic1@jhmi.edu

*Address all correspondence to: Ahmet.Kilic@osumc.edu

1 Department of Surgery, Johns Hopkins Hospital, Baltimore, MD, USA

2 Division of Cardiac Surgery, The Ohio State University College of Medicine, Columbus, OH, USA

References

[1] Shennan T. Dissecting aneurysms. Medical Research Council, Special Report Series, No 193. 1934.

[2] Shumacker Jr HB, King H. Surgical management of rapidly expanding intrathoracic pulsating hematomas.SurgGynecolObstet 1959; 109:155-164.

[3] Stanson AW, Kazmier FJ, Hollier LH, Edwards WD, Pairolero PC, Sheedy PF, Joyce JW, Johnson MC. Penetrating atherosclerotic ulcers of the thoracic aorta: natural history and clinicopathologic correlations. Ann VascSurg 1986; 1:15-23.

[4] Nienaber CA, Powell JT. Management of acute aortic syndromes. Eur Heart J 2012; 33: 26-35b.

[5] Meszaros I, Morocz J, Szlavi J, Schmidt J, Tornoci L, Nagy L, Szep L. Epidemiology and clinicopathology of aortic dissection. Chest 2000; 117:1271–1278.

[6] Vilacosta I, San Roman JA. Acute aortic syndrome. Heart 2001; 85:365 –368.

[7] Choi SH, Choi SJ, Kim JH, Bae SJ, Lee JS, Song KS, Lim TH. Useful CT findings for predicting the progression of aortic intramural hematoma to overt aortic dissection. J Comput Assist Tomogr2001; 25:295 –299.

http://dx.doi.org/10.5772/54107

[8] Botta L, Buttazzi K, Russo V, Parlapiano M, Gostoli V, Di Bartolomeo R, Fattori R. Endovascular repair for penetrating atherosclerotic ulcers of the descending thoracic aorta: early and mid-term results. Ann ThoracSurg 2008; 85: 987-992.

[9] Gottardi R, Zimpfer D, Funovics M, Schoder M, Lammer J, Wolner E, Czerny M, Grimm M. Mid-term results after endovascular stent-graft placement due to penetrating atherosclerotic ulcers of the thoracic aorta. Eur J CardiothoracSurg 2008; 33: 1019-1024.

[10] Brinster DR. Endovascular repair of the descending thoracic aorta for penetrating atherosclerotic ulcer disease. J Card Surg 2009; 24: 203-208.

[11] Hirst AE Jr, Barbour BH. Dissecting aneurysm with hemopericardium: report of a case with healing. N Engl J Med 1958; 258: 116-20.

[12] Lehman SJ, Abbara S, Cury RC, Nagurney JT, Hsu J, Goela A, Schlett CL, Dodd JD, Brady TJ, Bamberg F, Hoffmann U.Significance of cardiac computed tomography incidental findings in acute chest pain. Am J Med 2009; 122:543-549.

[13] Machaalany J, Yam Y, Ruddy TD, Abraham A, Chen L, Beanlands RS, Chow BJ. Potential clinical and economic consequences of noncardiac incidental findings on cardiac computed tomography. J Am CollCardiol 2009; 54: 1533-1541.

[14] Coady MA, Rizzo JA, Elefteriades JA. Pathologic variants of thoracic aortic dissections: penetrating atherosclerotic ulcers and intramural hematomas. CardiolClin 1999; 17:637–657.

[15] Cho KR, Stanson AW, Potter DD, Cherry KJ, Schaff HV, Sundt TM 3rd.Penetrating atherosclerotic ulcer of the descending thoracic aorta and arch.J ThoracCardiovascSurg 2004; 127:1393-1399.

[16] Hayashi H, Matsuoka Y, Sakamoto I, Sueyoshi E, Okimoto T, Hayashi K, Matsunaga N.Penetrating atherosclerotic ulcer of the aorta: imaging features and disease concept. Radiographics 2000; 20:995-1005.

[17] Quint LE, Williams DM, Francis IR, Monaghan HM, Sonnad SS, Patel S, Deeb GM. Ulcerlike lesions of the aorta: imaging features and natural history. Radiology 2001;218:719-723.

[18] Coady MA, Rizzo JA, Hammond GL, Pierce JG, Kopf GS, Elefteriades JA. Penetrating ulcer of the thoracic aorta: what is it? How do we recognize it? How do we manage it? J VascSurg 1998; 27:1006-1015.

[19] Tittle SL, Lynch RJ, Cole PE, Singh HS, Rizzo JA, Kopf GS, Elefteriades JA. Midterm follow-up of penetrating ulcer and intramural hematoma of the aorta. J ThoracCardiovascSurg 2002; 123:1051-1059.

[20] Ganaha F, Miller DC, Sugimoto K, Do YS, Minamiguchi H, Saito H, Mitchell RS, Dake MD. Prognosis of aortic intramural hematoma with and without penetrating atherosclerotic ulcer: a clinical and radiological analysis. Circulation 2002; 106:342-8.

[21] Tittle SL, Lynch RJ, Cole PE, Singh HS, Rizzo JA, Kopf GS, Elefteriades JA. Midterm follow-up of penetrating ulcer and intramural hematoma of the aorta J ThoracCardiovascSurg 2002; 123:1051-1059.

[22] Brinster DR, Wheatley GH 3rd, Williams J, Ramaiah VG, Diethrich EB, Rodriguez-Lopez JA.Are penetrating aortic ulcers best treated using an endovascular approach? Ann ThoracSurg 2006; 82:1688-1691.

[23] Patel HJ, Sood V, Williams DM, Dasika NL, Diener AC, Deeb GM. Late outcomes with repair of penetrating thoracic aortic ulcers: the merits of an endovascular approach. Ann ThoracSurg 2012; 94:516-522.

[24] Czerny M, Funovics M, Sodeck G, Dumfarth J, Schoder M, Juraszek A, Dziodzio T, Loewe C, Reineke D, Krähenbühl E, Grimm M, Ehrlich M. Results after thoracic endovascular aortic repair in penetrating atherosclerotic ulcers. Ann ThoracSurg 2011; 92:562-566.

[25] Eggebrecht H, Herold U, Schmermund A, Lind AY, Kuhnt O, Martini S, Kühl H, Kienbaum P, PetersJ, Jakob H, Erbel R, Baumgart D. Endovascular stent-graft treatment of penetrating aortic ulcer: results over a median follow-up of 27 months. Am Heart J 2006; 151:530-536.

Chapter 16

Fast – Track Total Arch Replacement

Tomoaki Suzuki and Tohru Asai

Additional information is available at the end of the chapter

http://dx.doi.org/10.5772/53600

1. Introduction

Total arch replacement (TAR) is still a challenging procedure for cardiovascular surgeons because of the high incidence of mortality and brain accident. We have developed a fast-track TAR technique which is completed within 3-4 hours. In the present chapter, we describe in detail our surgical procedure for improving TAR outcomes.

Historically, TAR has required deep hypothermic circulatory arrest (DHCA) or retrograde cerebral perfusion with DHCA during distal anastomosis. However, DHCA has been shown to have adverse effects upon multiple organ systems. Moreover, these techniques do not give the surgeon adequate time to complete the aortic arch repair, the safety margin for which is limited to 40 to 60 minutes.

The antegrade selective cerebral perfusion (SCP) technique has been applied worldwide with various modifications. However, there is no common guideline as to the temperature that should be achieved before extracorporeal circulation can be stopped and replaced by initiation of SCP. Many institutions have recently attempted to elevate body temperature and reported excellent results in SCP with mild to moderate hypothermic circulatory arrest. We have begun to use milder levels of hypothermia based on a tympanic temperature of 25-28℃. We present our experience of using an SCP technique with mild hypothermia in total arch replacement.

2. Preoperative evaluation

A contrast enhanced computed tomography of the chest and the abdomen was performed to evaluate systemic atherosclerotic disease. A coronary angiography was performed routinely to evaluate the coronary artery disease in elective cases and also magnetic resonance angiography of carotid, vertebral and intracranial arteries to evaluate potential cerebral ischemia.

3. Indication for open surgery

Our threshold diameter for the treatment of aneurysm was 5 cm, however, the presence of risk factors influenced the individual indication for surgery such as age, pain symptom, chronic obstructive pulmonary disease, renal insufficiency and the expansion rate of the aneurysm. A saccular type aneurysm was indicated for surgery regardless of the size.

4. Surgical technique

The arterial cannulation site is decided according to preoperative computed tomography (CT) and intraoperative epiaortic ultrasonography findings. Our first-choice site is the ascending aorta. If the ascending and arch aorta is severely atherosclerotic, we use axillary artery cannulation. Venous cannulae are inserted into the superior and inferior vena cava. A left ventricular vent cannula is inserted through the right superior pulmonary vein and systemic cooling is started immediately. The head is packed in ice to maintain cerebral hypothermia until cardiopulmonary bypass (CPB) is restarted. Myocardial protection is ensured by retrograde infusion of cold blood cardioplegia solution. Tympanic and bladder temperature are monitored; systemic cooling is considered adequate for circulatory arrest when the tympanic temperature falls to 25℃-28℃. Circulatory arrest is achieved at a tympanic temperature of 25-28℃, at which point the arch aorta is opened. SCP is always used in total arch replacement. A 14Fr balloon-tipped cannula is inserted into the brachiocephalic artery, and 12Fr cannulae into the left common carotid and left subclavian arteries. Antegrade SCP flow is 10-13ml/kg/min, brain oxygen monitoring is carried out using INVOS 5100C (Somanetics, Troy, Mich.), and bilateral radial artery pressure is monitored. Distal anastomosis is performed with a 4-0 monofilament continuous suture reinforced with Teflon felt strips. An ESTECH retractor is often used during the distal procedure to create a comfortable surgical field.(Fig 1) A sealed quadrifurcated Dacron graft is always used for arch repair. After completion of the distal repair, the vascular prosthesis is clampe, antegrade systemic circulation restarted through the side-branch of the prosthesis, and rewarming begun. Next, proximal anastomosis is performed with Teflon felt strip reinforcement approximately 1 cm above the sinotubular junction after completion of which, coronary circulation is started. Finally, the three arch vessels are reconstructed using 5-0 monofilament continuous sutures from the left subclavian artery to the brachiocephalic artery.(Fig 2,3) When this is completed, systemic rewarming and heart-beat adequate for weaning from CPB can be achieved.

Sequence of surgical procedure

1. CPB establishment with ascending aortic cannulation and bicaval venous drainage
2. Systemic cooling with topical head cooling in ice pack
3. Circulatory arrest at tympanic temperature of 25-28℃
4. SCP insertion into three arch vessels

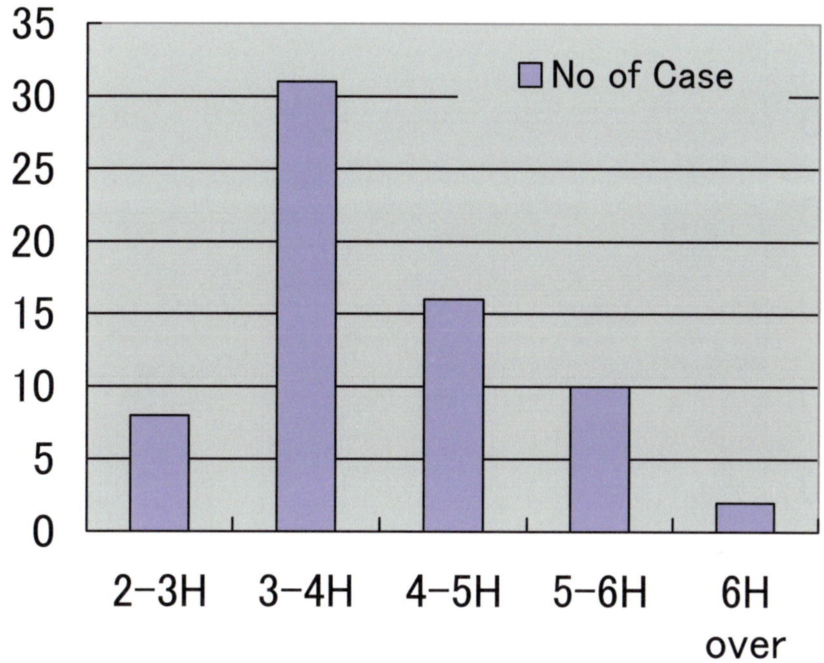

Figure 1. Operation Time (Hours)

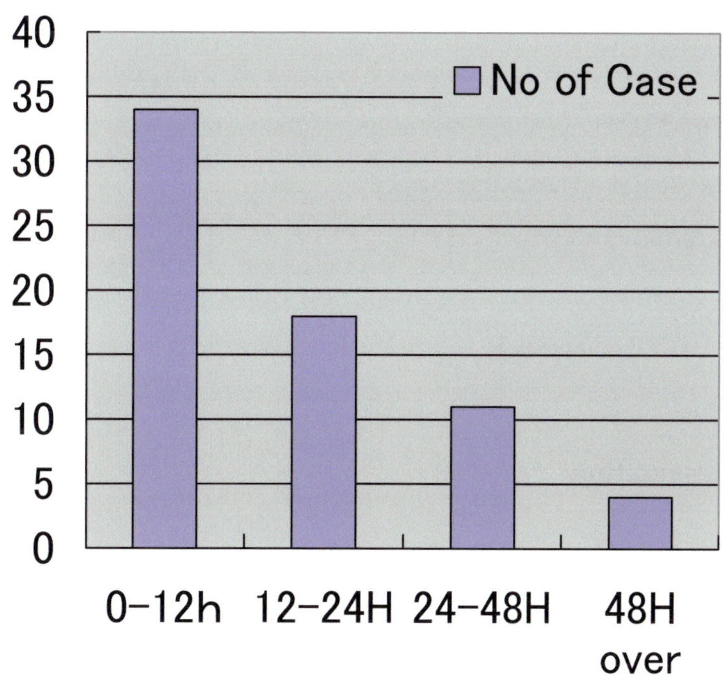

Figure 2. Postoperative Intubation Time (Hours)

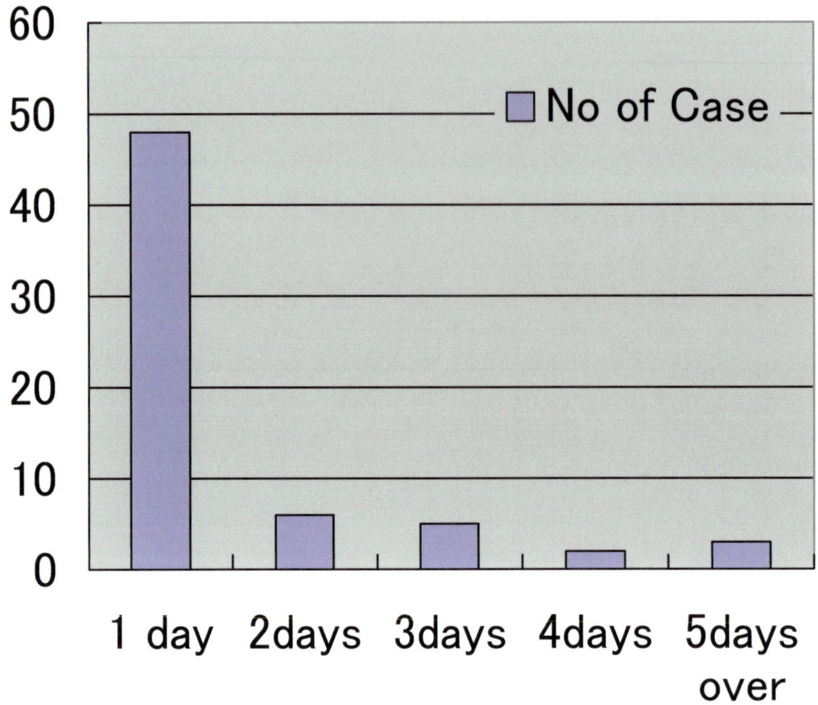

Figure 3. Stay of Intensive Care Unit (day)

5. Distal anastomosis using ESTECH retractor to create good surgical field
6. CPB restart from side branch and start of systemic rewarming to 35℃
7. Proximal anastomosis to ascending aorta
8. Coronary reperfusion and heartbeat start
9. Arch vessel reconstruction from subclavian artery to brachiocephalic artery
10. Weaning from CPB immediately after reconstruction of arch vessels

5. Clinical presentation

From January 2008 to July 2012, a total of 112 patients underwent total arch replacement under a single surgeon (A.T.) at Shiga Medical University Hospital. Of these 112 patients, the 45 requiring concomitant procedures were excluded and the remaining 67 isolated TAR patients (including 11 emergent cases), whose mean age was 73.3 years were admitted as subjects. The type of aortic disease was aortic dissection in thirteen (including three emergent) cases and atherosclerotic true aneurysm in 54 (including eight emergent) cases.

The operation time was 2.5 to 3 hours in eight cases, 3 to 4 hours in 31 cases, 4 to 5hours in 16 cases, and more than 5 hours in 12 cases. The CPB time was 82-268 minutes (mean 140 ± 36), the coronary ischemic time 38-158 minutes (mean 76 ± 26), the circulatory arrest time 28-137minutes (mean 45 ± 21), and the SCP time 57-212 minutes (mean 83 ± 29). (Fig 4)

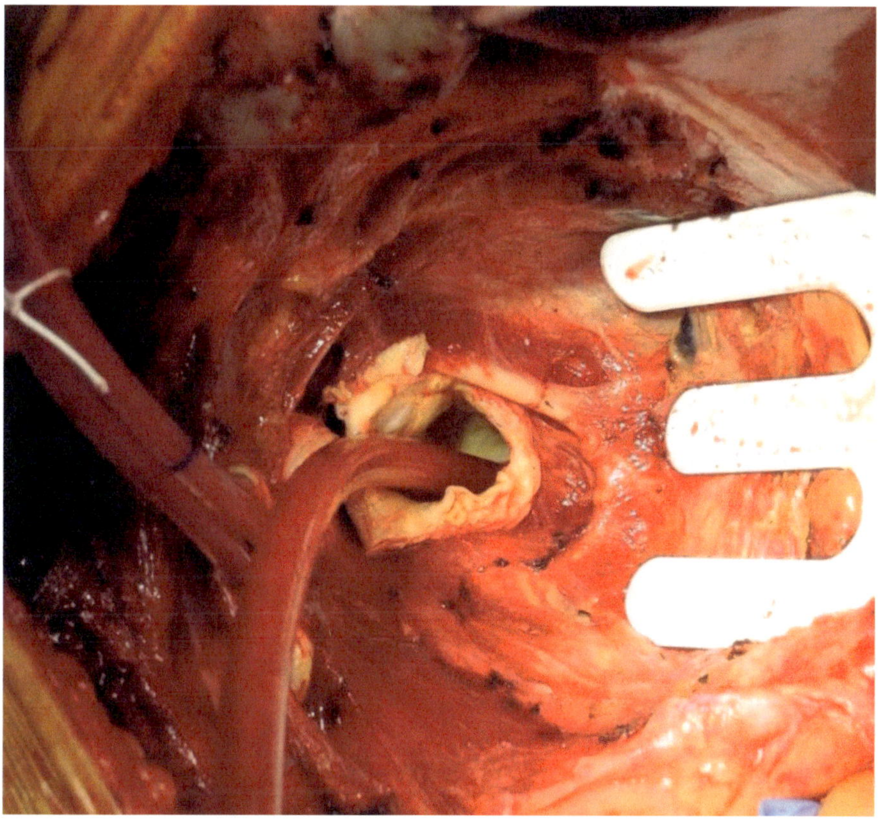

Figure 4. Surgical view of distal anastomose site using ESTECH retractor

5.1. Early morbidity

Hemorrhage requiring rethoracotomy occurred in three patients (4.5%), cerebrovascular deficit in three patients (4.5%), mediastinitis in two patients (3%), pulmonary failure in four patients (6%), and acute renal failure in four patients (6%). Prolonged intubation (>48H) was required in four patients (6%), and prolonged intensive care unit stay (>72H) in five.(Fig 5,6) The hospital stay from surgery to discharge was from 9 to 102 days with a mean of 14 days.

5.2. Mortality

No thirty-day mortality occurred. Two hospital mortalities occurred (3%), one due to multisystem organ failure following emergent rupture and the other to cerebrovascular accident.

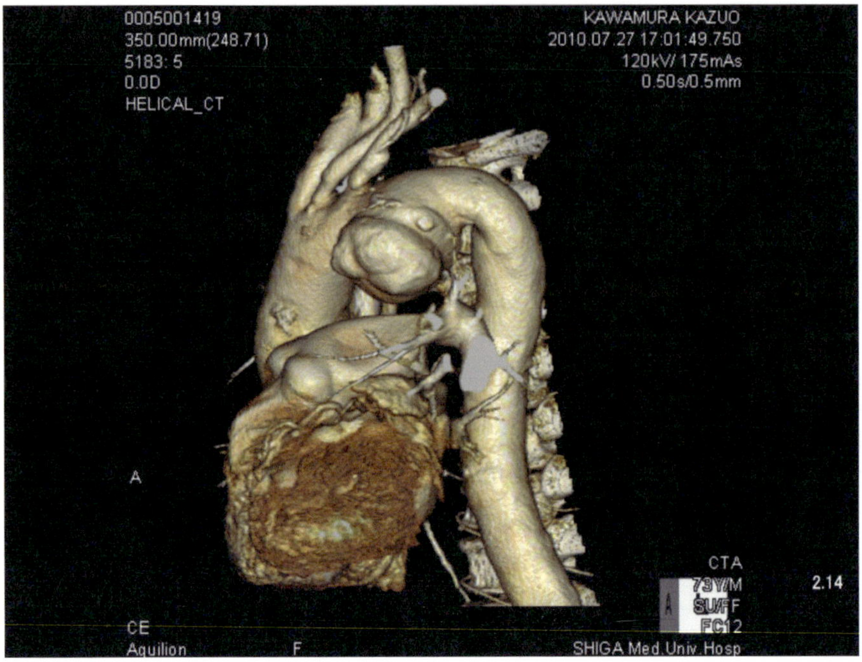

Figure 5. CT finding of distal arch aneurysm of thoracic aorta

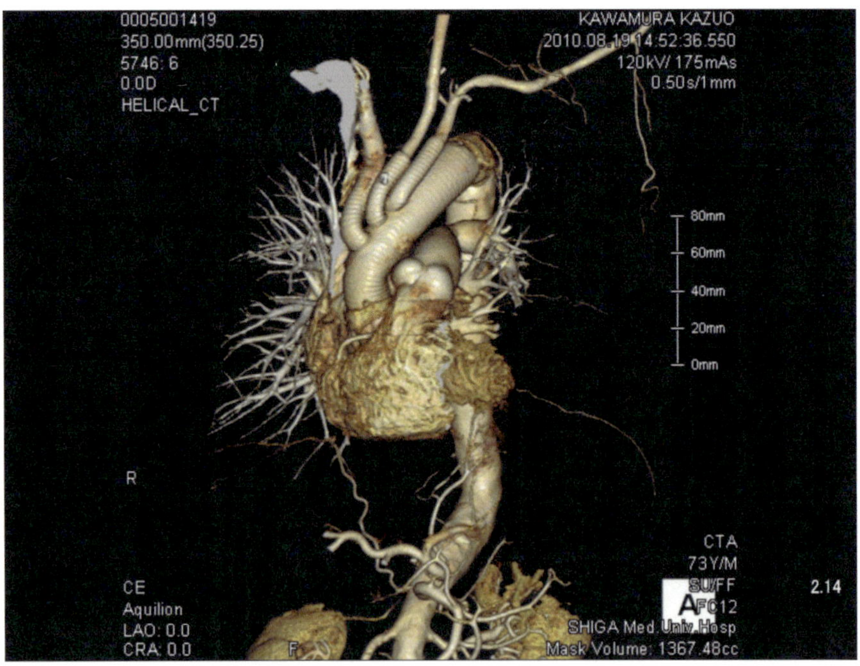

Figure 6. CT finding of repaired arch with a sealed quadrifurcated Dacron graft

6. Comment

6.1. Moderate hypothermia

Historically, total arch replacement has required deep hypothermic circulatory arrest (DHCA) or retrograde cerebral perfusion with DHCA during distal anastomosis.[1,2] However, these techniques do not give the surgeon adequate time to complete the aortic arch repair. The SCP technique, which extends the safe limits of time for arch surgery, has now gained acceptance.[4,5,6] As reliable SCP allows a high temperature setting during distal anastomosis, we have begun to use more moderate levels of hypothermia based on a tympanic temperature of 25-28℃. Core temperature based on bladder or rectal temperature has generally been used as the minimum setting and the safety of using tympanic temperature as the minimum setting is controversial. Ehrlich and coworkers [7] showed that brain oxygen consumption is reduced to 50% of baseline values if the patient is cooled systemically to a core temperature of 28C, while Zierer and coworkers [6] showed that SCP in combination with mild hypothermia (core temperature of 30C) offers sufficient cerebral protection and may be safely applied to aortic arch surgery requiring SCP time of up to 90 minutes or more. Our minimum temperature setting is tympanic temperature of 25-28℃. In almost all cases, when the tympanic temperature reaches 25℃, which takes approximately 10-20 minutes, the core temperature is still at 30-32℃. Our clinical outcomes show a low incidence of neurologic deficits and suggested that the application of this perfusion and temperature management protocol to aortic arch surgery was safe.

6.2. Sequence of reconstruction procedure

After completion of distal anastomosis, CPB was restarted from the side branch of the graft and rewarming initiated immediately. This early rewarming protocol with SCP is also controversial. Okada, who also used the INVOS system for monitoring brain oxygenation and increased SCP flow to maintain the INVOS index at preoperative values, reported that early rewarming can minimize CPB time, but that monitoring of brain oxygenation during rewarming is particularly important. [8]

After restart of CBP and rewarming, the proximal anastomosis is performed next and coronary perfusion restarted. Infusion of cardioplegic solution is thus needed only once. During arch vessel reconstruction, the heart-beat and progress of rewarming were sufficient to allow weaning from CPB, so that CPB could be discontinued immediately after reconstruction of the brachiocephalic artery. This sequence of reconstruction procedures minimizes CPB time and coronary ischemic time.

Recently, a number of studies have reported the safety of SCP with mild-moderate hypothermia for protection of the brain and visceral organs. In the present chater, the excellent surgical results also indicate the safety of SCP under mild hypothermia.

Operative Data	Total arch replacement (n=67)
Operative time	156~419 minutes (mean 238 ± 64)
CPB time	82-268 minutes (mean 140 ± 36)
Coronary ischemic time	38-158 minutes (mean 76 ± 26)
Circulatory arrest time	28-137minutes (mean 45 ± 21)
SCP time	65-212 minutes (mean 83 ± 29).
(Postoperative Data)	
Reoperation for bleeding	3 (4%)
Deep sternal infection	2 (3%)
Permanent stroke	3 (4%)
Respiratory failure*	4 (6%)
Mortality	
30days	0 (0%)
Hospital	2 (3%)

CPB = cardiopulmonary bypass

*Requiring prolonged ventilation support of more than 48 hours

ICU = intensive care unit

Table 1. Operative and Postoperative Data

Author details

Tomoaki Suzuki* and Tohru Asai

*Address all correspondence to: suzukikatuta@yahoo.co.jp

Department of Cardiovascular Surgery, Shiga University of Medical Science, Setatsukinowa, Ootsu, Shiga, Japan

References

[1] Ergin, M. A, Galla, J. D, Lansman, L, et al. Hypothermic circulatory arrest in operations on the thoracic aorta. Determinants of iperative mortality and neurologic outcome. J Thorac Cardiovasc Surg (1994). , 107, 788-97.

[2] Griepp, R. B, Stinson, E. B, Hollingaworth, J. F, et al. Prosthetic replacement of the aortic arch. J Thorac Cardiovasc Surg (1975). , 70, 1051-63.

[3] Hagl, C, Ergin, M. A, Galla, J. D, et al. Neurologic putcome after ascending aorta-aortic arch operations; effect of brain protection technique in high-risk patients. J Thorac Cardiovasc Surg (2001). , 121, 1107-21.

[4] Kamiya, H, Hagl, C, Kropivnitskaya, I, et al. The safety of moderate hypothermic lower body arrest with selective cerebral perfusion: A propensity score analysis. J Thorac Cardiovasc Surg (2007). , 133, 501-509.

[5] Minatoya, K, Ogino, H, Matsuda, H, et al. Evolving selective cerebral perfusion for aortic arch replacement : High flow rate with moderate hypothermic circulatory arrest. Ann Thorac Surg (2008). , 86, 1827-32.

[6] Zierer, A, Detho, F, Dzemali, O, et al. Antegrade Cerebral perfusion with mild hypothermia for aortic arxh replacement: Single center experience in 245 consecutive patients. Ann Thorac Surg (2011). , 91, 1868-74.

[7] Ehrlich, M. P, Mccullough, J. N, Zhang, N, et al. Effect of hypothermia on cerebral blood flow and metabolism in the pig. Ann Thorac Surg (2002). , 73, 191-7.

[8] Olsson, C, & Thelin, S. Resional cerebral saturation monitoring with near-infraed spectroscopy during selective antegrade cerebral perfusion: Diagnostic performance and relationship to postoperative stroke. J Thorac Cardiovasc Surg (2006). , 131, 371-79.

Chapter 17

Contemporary Surgical Management of Acute Massive Pulmonary Embolism

Dawn S. Hui and P. Michael McFadden

Additional information is available at the end of the chapter

http://dx.doi.org/10.5772/53969

1. Introduction

Pulmonary embolism (PE) is the most lethal pulmonary condition in the United States and internationally. It is also the third most common cause of death in hospitalized patients. Since the introduction of computed tomographic pulmonary angiography (CT-PA), the estimated incidence of PE has risen from 62.1 to 112.3 cases per 100,000 [1]. Untreated, the associated mortality of PE is as high as 30% with recurrent embolism being the most common cause. Globally, systemic anticoagulation is the mainstay of treatment for both chronic and acute PE. In the case of acute massive PE (presenting with hypotension and systolic arterial pressure less than 90 mm Hg) the prognosis is much graver and associated with a mortality of 30-60%, second only to sudden cardiac death as a cause of sudden death. This condition mandates a more aggressive and urgent algorithm for diagnosis and treatment. Prompt and appropriate treatment, which may include surgical pulmonary embolectomy, can be life-saving.

2. Historical developments

The history of venous thrombosis and PE is intertwined with landmark developments in the disciplines of anatomy, pathology, hematology, and surgery [2]. While pathologic observations of postmortem pulmonary thrombi were detailed by Morgagni [3], Laennec [4], and Cruveilhier [5] in the 18th and 19th centuries, it was not until the late 19th century that the concept of thromboembolism was by recognized by Virchow. Virchow wrote "A plug may extend into the vena cava as thick as the last phalanx of the thumb. These are the thrombi that constitute the source of real danger; it is in them that ensues the crumbling away which leads to secondary occlusion in remote vessels" [6]. He was thus the first to ascribe a single pathophysiologic mechanism to these anatomically separate phenomena (Figures 1 and 2).

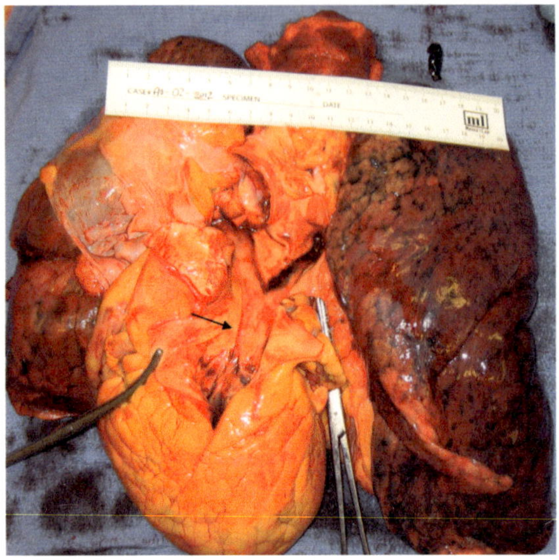

Figure 1. Autopsy photo demonstrating a sudden fatal saddle embolism which occurred six days following pulmonary lobectomy.

The surgical treatment of pulmonary embolism was first proposed by Friedrich Trendelenburg, a German professor of surgery from Leipzig. Having studied the cases of nine patients who died from acute pulmonary embolism, he developed a technique of pulmonary embolectomy through animal experimentation. His first two human patients died at 15 hours and 37 hours, from heart failure and hemorrhage of the internal mammary artery respectively [7]. Trendelenburg's student Martin Kirschner reported the first successful pulmonary embolectomy to the German Surgical Conference in Berlin in 1924 [8]. In Europe this became a popular emergent bedside operation for patients in whom PE was strongly suspected. Surgical residents were relegated to a bedside vigil and watched for sudden circulatory collapse and respiratory compromise in high-risk patients. Fewer than 10 patients survived the operation in 300 cases over a decade [2]. Though popular in Europe, the first successful pulmonary embolectomy was not reported in the United States until 1958 [9]. Operative mortality was frequently due to myocardial ischemia resulting in ventricular fibrillation and death at anesthetic induction [10]. The development of extracorporeal circulation by John Gibbon was in fact stimulated by his reflections while keeping vigil over a patient who underwent an unsuccessful attempt at pulmonary embolectomy: "...During the hours that night, John watched the patient's distended veins and recorded the faltering pulse, respirations and blood pressure, the thought occurred to him and constantly recurred to him that her conditions could surely be improved if only there were some form of continuously withdrawing some of the blue blood from the swollen veins into an apparatus where the blood could pick up oxygen and discharge carbon dioxide, and then be pumped back into the patient's arteries" [11]. This stimulated his work over the next twenty years to develop the heart-lung machine, ultimately opening the doors to modern cardiac surgery and to the first successful pulmonary embolectomy on cardiopulmonary bypass (CPB) by Edward Sharp in 1962 [10].

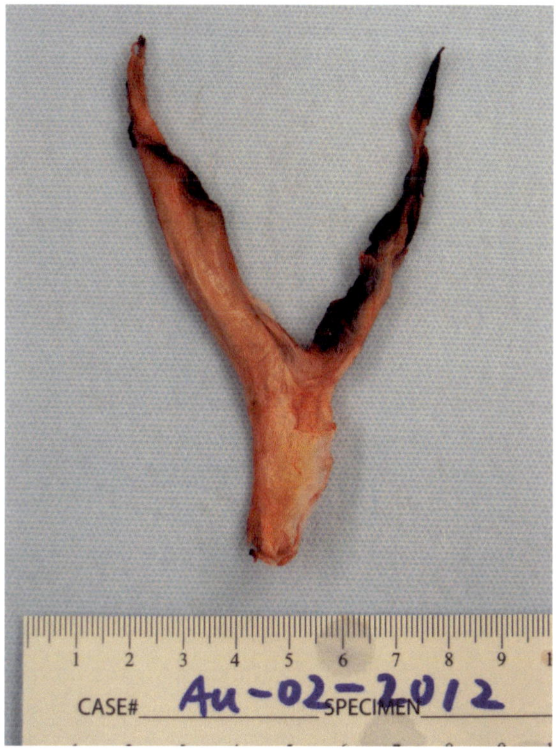

Figure 2. The saddle embolism isolated

Other surgical developments benefited from Virchow's legacy by attacking the problem at its more proximate source. The American surgeon Alton Ochsner, who had been present at Kirschner's 1924 address, proposed with Michael DeBakey to ligate the IVC in 1932 [12, 13]. John Homans, a general surgeon focused on venous disease, performed prophylactic lower extremity vein ligation [14]. Caval interruption commonly resulted in chronic lower extremity edema with the complications of varices, edema, and ulceration. As Spencer stated, "Because of the morbidity often following ligation of the vena cava, it is probably used too seldom and too late, being reserved as last resort..." [15]. Narrowing of the IVC via a right flank incision as an adjunct to pulmonary embolectomy has also been described, with the authors abandoning this technique due to impaired venous return [16]. Refinement of venous interruption came in the form of the Miles clip [17], partial caval plication, and finally percutaneous intraluminal occlusive devices (Figure 3). Early occlusive devices were hampered by complications of migration, embolization, vena cava wall rupture, and the need for femoral cutdown. Current filters have evolved in ease of insertion, lower complication rates, and efficacy with long-term patency rates of 98% and 3% recurrent embolism rates [18,19] (Figure 4).

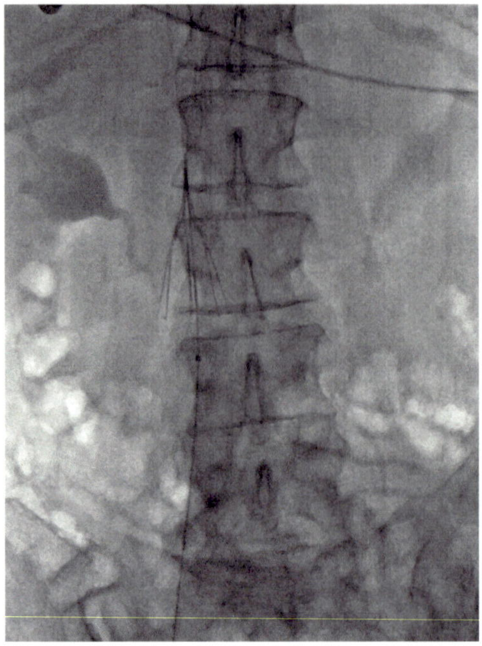

Figure 3. Vena Cava Filter.

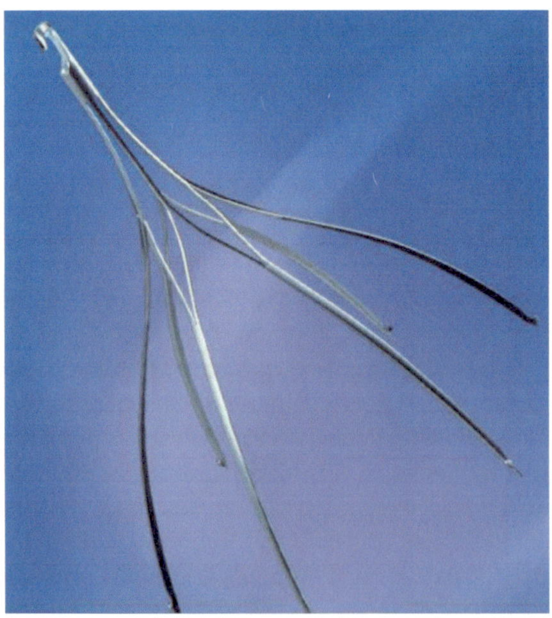

Figure 4. Nitinol Option™ Vena Cava Filter (Argon Medical Devices, Plano, TX). Features of contemporary filters include retrievability, MRI compatibility, and percutaneous insertion.

Concurrent with the developments in surgical techniques to treat PE were discoveries in anticoagulation. Heparin, discovered by McLean [20] and validated by Murray [21], has become the workhorse of initial therapy of PE. The discovery of oral dicumerol in the 1940s has led to the use of anticoagulation as the mainstay of both prevention of and therapy for venous thrombosis and PE. The efficacy of anticoagulants, thrombolytics, and vena caval filters combined with the high mortality rate of pulmonary embolectomy, had led to a paradigm shift towards nonoperative management of acute massive PE.

3. Contemporary management: diagnosis and prognostication

Classification of PE was historically based on the angiographic burden, using the Miller Index [22]. Current classification by American Heart Association differentiates between massive PE (sustained hypotension for at least 15 minutes or requiring inotropic support, pulselessness, or persistent profound bradycardia) from submassive (acute PE without systemic hypotension but with either RV dysfunction or myocardial necrosis) (Table 1) [23]. Early identification and risk stratification is mandatory at the time of diagnosis in order to coordinate multimodality treatment strategies. Prompt diagnosis and initiation of treatment can reverse RV failure and reduce mortality. Current tools for prognostication include clinical parameters, radiographic findings, and laboratory markers.

Massive PE	Acute PE with sustained hypotension (Systolic blood pressure <90 mm Hg for at least 15 minutes or requiring inotropic support)
	Not due to a cause other than PE, such as arrhythmia, hypovolemia, sepsis, or left ventricular [LV] dysfunction
	Pulselessness
	Persistent profound bradycardia (heart rate<40 bpm with signs or symptoms of shock)
Submassive PE	Acute PE without systemic hypotension (systolic blood pressure <90 mm Hg) but with either right ventricular (RV) dysfunction or myocardial necrosis
	RV dysfunction means the presence of at least 1 of the following:
	RV dilation (apical 4-chamber RV diameter divided by LV diameter > 0.9) or RV systolic dysfunction on echocardiography
	RV dilation (4-chamber RV diameter divided by LV diameter > 0.9) on computed tomography
	Elevation of beta-natriuretic peptide (BNP >90 pg/mL)
	Elevation of N-terminal pro-BNP (> 500 pg/mL)
	Electrocardiographic changes (new complete or incomplete right bundle-branch block, anteroseptal ST elevation or depression, or anteroseptal T-wave inversion)
	Myocardial necrosis is defined as either of the following:
	Elevation of troponin I (>0.4 ng/mL) or
	Elevation of troponin T (>0.1 ng/mL)

Table 1. American Heart Association Classification of Pulmonary Embolism [23].

Clinical signs consistent with major PE include transient syncope, cyanosis, elevated jugular venous pressure, tachypnea, unilateral restriction of chest wall movement, fever, and signs of RV dysfunction (Table 2).

Clinical Signs of RV dysfunction	Left parasternal heave
	Accentuated P2
	Murmur of tricuspid regurgitation
	Distended neck veins
	Unilateral restriction of chest wall
Electrocardiogram Signs of Right Heart Strain	RBBB
	Right axis deviation
	T-wave in V1-V4
	Qr pattern in V1
P2 = pulmonic second heart sound	
RBBB = right bundle branch block	
RV = right ventricle	

Table 2. Clinical and Electrocardiographic Signs of RV dysfunction [24]

Several scoring systems including the Pulmonary Embolism Severity Index [25] and Revised Geneva Score [26] have been developed based primarily on clinical signs and history (Tables 3 & 4). They have been shown to have prognostic value [23] and do not require diagnostic studies, making them a valuable tool for early prognostication.

Pulmonary Embolism Severity Index	**Score**
Age	1 point per year
Male Sex	10
History of Cancer	30
History of Heart Failure	10
History of Chronic Lung Disease	10
Pulse > 110 beats/min	20
Systolic Blood Pressure < 100 mm Hg	30
Respiratory Rate > breaths/min	20
Temperature < 35 °C	20
Altered Mental Status	60
Arterial oxyhemoglobin saturation level <90%	20
Class	**Mortality Risk**
Class I - < 65 points	0 - 1.6%
Class II - 65-85 points	1.7 - 3.5%
Class III - 85-105 points	3.2 - 7.1%
Class IV - 106-125 points	4.0 - 11.4%
Class V - >125 points	10.0 - 24.5%

Table 3. Pulmonary Embolism Severity Index [25]

Revised Geneva Score	Points
Age > 65 years	1
Previous DVT or PE	3
Surgery under general anesthesia or lower limb fracture within 1 month	2
Active malignant condition (solid or hematologic, currently active or considered cured < 1 year)	2
Unilateral lower limb pain	3
Hemoptysis	2
Heart rate 75-94 beats/min	3
Heart rate > 94 beats/min	5
Pain on lower limb deep venous palpation and unilateral edema	4
Clinical Probability	
Low: 0 - 3 points	
Intermediate: 4-10 points	
High: >10 points	

Table 4. Revised Geneva Score [26]

Biomarkers assessing the degree of right ventricular dysfunction associated with massive PE that have been studied include troponin and beta-natriuretic peptide (BNP). Right ventricular strain results in elevated troponin levels through acute shear stress causing microinjury and microinfarction, as well as increased oxygen demand and diminished perfusion from an acutely dilated and overloaded RV. Troponin levels have been found to correlate with the presence of RV dysfunction [27,28], and cutoff values for troponin prognostication in PE are identical to those in acute MI [29] while cutoff values for BNP are lower than those in congestive heart failure. Negative predictive value for both troponin and BNP are 97-100%; however the positive predictive values are low, with a wide range of sensitivities and low specificity for adverse events.

While most patients with suspected PE will have computed tomography angiography of the chest, on occasion concerns for acute renal injury will prompt workup with ventilation-perfusion scans. RV enlargement, defined as RV to LV dimension ratio > 0.9 on a reconstructed CT 4-chamber view, has been found to correlate with echocardiographic findings of RV dysfunction [30]. Subsequently, a study of 431 consecutive patients with acute PE found that RV enlargement predicted 30-day mortality (15.6% vs 7.7%, hazard ratio 5.17) as well as the composite end-point of death and in-hospital complications [31]. Dynamic CT assessment of right ventricular response to reperfusion therapy or surgical embolectomy found that although RV enlargement persisted in 43%, significant reductions in mean RV dimension and RV/LV ratio and significant increases in mean LV occurred with therapy, and did so equally in patients treated with thrombolysis versus embolectomy. Patients presenting with cardiogenic shock had a greater degree of initial RV enlargement and a greater reduction post-therapy [32]. Echocardiography may demonstrate the McConnell sign of acute pulmonary embolism, a characteristic pattern of akinesis of the mid free wall and normal motion of the apex [33]. Other signs include right ventricular hypokinesis, right ventricle dilation, and signs of pulmonary hypertension. In normotensive patients, RV dilation is present in 30-40% and predicts in-hospital mortality as well higher non-resolution and recurrence of pulmonary thrombus burden [34].

4. Contemporary multimodality management

While chronic conditions such as heart failure and malignancy are responsible for most of the late deaths in acute PE, early 30-day mortality results primarily from right ventricular failure [31]. Contemporary diagnostic modalities such as computed tomography and echocardiography allow for improved risk stratification and patient selection for pulmonary embolectomy, while evolution of surgical techniques has prompted a renewed enthusiasm for surgical pulmonary embolectomy as part of a multimodality approach to massive acute PE (Figure 5). The indications for open surgical embolectomy have traditionally been for clearly documented acute massive pulmonary embolism with persistent hypotension refractory to maximal pharmacological support.

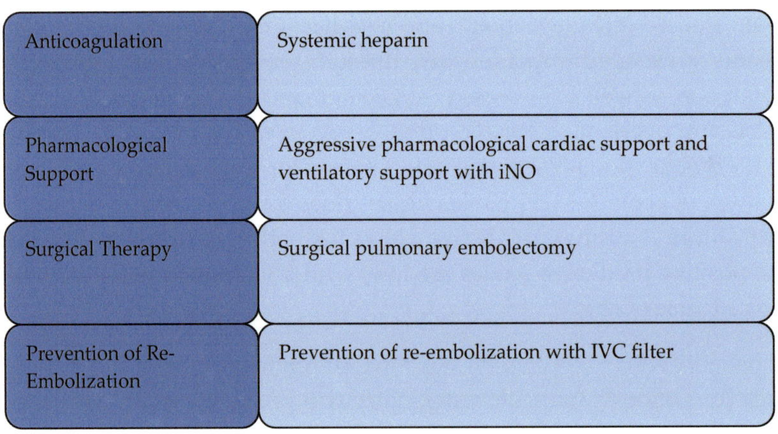

Figure 5. Contemporary multimodality approach to treatment of acute massive PE

Multimodality treatment begins with immediate systemic heparinization at diagnosis, cardiogenic support with inotropic agents and vasopressors as indicated, and correction of hypoxemia with supplemental oxygen or ventilatory support with pulmonary arterial vasodilation using inhaled nitric oxide. The underlying critical pathology is acutely elevated pulmonary vascular resistance (PVR) leading to pressure overload of the right ventricle and acute RV distention. Through ventricular interdependence, LV filling is reduced, compromising cardiac output and oxygen delivery. (Figure 6). The initial goals of medical management are optimization of RV preload and systolic function, reduction of pulmonary vascular resistance, and maintenance of right coronary perfusion pressure by adequate aortic root pressure [35]. Acute massive pulmonary embolism is initially a pressure overload problem of the RV. Higher filling pressures may be required; however an altered Frank-Starling curve in the setting of RV dysfunction may lead to volume overload as well. For patients with low cardiac output and normal blood pressure, modest fluid challenges may be beneficial, and the use of dobutamine and dopamine is a class IIa recommendation. Class I recommendations include correction of systemic hypotension and use of vasopressors, although the use of norepinephrine lacks clinical data, while the beneficial use of epinephrine in PE with shock has been reported [36].

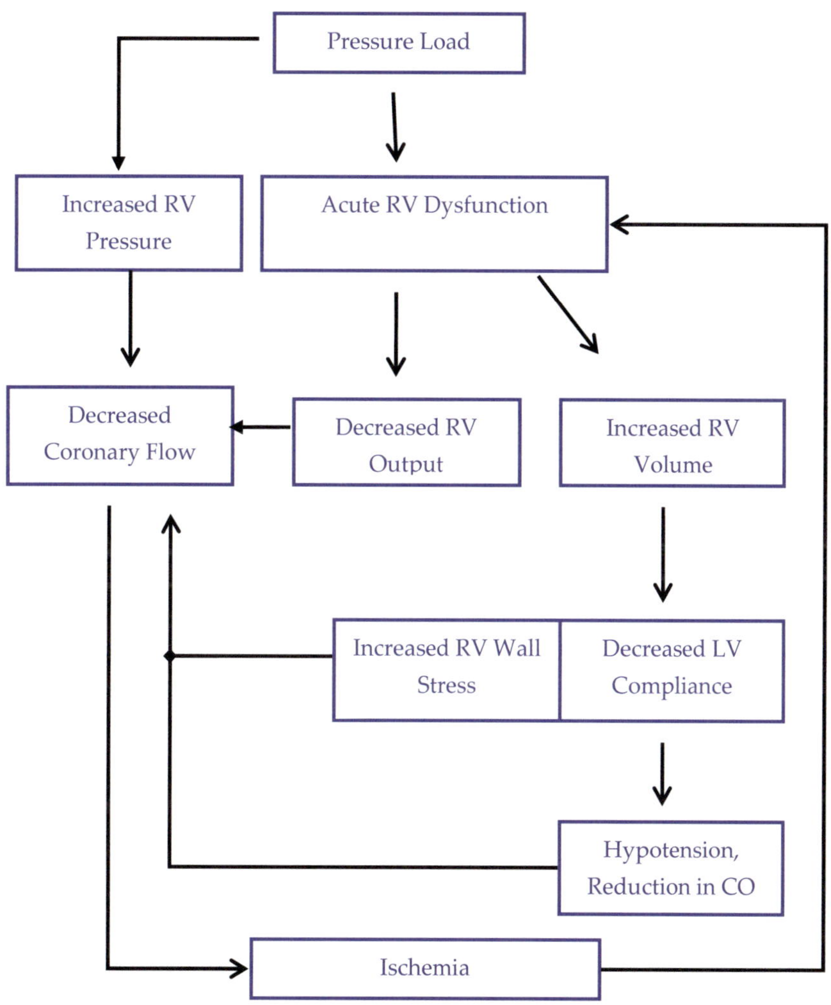

Figure 6. Hemodynamic effects of acute massive PE

RV function is coupled to pulmonary vascular resistance. Agents to reverse elevated PVR may be intravenous, inhaled, or oral. All intravenous forms (prostacyclin, iloprost, sildenafil, milrinone, and adenosine) carry the risk of systemic hypotension and should be instituted only after resuscitation and adequate perfusion of the RV. These agents may worsen the ventilation/perfusion ratio, increasing the degree of pulmonary shunt. Inhalational agents target the therapy to well-ventilated regions of the pulmonary bed, improving V/Q ratio and decreasing shunt fraction. Inhaled nitric oxide (iNO) has been studied in ARDS, pulmonary hypertension, and post mitral valve surgery, while evidence of its use in pulmonary embolism is limited to case reports and small case series. [37, 38, 39, 40]. While controlled studies supporting its routine use as an adjunct are lacking, anecdotal evidence based on timing of the institution of iNO seems to point to reductions in mean pulmonary artery pressures, increases in arterial oxygenation, and improvement in hemodynamics [38].

4.1. Surgical pulmonary embolectomy

The Trendelenburg operation was performed through a second transthoracic incision with resection of the second rib, occlusion of the aorta and pulmonary artery with an encircling rubber tube, and rapid removal of the embolism through a limited arteriotomy. Occlusion was limited to "forty-five seconds to two minutes, beyond that, death occurs" [7]. Modern surgical approach is by median sternotomy. After systemic heparinization, normothermic CPB is instituted via aortic and bicaval cannulation. The vena cavae are encircled with umbilical tapes. The operation is performed either with a beating heart and vacuum-assisted venous drainage or with the heart arrested. Deep hypothermic circulatory arrest has also been used in cases to optimize visualization for complete embolectomy [41]. The cavae are snared to isolate right heart inflow. A longitudinal incision of the pulmonary trunk is made two cm above the pulmonary valve. The extent of pulmonary arteriotomy is tailored to the location of thrombus. The incision can be carried in a hockey-stick fashion onto the left main pulmonary artery (Figure 7). For right-sided embolectomy, the right pulmonary artery is incised between the superior vena cava and the aorta. A variety of techniques of thrombus extraction have been described. Large clot can be retrieved with Randall stone forceps, vigorous suction, and Fogarty embolectomy catheters passed into branch arteries. Opening of the bilateral pleura and manual compression of the lungs to extrude peripheral clot has been described but has the drawbacks of mechanical injury to the arterial walls and lung parenchyma, as well as possibly causing endobronchial bleeding [42].

Retrograde flushing via direct cannulation of the pulmonary veins from the left atrium has been described to remove not only residual thrombotic material but air embolism as well. As described by Zarrabi et al, if the right atrium is opened to look for suspected clot, a septal incision through the fossa is then made, the left atrium entered, and the pulmonary veins identified. A cannula is attached to the pump oxygenator, inserted into each pulmonary vein sequentially, and flushed for 60-80 seconds with a mean pressure of 15-17 mm Hg. Clot and debris thus flushed retrograde through the pulmonary veins is extracted through the pulmonary arteriotomy [43]. If the right atrium is not entered, retrograde flushing of the left atrium can be performed via a 20 Fr cannula. This is inserted through the right superior pulmonary vein and attached to the arterial line through a Y connector [44]. Finally, adequate visualization of the distal arterial tree can be extended with use of an arterioscope. Postoperative mortality in these patients is felt to be due to eventual right ventricular failure from residual thrombus causing persistent pulmonary hypertension and interstitial pulmonary edema [41]. However, data concerning which of the above techniques is best to remove thrombus burden in the lungs, reduce RV strain, or improve outcomes is lacking. Intraoperative use of TEE during pulmonary embolectomy is recommended and can identify intrathoracic extrapulmonary thromboemboli which may alter planned surgical maneuvers [45]. Reflecting back towards the original Trendelenburg procedure, inflow occlusion pulmonary embolectomy is an option where CPB is not immediately available. This technique consists of caval occlusion for 3-minute maximal periods, beyond which there is great risk of cardiac and neurologic complications [46].

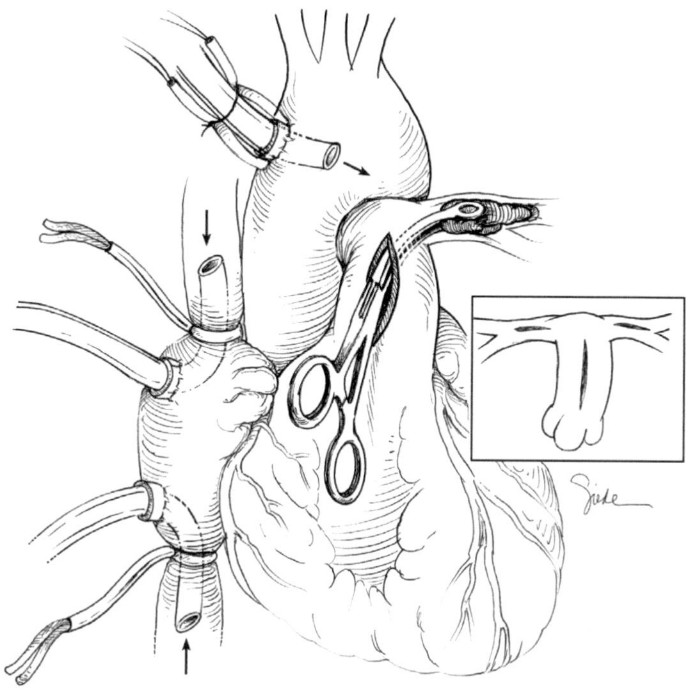

Figure 7. Technique of cardiopulmonary bypass with bicaval cannulation, arrows indicating direction of blood flow. Randall stone forceps are inserted through the main pulmonary arteriotomy to extract a portion of embolus from the left pulmonary artery. Inset: The three arteriotomy sites: main pulmonary artery, left and right pulmonary arteries

4.2. Contemporary surgical outcomes and expanded indications

A systematic review of pulmonary embolectomies in the period from 1961 to 2006 showed the average mortality to be 30%. Several important factors in mortality included the time period, with higher mortality reported in studies before 1985 (32% vs 20%) and in patients with preoperative cardiac arrest (59% vs 29%) [47]. Prospectively studied patients that have failed an initial course of thrombolytics have lower mortality with embolectomy than with a second course of thrombolysis (7% vs. 38%) [48]. More recent studies have begun to examine results in patients not meeting strict criteria of sustained hypotension or cardiogenic shock, but rather using evidence of RV dysfunction as an expanded criteria for pulmonary embolectomy, with operative mortality in contemporary series being 6-8% [49-53]. Expediency of operation has also found to have improved outcomes, particularly with surgical therapy occurring within 24 hours of diagnosis [54]. The improvement in operative mortality in the modern era may be due to several factors: improved patient selection, early identification of RV dysfunction with contemporary diagnostic modalities, extent of pulmonary thrombectomy to prevent residual thrombus and thus pulmonary hypertension, the prophylactic use of IVC filters, and early operation before the development of cardiogenic shock or the need for cardiopulmonary resuscitation, both of which confer a significantly increased in-hospital mortality (25% and 65%, respectively vs 8.1%) [55]. By instituting a criteria of RV dysfunction as an indication for pulmonary embolectomy, the population to be considered expands to include patients with submassive PE.

4.3. Thrombolytics, special populations, catheter-based therapy, and IVC filters

The benefit of thrombolytic therapy in the treatment of acute PE has been controversial. A meta-analysis showed that overall, there was no significant reduction in PE or death when comparing thrombolysis with heparin; neither was the risk of major bleeding significantly increased. Subgroup analysis showed a significant reduction in PE and death in the trials that included patients with major (i.e. hemodynamically unstable) PE and no benefit in those trials that excluded those patients [56]. A review of current evidence concluded that, "Despite the lack of a verifiable mortality benefit associated with thrombolytic therapy in patients with massive PE resulting in hemodynamic instability, most clinicians accept this clinical scenario as indication for thrombolytics and it is guideline based" [57]. In the most recent guidelines (2012), The American College of Chest Physicians evidence for thrombolytic administration is graded 2C for unstable patients without high bleeding risk; recommendations are against thrombolytics in stable patients (Grade 1C) [58].

Because the effects are systemic, thrombolytics poses a risk of serious perioperative bleeding and should be approached with caution in patients with acute massive PE that may be considered for surgical embolectomy.

This decision is of particular interest in populations whose underlying disease places them at increased risk of bleeding elsewhere. Trauma patients with immobility and/or traumatic brain injury are prone to DVT and PE; sites of bleeding risk include concomitant solid organ injury and intracranial hemorrhage. Reluctance to place prophylactic IVC filters has been due to filter-related complications and inconsistent follow-up; this has been tempered by more recent studies showing low complication rates and safe retrievability at greater intervals. Limited data consisting of matched-control trials have shown reduced PE and PE-related mortality rates with prophylactic filters [59]. Yet, prophylactic IVC filter placement in at-risk patients remains a Level III recommendation by the Eastern Association for the Surgery

Trauma guidelines [60]. Increased risk of both thromboembolic disease and intracranial hemorrhage is seen also in patients with brain tumors. Successful pulmonary embolectomy has been reported in a patient with advanced glioblastoma multiforme, suggesting that this clinical scenario may represent an extended indication for surgery [61]. In patients with significant cardiac disease, pulmonary symptoms are often ascribed to cardiac etiology, but rarely concomitant PE may be discovered [62], in which case surgical pulmonary embolectomy may be combined with the operation to treat the primary cardiac disease.

Catheter-based techniques include aspiration thrombectomy, fragmentation, and rheolytic thrombectomy. Rheolytic thrombectomy using the AngioJet and Rotarex devices has been shown to be technically feasible with success rates of 92.2% to 100%, with significant improvements in both angiographic indices and clinical indices (i.e, Miller Index, obstruction index, perfusion index, mean pulmonary artery pressures, partial arterial pressures) [63, 64]. Data is limited to small series, and this therapy requires experienced laboratories. Its role as primary therapy is for patients with contraindications to thrombolysis, failed thrombolysis, or impending death from shock prior to thrombolysis when no other intervention is available [58].

The placement of IVC filters is prudent even after treatment with pulmonary embolectomy to prevent recurrent embolism from lower extremity sources. In several series, this has resulted in a zero recurrence rate [53, 65], while a 23% recurrence rate was noted in a series of patients without IVC filter placement after embolectomy [48].

5. Conclusion

Acute massive pulmonary embolism is a disease best treated by multimodality therapy, beginning with systemic heparinization and IVC filter placement. A multitude of diagnostic modalities, including transesophageal echocardiography and computed chest tomography, are available in the contemporary setting to guide risk-stratification and to assess RV dysfunction. Contemporary series of pulmonary embolectomy have demonstrated low operative mortality with improved surgical techniques, and survival is increased when operative therapy occurs before the development of hemodynamic collapse. Thus, the modified Trendelenburg procedure with extended distal pulmonary embolectomy should be part of an aggressive approach to an otherwise lethal problem in the current age.

Author details

Dawn S. Hui and P. Michael McFadden

Department of Cardiothoracic Surgery, University of Southern California Keck School of Medicine, Los Angeles, California, USA

References

[1] Wiener RS, Schwartz LM, Woloshin S. Time trends in pulmonary embolism in the United States: evidence of overdiagnosis. Arch Intern Med. 2011;171(9):831.

[2] McFadden PM, Ochsner JL. A history of the diagnosis and treatment of venous thrombosis and pulmonary embolism. Ochsner J. 2002; 4(1): 9-13.

[3] Westaby S. The foundations of cardiac surgery. In: Landmarks in cardiac surgery. Oxford, UK: Isis Medical Meia; 1997. p. 1-47.

[4] Laennec RTH. De l'auscultation medicale ou traité du diagnostic des maladies des poumons et du couer. Paris, France: Brossen et Claude; 1819.

[5] Cruveilhier J. Anatomie pathologique du corps humain: ou description, avec figures lithographiées et colorieés, des diverses alterations morbides dont le corps humain est susceptible. Paris, France: JB Bailliere; 1829-1842.

[6] Virchow R. Die cellularpathologic in ihrer begrudung auf physiologische und gewebelehre. Berlin, Germany: A Hirschwald; 1858).

[7] Trendelenburg F. General surgery, pathology and therapy. I. Operative interference in embolism of the pulmonary artery. Annals of Surgery 1908 Nov; 48 (5): 772-786.

[8] Kirschner M. Ein durch die trendelenburgsche operation geheilter fall von bolie der arterien pulmonalis. Arch Klin Chir. 1924; 133:312.

[9] Steenburg, RW, R. Warren, R E Wilson, and Le Rudolf: A new look at pulmonary embolectomy. Surg., Gynec & Obst.1958; 107:214.

[10] Sharp EH. Pulmonary embolectomy: successful removal of a massive pulmonary embolus with the support of cardiopulmonary bypass - case report. Annals of Surgery 1962; 156(1): 1-4.

[11] Litwak, R.S. The growth of cardiac surgery: historical notes. Cardiovascular Clinics 1971; 3: 5-50.

[12] Ochsner A, Ochsner JL, Sanders HS. Prevention of pulmonary embolism by caval ligation. Ann Surg 1970; 171: 923-938.

[13] Ochsner A, Ochsner JL. Prevention of pulmonary embolism. Milit Med 1971; 136: 829-835.

[14] Homans J. Thrombosis of deep veins of the lower leg, causing pulmonary embolism. New Engl J Med 1934; 211: 993-997.

[15] Spencer FC, Quattlebaum JK, Sharp EH, Jude JR. Plication of the inferior vena cava for pulmonary embolism: a report of 20 cases. Annals of Surgery 1962; 155(6): 827-35.

[16] Blake DB. Pulmonary embolectomy re-evaluated. Ann Royal College of Surgeons of England 1981; 63: 18-24.

[17] Miles RM, Chappell F, Renner O. A partially occluding caval clip for the prevention of pulmonary embolism. Am Surg 1964; 30: 40-47.

[18] Greenfield LJ, Zocco J, Wilk J, Schroeder TM, Elkins RC. Clinical experience with the Kim-Ray Greenfield vena cava filter. Ann Surg 2977; 185: 692-698.

[19] Roehm JOF Jr, Gianturco C, Barth MH, Wright KC. Percutaneous transcatheter filter for the inferior vena cava: a new device for treatment of patients with pulmonary embolism. Radiology 1984; 150: 255-257.

[20] McLean J. The thromboplastin action of cephalin. Am J Physiol 1916; 41: 250.

[21] Murray DWG, Jacques LB, Perrett TS, Best CH. Heparin and thrombosis of veins following injury. Surgery 1937; 2:163-187.

[22] Miller GA, Sutton GC, Kerr IH, Gibson RV, Honey M. Comparison of streptokinase and heparin in treatment of isolated acute massive pulmonary embolism. Br Med J. 1971; 2: 681– 684.

[23] Jaff MR, McMurtry MS, Archer SL, Cushman M, Goldenberg NA,

[24] Goldhaber SZ, Jenkins JS, Kline JA, Michaels AD, Thistlethwaite P, Vedantham S, White RJ, Zierler BK; on behalf of the American Heart Association Council on Cardiopulmonary, Critical Care, Perioperative and Resuscitation, Council on Peripheral Vascular Disease, and Council on Arteriosclerosis, Thrombosis and Vascular Biology. Management of massive and submassive pulmonary embolism, iliofemoral deep vein thrombosis, and chronic thromboembolic pulmonary hypertension: a scientific statement from the American Heart Association. Circulation. 2011;123:1788 –1830.

[25] Goldhaber SZ. Cardiac biomarkers in pulmonary embolism. Chest 2003; 123: 1782-84.

[26] Aujesky D,Obrosky DS,Stone RA, Auble TE, Perrier A, Cornuz J et al. Derivation and validation of a prognostic model for pulmonary embolism. Am J Respir Crit Care Med Year 2005: 172 (8); 1041-1046.

[27] Le Gal G, Righini M, Roy PM, Sanchez O, Aujesky D, Bounameaux H, Perrier A. Prediction of pulmonary embolism in the emergency department: the revised Geneva score. Ann Intern Med. 2006 Feb 7;144(3):165-71.

[28] Meyer T, Binder L, Hruska N, Luthe H, Buchwald AB. Cardiac troponin I elevation in acute pulmonary embolism is associated with right ventricular dysfunction. JACC 2000; 36: 1632-1636

[29] Giannitsis E, Muller-Bardorff M, Kurowski V, Weidtmann B, Wiegand U, Kaampmann M, Katus HA. Independent prognostic value of cardiac troponin T in patients with confirmed pulmonary embolism. Circulation. 2000;102:211-217.

[30] Piazza G, Goldhaber SZ. The acutely decompensated right ventricle: pathways for diagnosis and management. Chest 2005; 128 (3): 1836-1852.

[31] Quiroz R, Kucher N, Schopef UJ, Kipfmueller F, Solomon SD, Costello P, Goldhaber SZ. Right ventricular enlargement on chest computed tomography: prognostic role in acute pulmonary embolism. Circulation 2004; 109: 2160-2167.

[32] Schoepf JU, Kucher N, Kipfmueller F, Quiroz R, Costello P, Goldhaber SZ. RV enlargement on chest computed tomography: a predictor of early death in acute pulmonary embolism. Circ 2004; 110: 3276-80

[33] Kipfmueller F, Quiroz R, Goldhaber SZ, Schoepf UJ,Costello P, Kucher N. Chest CT assessment following thrombolysis or surgical embolectomy for acute pulmonary embolism. Vasc Med 2005; 10; 85-89.

[34] McConnell MV, Solomon SD, Rayan ME, Come PC, Goldhaber SZ, Lee RT. Regional right ventricular dysfunction detected by echocardiography in acute pulmonary embolism. Am J Cardiol. 1996; 78: 469–473.

[35] Masotti L, Righini M, Vuilleumier N, Antonelli F, Landini G, Cappelli R, Ray P. Prognostic stratification of acute pulmonary embolism: focus on clinical aspects, imaging, and biomarkers. Vasc Health Risk Manag. 2009; 5: 567–575.

[36] Price LC, Wort SJ, Finney SJ, Marino PS, Brett SJ. Pulmonary vascular and right ventricular dysfunction in adult critical care: current and emerging options for management: a systematic literature review. Critical Care 2010; 14(5): R169

[37] Guidelines on the diagnosis and management of acute pulmonary embolism: The Task Force for the Diagnosis and Management of Acute Pulmonary Embolism of the European Society of Cardiology (ESC) Eur Heart J (2008) 29(18): 2276-2315. doi: 10.1093/eurheartj/ehn310

[38] Capellier G, Jacques T, Balvay P, Blasco G, Belle E, Baralle F. Inhaled nitric oxide in patients with pulmonary embolism. Intensive Care Med 23: 1089-1092.

[39] Szold O, Khoury W, Biderman P, Klausner JM, Halper P, Weinbroum AA. Inhaled nitric oxide improves pulmonary functions following massive pulmonary embolism: a report of four patients and review of the literature. 2006 Lung 184: 1-5.

[40] Schenk P, Mittermayer C, Ratheiser K. Inhaled nitric oxide in a patient with severe pulmonary embolism. Ann Emerg Med 1999; 33: 710-714.

[41] Trummer G, Berchtold-Herz M, Martin J, Beyersdoff F. Successful treatment of pulmonary hypertension with inhaled nitric oxide after pulmonary embolectomy. Ann Thoracic Surg 2002; 73: 1299-1301.

[42] Van Putte BP, Bantal N, Snijder R, Morshuis WJ, Van Boven W-J. Interact CardioVasc Thorac Surg 2008 (7): 412-414.

[43] Kadner A, Schmidli, Schönhoff F, Krähenbühl E, Immer F, Carrel T, Eckstein F. Excellent outcome after surgical treatment of massive pulmonary embolism in critically ill patients. JTCVS 2008 Aug; 136: 448-51.

[44] Zarrabia K, Yarmohammadi H, Ostova MA. Retrograde pulmonary embolectomy in massive pulmonary embolism. Eur J Cardiothorac Surg 2005; 28(6): 897-899.

[45] Spagnolo S, Grasso MA, Tesler UF. Retrograde pulmonary perfusion improves results in pulmonary embolectomy for massive pumonary embolism. Tex Heart Inst J. 2006; 33: 473-6.

[46] Rosenberger P, Shernan SK, Mihaljevic T, Eltzschig HK. Transesophageal echocardiography for detecting extrapulmonary thrombi during pulmonary embolectomy. Ann Thoracic Surg 2004; 78: 862-866.

[47] Bobadilla J, Wigfield CH, Chopra PS. Inflow occlusion pulmonary embolectomy in the modern era of cardiac surgery. J Thorac Cardiovasc Surg 2006;131:484-486.

[48] Stein PD, Alnas M, Beemath A, Patel NR. Outcome of pulmonary embolectomy. Am J Cardiol 2007; 99: 421-423.

[49] Meneveau N, Séronde M, Blonde M, Legalery P, Didier-Petit K, Briand F et al. Management of unsuccessful thrombolysis in acute massive pulmonary embolism. Chest 2006; 129: 1043-1050.

[50] Yalamanchili K, Fleisher AG, Lehrman SG, Axelrod HI, Lafaro RJ, Sarabu MR et al. Open pulmonary embolectomy for treatment of major pulmonary embolism. Ann Thorac Surg 2004; 77: 819-23.

[51] Carvalho EM, Macedo FIB, Panos AL, Ricci M, Salerno TA. Pulmonary embolectomy: recommendation for early surgical intervention. J Card Surg 2010; 25:261-26.

[52] Leacche M, Unic D, Goldhaber SZ, Rawn JD, Aranki SF, Couper GS et al. Modern surgical treatment of massive pulmonary embolism: results in 47 consecutive patients after rapid diagnosis and aggressive surgical approach. JTCVS 2005; 129:1018-23.

[53] Aklog L, Williams CS, Byrne JG, Goldhaber SZ. Acute pulmonary embolectomy: a contemporary approach. Circ 2002; 105:1415-1419.

[54] Sareyyupoglu B, Greason KL, Suri RM, Keegan MT, Dearani JA, Sundt TM. A more aggressive approach to emergency embolectomy for acute pulmonary embolism. Mayo Clin Proc 2010; 85 (9): 785-790.

[55] Ahmed P, Khan AA, Smith A, Pagala M, Abrol S, Cunningham JN, Vaynblat M. Expedient pulmonary embolectomy for acute pulmonary embolism: improved outcomes. Interact CardioVasc Thorac Surg 2008; 7: 591-4.

[56] Kasper W, Konstantinides S, Geibel A, Olschewski M, Heinrich F, Grosser KD, Rauber K, Iversen S, Redecker M, Kienast J. Management strategies and determinants of outcome in acute major pulmonary embolism: results of a multicenter registry. J Am Coll Cardiol. 1997;30:1165–1171.

[57] Wan S, Quinlan DJ, Agnelli G, Eikelboom JW. Thrombolysis compared with heparin for the intial treatment of pulmonary embolism: a meta-analysis of the randomized controlled trials. Circ 2004; 110: 744-749.

[58] Todd JL, Tapson VF. Thrombolytic therapy for acute pulmonary embolism: a critical appraisial. Chest 2009; 135: 1321-1329.

[59] Kearon C, Akl EA, Comerota AJ, Prandoni P, Bounameaux H, Goldhaber SZ, et al. Antithrombotic therapy for VTE disease: antithrombotic therapy and prevention of thrombosis, 9th ed: American College of Chest Physicians evidence-based clinical practice guidelines. Chest 2012 Feb; 141 (2 Suppl): e419s-494s.

[60] Kidane B, Madani AM, Vogt K, Girotti M, Maltaner RA, Parry NG. The use of prophylactic inferior vena cava filters in trauma patients: a systematic review. Injury 2012; 43: 542-547.

[61] Rogers FB, Cipolle MD, Velmahos G, Rozycki G, Luchette FA. Practice management guidelines for the prevention of venous thromboembolism in trauma patients: the EAST practice management guidelines work group. J Trauma 2002; 53: 142-64.

[62] Firstenberg MS, Blais D, Abel E, Newton HB, Crestanello J. Emergent pulmonary embolectomy and advanced glioblastoma multiforme. Case Reports in Medicine 2010: 2010: 862028.

[63] Firstenberg MS, Abel E, Higgins RA, Sirak JH, Sai-Sudhakar CB, Kilic A, Crestanello J. Shortness of breath: pulmonary embolism, ischemic heart failure, or both? The role of concomitant surgery. The Heart Surgery Forum 2012; 15: E56-58.

[64] Chechi T, Vecchio S, Spaziani G, Giuliani G, Giannotti F, Arcangeli C, et al. Rheolytic thrombectomy in patients with massive and submassive acute pulmonary embolism. Catheterization and Cardiovascular Interventions 2009; 73: 506-513.

[65] Liu S, Shi HB, Gu JP, Yang ZQ, Chen L, Lou WS, et al. Massive pulmonary embolism: treatment with the Rotarex thromboectomy system. Cardiovasc Intervent Radiol 20101 Feb; 34(10): 106-113.

[66] Kucher N, Rossi E, De Rosa M, Goldhaber ASZ. Massive pulmonary embolism. Circulation 2006; 113 (4): 577-582.